PENGUIN CANADA

LESLIE BECK'S NUTRITION GUIDE TO A HEALTHY PREGNANCY

Leslie Beck, a registered dietitian, is a leading nutritionist who has helped over 2000 individuals achieve their nutrition and health goals. She is the bestselling author of *Leslie Beck's Nutrition Guide to Menopause, Leslie Beck's 10 Steps to Healthy Eating, Leslie Beck's Nutrition Guide for Women,* and *Leslie Beck's Nutrition Encyclopedia*, and is a contributing author in *Rose Reisman's Sensationally Light Pasta & Grains*. Leslie writes nutrition articles for national magazines, is the nutrition expert for CTV's *Canada AM*, and is the host of Discovery Channel's *Foodstuff*, a daily nutrition program aired nationally. She can also be heard two mornings a week on CFRB's *Ted Woloshyn Show*. Leslie runs a private practice at the Medcan Clinic in Toronto.

Leslie has worked with many of Canada's leading businesses and international food companies. She regularly delivers nutrition workshops to corporate groups across Canada and the United States. Having a strong interest in sports nutrition, Leslie acts as nutrition consultant to the Toronto Raptors and has worked with the Canadian International Marathon (1995–1997). She often holds nutrition workshops for Toronto's marathon and running clinics. Leslie keeps fit herself by running, cycling, and weight training.

Born and raised in Vancouver, B.C., Leslie obtained her bachelor of science (dietetics) from the University of British Columbia and proceeded to complete the dietetic internship program at St. Michael's Hospital in Toronto. She is a member of the Dietitians of Canada, the College of Dietitians of Ontario, and the Consulting Dietitians of Ontario. She lives in Toronto.

Visit Leslie Beck's website at **www.lesliebeck.com**.

Also by Leslie Beck

Leslie Beck's 10 Steps to Healthy Eating

Leslie Beck's Nutrition Encyclopedia

Leslie Beck's Nutrition Guide for Women

Leslie Beck's Nutrition Guide to Menopause

leslie beck's
nutrition guide to a
healthy pregnancy

what to eat before, during,
and after your pregnancy

leslie beck RD

Associate Researcher Anne von Rosenbach, B.A., M.L.S.

PENGUIN
CANADA

PENGUIN CANADA

Penguin Group (Canada), a division of Pearson Penguin Canada Inc.,
   10 Alcorn Avenue, Toronto, Ontario M4V 3B2

Penguin Group (U.K.), 80 Strand, London WC2R 0RL, England
Penguin Group (U.S.), 375 Hudson Street, New York, New York 10014, U.S.A.
Penguin Group (Australia) Inc., 250 Camberwell Road, Camberwell, Victoria 3124, Australia
Penguin Group (Ireland), 25 St. Stephen's Green, Dublin 2, Ireland
Penguin Books India (P) Ltd, 11, Community Centre, Panchsheel Park, New Delhi – 110 017, India
Penguin Group (NZ), cnr Airborne and Rosedale Roads, Albany, Auckland 1310, New Zealand
Penguin Books (South Africa) (Pty) Ltd, 24 Sturdee Avenue, Rosebank 2196, South Africa

Penguin Group, Registered Offices: 80 Strand, London WC2R 0RL, England

First published 2004

(WEB) 10 9 8 7 6 5 4 3 2 1

This publication contains the opinions and ideas of its author and is designed to provide useful advice
in regard to the subject matter covered. The herbs and other treatments in this book are described for the
information and education of readers. They are not a replacement for diagnosis and treatment by qualified
health professionals. The author and publisher are not engaged in rendering health or other professional
services in this publication. This publication is not intended to provide a basis for action in particular
circumstances without consideration by a competent professional. The author and publisher expressly
disclaim any responsibility for any liability, loss, or risk, personal or otherwise, which is incurred as
a consequence, directly or indirectly, of the use and application of any of the contents of this book.

Manufactured in Canada.

NATIONAL LIBRARY OF CANADA CATALOGUING IN PUBLICATION

Beck, Leslie
   Leslie Beck's nutrition guide to a healthy pregnancy / Leslie Beck.

Includes index.
ISBN 0-14-301632-6

1. Pregnancy—Nutritional aspects. I. Title. II. Title: Nutrition guide to a healthy pregnancy.

RG559.B42 2004   618.2'42   C2004-900818-8

Visit the Penguin Group (Canada) website at **www.penguin.ca**

The moment a child is born,
the mother is also born.
She never existed before.
The woman existed, but the mother, never.
A mother is something absolutely new.

—Rajneesh

Contents

Acknowledgments

Many people have helped make this book become a reality. I am so grateful to be surrounded by a team of people who support me—individuals who have given their time, their hard work, and emotional support. It is with heartfelt thanks and gratitude that I thank the following people for their invaluable contributions:

Anne von Rosenbach, a dedicated and thorough researcher who has helped me enormously. Without Anne's assistance, I am certain this book would still be in the making. Anne spent months and months gathering and organizing studies and articles on nutrition during pregnancy and breastfeeding. And she was kind enough to put her own experience with pregnancy into words on the pages of this book.

Donna Bartolini and The Canadian Living Test Kitchen, for their time and effort in helping me put together a meal plan with so many delicious and nutritious recipes.

Andrea Crozier at Penguin Canada, for encouraging me to write this book.

Professor Hélène Delisle of the University of Montreal's Faculty of Medicine for her valuable feedback on the manuscript.

My mother, Janet, for sharing her pregnancy and postpartum stories with me. As an expecting mother in the 1960s, her experiences were very different from those of pregnant women today. Speaking with her made me realize how much our knowledge has progressed over the past two generations.

My close friends and clients who are mothers, who so generously answered my some-times intruding questions about their pregnancies and breastfeeding. Their stories brought to life so many aspects of pregnancy.

My clients who, over the years, have stimulated my continued learning. In the field of nutrition, there is something new to learn every day. I hope that never changes, for it is what keeps me motivated (and writing books!).

My female clients, who made it clear that, despite its benefits, breastfeeding remains a mother's personal decision and one that they should not be made to feel guilty for, whichever method of feeding they choose.

My colleague and registered dietitian, Janice Daciuk, for offering her personal tips on making baby food.

My assistants, Kelly Thompson and Victoria McCowan, for keeping my practice running smoothly as my deadline for this book drew nearer—and for allowing me to interrupt their own work for so many last minute research requests.

And finally, my family and friends, who have not seen much of me for the last few months of writing this book. Thanks for hanging in and supporting me along the way. Your emotional support means the world to me.

Introduction

Our knowledge about pregnancy and nutrition has come a long way over the past 50 years. It used to be that when a woman became pregnant, she didn't alter her habits much. When my mother was pregnant with me, she wasn't told to cut out alcohol, watch her caffeine intake, or get more omega-3 fats. And there was certainly no mention of folic acid. Once I was born, she wasn't even advised to breastfeed. Instead, her breasts were bound in bandages and she suffered through a few days of pain while her milk supply dried up. She was then advised to feed me a homemade concoction of evaporated milk.

Today we have a wealth of scientific knowledge and medical expertise at our fingertips. And new research continues to emerge every day. But even with all the high-tech equipment and diagnostic tests available, good nutrition is still the key factor in giving your baby a healthy start in life. Over the past few generations, we've learned that how and what you eat before and during pregnancy is critical for producing a healthy baby. From the moment of conception and even before, the choices you make about diet, exercise, and health care will have a profound effect on the growth and development of your baby and can influence your child for the rest of his life.

This book is a must-read for women who are contemplating pregnancy, who are already expecting, and who are brand-new mothers. You'll find plenty of practical advice that translates the most up-to-date research into healthy eating strategies. No matter how well you eat right now, there is always room to fine-tune your diet. And no matter how far you are in your pregnancy, it's never too late to make healthy changes. Whether your eating habits need a tune-up or a complete overhaul, you'll get all the information you need in the chapters that follow—information that's translated into real food choices.

How to Use this Book

Eat Healthy Before, During, and After Your Pregnancy

This book allows you to jump in and follow my nutrition advice no matter what stage of pregnancy you're in. If you're not yet pregnant, you'll learn how to improve your diet to get your body ready for the physical demands of pregnancy. You'll have the opportunity to assess your eating and lifestyle habits and determine what needs improvement. I've even given you a pre-pregnancy checklist to help you prepare for the new venture you are about to embark on. Getting a head start on healthy eating, exercise, and weight control will make the eating-right part of pregnancy much easier. There will be no big adjustments to make, just a little fine-tuning here and there as your pregnancy progresses.

I've also given you a trimester-by-trimester guide to your calorie, protein, vitamin, and mineral requirements. You'll find advice on weight gain, prenatal supplements, and food safety. And I've included a chapter that will help you exercise your way through pregnancy, whether you're new to exercise or a veteran. This book also explains the facts of common discomforts and disorders associated with pregnancy, and offers plenty of nutrition strategies to help you feel your best. And at every stage along the way, I tell you what's happening inside your body and how your baby is developing.

You'll find a nutrition plan for breastfeeding for once your baby is born, along with plenty of tips to help you nurse your baby. For those of you who decide not to breastfeed, I've included a chapter that will help you navigate the world of infant formulas. As your baby grows, you'll learn when to introduce her to solid foods—what foods first, how much, and how to avoid allergic reactions.

This book wouldn't be complete without a chapter that helps you lose those pregnancy pounds. Whether or not you're breastfeeding, you'll find weight loss advice to help you get back to your pre-pregnancy weight, gradually and safely. I've included weight loss plans, exercise tips, and strategies to help you keep the pounds off.

A Two-Week Meal Plan to Get You Started

I know all too well how busy life can be. Preparing healthy meals day after day and week after week can be a challenge. And you may not have the energy or inclination to plan a meal in the early stages of your pregnancy. That's why I've made it easy by giving you a starter kit. With help from the experts at The Canadian Living Test Kitchen, I've mapped out a 14-day plan for you—a meal plan based on the same nutrition principles you'll read about throughout this book. If you don't want to follow a structured meal plan, enjoy the recipes—there are over 75 of them—on their own. Incorporate them as you please into your mealtimes. Each recipe in this book was developed and tested by the folks at The Canadian Living Test Kitchen. The dishes taste great, they're easy to prepare, and, of course, they're good for you and your developing baby. Each recipe is accompanied by a per-serving nutrient analysis: a breakdown of its calories, protein, fat, carbohydrate, fibre, cholesterol, sodium, calcium and iron content, among others. In addition to 14 days' worth of breakfast, lunch, and dinner ideas, you'll find recipes for great tasting vegetables, whole grains, snacks, and desserts (healthy ones, of course).

Pregnancy is a time of tremendous change in a woman's life. It's a time of excitement and joy, but these emotions are also accompanied by feelings of fatigue, anticipation, and fear. Paying attention to your nutrition and fitness, from preconception to motherhood, will allow you to feel confident that you are doing the very best for you and your baby. There is no greater gift you can give your child than to live a healthy lifestyle every day, during your pregnancy and beyond.

Enjoy your journey to motherhood and the joys of raising your child.

Leslie Beck, RD
Toronto, 2004

Part One

Preparing for
a Healthy Pregnancy

1

———✥———

Getting Ready for Pregnancy:
Assess Your Diet and Lifestyle

If you're reading this book, chances are you're planning a family. Whether it's your first pregnancy or second (or third or fourth), this chapter will help get you started preparing your body for conception. Or perhaps you're already pregnant. Congratulations—that's wonderful news! Regardless of where you are in your pregnancy, it is never too late to make healthy changes to your diet. There's no question that your current eating habits can influence your pregnancy. Here are just a few examples:

- Getting enough folic acid (an important B vitamin you'll learn all about in the chapters that follow) before pregnancy and during the first trimester is critical for the healthy formation of your baby's spinal column (neural tube). It's estimated that up to 70 percent of neural tube defects can be prevented by consuming an adequate amount of folic acid.

- Boosting your iron intake when you are *considering* getting pregnant can prevent anemia during pregnancy.

- Overweight women are more likely to give birth to heavier babies. Studies suggest that a high birth weight is linked to a greater risk of weight problems in adulthood. Getting your body in shape before you conceive can enhance your baby's future health.

- Women with pre-existing diabetes are much more likely to have a baby with birth defects than non-diabetic women. Research suggests that a daily multivitamin can offset some of this risk.

- Women who exercise before and during their pregnancies are better able to cope with the physical stresses of pregnancy and labour.

Before you set out to change your diet, you need to know what areas need improvement the most. Chances are, you're already doing a lot of things right. The quizzes in this chapter will help you evaluate your diet and lifestyle habits, spot your strengths, and identify your weaknesses. You'll determine nutritional needs to start working on right now.

Take a few minutes to assess your current eating habits. Your answers to the questions below will determine what you need to focus on to ensure you are eating right *before* you become pregnant. And if you are happily expecting as you read this chapter, your answers will pave the way for a nutrient-packed diet and a healthy pregnancy.

Score Your Eating Habits

Does your pre-pregnancy diet need some fixing up? Circle Yes or No after each statement, then see how you score. I recommend that if the baby's father is involved with your pregnancy, he can take this quiz, too. As you'll learn later on in this book, healthy sperm production requires key nutrients from a healthy diet.

1. I am at a healthy weight.
   My body mass index (BMI) is between 20 and 25. (Turn to page 7 to calculate your body mass index.) If you are pregnant, omit this question.   YES   NO

2. I am not following a fad diet or a very low calorie weight loss plan.   YES   NO

3. I don't skip meals; I always eat three meals each day.   YES   NO

4. I plan for midday snacks when my meals are more than four to five hours apart.   YES   NO

5. I include a wide variety of foods in my diet.   YES   NO

6. I include at least three whole-grain foods in my daily diet (e.g., barley, brown rice, bulgur, flaxseed, kamut, millet, oatmeal, oat bran, quinoa, ready-to-eat cereal with whole grains, whole-wheat or whole-rye bread).   YES   NO

7. I include protein-rich foods in two meals each day
    (e.g., lean meat, poultry, fish, eggs, cottage cheese, tofu,
    cooked beans, lentils).   YES   NO

8. I eat oily fish at least two times per week
    (e.g., salmon, trout, sardines, herring).   YES   NO

9. I limit my intake of swordfish, tuna steak, king mackerel,
    and shark to once per month.   YES   NO

10. I limit my intake of animal fat by choosing lean cuts of meat,
    poultry breast, and low-fat dairy products.   YES   NO

11. I add fats and oils sparingly to my foods.   YES   NO

12. When I do use vegetable oil, I choose healthy products
    (e.g., olive, canola, peanut, safflower, and flaxseed oils). YES   NO

13. I try my best to avoid foods made with partially hydrogenated
    vegetable oil or shortening (e.g., commercial baked goods,
    fried fast foods, potato chips, stick or tub margarine).   YES   NO

14. I eat at least two or three fruit servings each day
    (one serving equals one medium-sized fruit, 3/4 cup or 175 ml
    unsweetened fruit juice, 1 cup or 250 ml berries or fruit salad). YES   NO

15. I eat at least three vegetable servings each day
    (one serving equals 1/2 cup or 125 ml cooked or raw vegetables,
    1 cup or 250 ml green salad, 3/4 cup or 175 ml vegetable juice). YES   NO

16. I rinse fruits and vegetables before eating to remove dirt
    and pesticide residue.   YES   NO

17. I get three servings of dairy or calcium-enriched beverage
    each day
    (one serving equals 1 cup or 250 ml milk, yogurt, calcium-enriched
    soy or rice beverage, or calcium-enriched fruit juice).   YES   NO

18. I include other high-calcium foods in my daily diet
    (e.g., tofu, almonds, green leafy vegetables, canned
    salmon with bones).   YES   NO

19. I drink at least 5 cups (1.25 litres) of plain water each day.   YES   NO

20. I limit my intake of alcohol to no more than seven drinks
    per week or one a day. (Men: no more than nine per week.)   YES   NO

21. I limit my intake of caffeine to no more than three small
    (6 ounce) cups of coffee each day.   YES   NO

22. I eat sugary foods such as cakes, pastries, cookies, ice cream,
    candy, chocolate bars, and soda pop on occasion only (no more
    than twice per week).   YES   NO

23. I limit my intake of salty foods and buy low-sodium products
    (e.g., snack foods, crackers, commercial soups, pre-packaged
    luncheon meat, packaged noodles or rice and sauce,
    frozen dinners).   YES   NO

24. I take a multivitamin and mineral supplement that supplies
    0.4 milligrams of folic acid and 18 milligrams of iron (women only).   YES   NO

So, how healthy are you eating? Add up your Yes answers to get your score:

20 to 24: **Excellent.** You're a nutrition pro. Your diet is ready for pregnancy. Take a look at your No answers to fine-tune your eating habits.

15 to 19: **Fair to good.** Pick three areas to improve on over the next few months. Your goal is to boost your score to Excellent.

Less than 15: **Needs improvement.** You need to actively work on eating better. Chapter 2 offers nutrition advice that will help you overhaul your diet before beginning your healthy pregnancy.

How Healthy Is Your Weight?

Researchers, nutritionists, and doctors use the body mass index (BMI) to assess your weight. The BMI is a mathematical formula that takes into account your weight and your height and determines whether your weight is putting your health at risk. It's used for adults aged 20 to 65. The BMI is not to be used for children, teens, pregnant or breast-feeding women, endurance athletes, or very muscular people.

You'll read in Chapter 2 how being underweight or overweight during your pregnancy can affect the health of your future baby. Now's the time to evaluate your weight so that if you need to, you can make the necessary adjustments to achieve a healthy weight.

Take a moment to calculate your BMI as follows (you will need a calculator):

Determine your weight in kilograms (kg)
(Divide your weight in pounds by 2.2) _____ Weight in kg

Determine your height in centimetres (cm)
(Multiply your height in inches by 2.54) _____ Height in cm

Determine your height in metres (m)
(Divide your height in centimetres by 100) _____ Height in metres

Square your height in metres (m)
(Multiply your height in metres by your height in metres) _____ Height in metres^2

Now, calculate your BMI.
(Divide your weight [in kg] by your height [in m^2]) _____ Your BMI

But what does a BMI mean? Long-term studies show that the overall risk of developing heart disease, diabetes, and high blood pressure is generally related to your BMI as follows:

BMI under 20	You may be more likely to develop certain health problems due to malnutrition, including anemia, osteoporosis, and irregular heart rhythms.
BMI 20–25	A healthy weight for most people. Your risk for health problems is very low.
BMI 25–29.9	Overweight. Having a BMI in this range is a call to action. Your risk for future health problems is starting to increase.
BMI 30 or higher	Obese. You are at high risk for weight-related health problems.

Pre-Pregnancy Weight and Fertility

If you are considering pregnancy, you should be aware that your body weight can affect your ability to become pregnant. Having a BMI greater than 27 is associated with reduced fertility. Being overweight means that your fat cells can produce enough estrogen to interfere with your ability to conceive. High estrogen levels tell your brain to stop stimulating the development of follicles (eggs) and, as result, ovulation doesn't occur. This is common in women with polycystic ovary syndrome. Studies show that losing weight and reducing body fat can lead to ovulation and pregnancy.

Weighing too little is not healthy either. Menstruation occurs at a critical level of fatness. If you lose too much weight, or you are already thin, your body fat diminishes, hormone levels are affected, and this, in turn, can lead to the inability to ovulate.

Pre-Pregnancy Weight and Your Baby's Health

Your pre-pregnancy weight is an important factor in your future baby's health. To have the healthiest pregnancy possible, start it at a healthy weight. That means your BMI should be between 20 and 25. Scientists are learning that some adult health problems, such as heart disease and cancer, may be shaped in the womb. The nutrients and hormones that flow to your unborn baby are partially influenced by your diet, your pre-pregnancy weight, and your rate of weight gain during pregnancy. Positive or negative conditions, at sensitive times of development, may have long-lasting effects on your baby's future risk of disease. Although this area of research is only just beginning, studies do suggest that it's possible to eat for your child's future health.

If you are underweight before pregnancy, there is a greater chance that your baby will be born underweight. Evidence suggests that full-term babies born underweight have a higher risk of diabetes, high blood pressure, heart disease, and stroke in adulthood. It seems that a child with a low birth weight is more likely to have an apple-shaped figure as an adult. And we know that carrying extra weight around your waistline increases your risk for diabetes and heart disease.

Being overweight before you become pregnant may have consequences, too. I mentioned earlier that overweight moms-to-be are more likely to deliver babies heavier than normal. And there is good evidence that birth weight is related to BMI and overweight in children and young adults.[1] According to the Nurses' Health Study from Harvard University, women who weighed more than 10 pounds (4.5 kilograms) at birth had a 62 percent chance of becoming overweight adults. Even those who weighed between 8.6 and 10 pounds (3.9 and 4.5 kilograms) at birth had an almost 20 percent chance of becoming overweight.[2] Some research even suggests that the higher the birth weight, the higher the risk of breast cancer later in life.[3]

The take-home message is clear: it is prudent to achieve a healthy weight *before* you conceive. In Chapter 2, I discuss how to lose those extra pounds or gain weight safely. If you are already pregnant and your pre-pregnancy BMI was outside the healthy zone, there's no need to worry. What's important now is that you gain the appropriate amount of weight, at the appropriate rate, during your pregnancy. In the chapters that follow, I will tell you how much weight you need to gain in each trimester and how to go about doing that.

Beyond Diet: Assess Your Lifestyle

Diet is not the only factor that can influence your pregnancy. Other lifestyle factors play important roles, too. By taking stock of your habits and the environment in which you live and work, you can correct problem areas before you conceive. Be honest when you evaluate your habits. If you answer True to any of the following questions, speak to your health care provider about making positive changes for a healthy pregnancy.

1. I am a smoker.   TRUE   FALSE

    Smoking during pregnancy is clearly linked to having a small or preterm baby (born before 37 completed weeks of pregnancy), and it may even harm your fetus. But smoking, even if only now and again, can also make it harder for you to get pregnant. And if the father-to-be smokes, his fertility is at risk, too, since smoking can damage his sperm.
      Now is the time to stop smoking. Ask your doctor about smoking cessation programs in your community. Studies reveal that quitting by your 16th week of pregnancy lessens the chance your baby will be born too early. Research also shows that cutting down on how much you smoke while pregnant can increase your baby's birth weight.

2. I live or work in an environment that exposes me to
    second-hand smoke.   TRUE   FALSE

    Living with someone who smokes means that you can breathe in harmful amounts of second-hand smoke—and that means your developing baby does, too. A growing body of research supports the notion that babies and children are harmed by second-hand smoke. Planning for pregnancy includes planning for your newborn's environment.

3. I take drugs: prescription drugs, over-the-counter medications,
    recreational drugs, or herbal remedies.   TRUE   FALSE

    Almost any drug can cross the placenta, an organ in the uterus that serves to nourish your unborn baby, and enter his bloodstream. Using illegal street drugs at any time during your pregnancy can harm your baby. Regular use of some street drugs can also cause him to be born with an addiction. If you use street drugs, stop before you become pregnant. If you learn you are pregnant while using such drugs, be sure to tell your doctor so you can get the prenatal care you need.
      Although few medications are *known* to harm your growing baby, most have not been studied for this, so we don't know for sure. Ideally, avoid all medications when

you become pregnant. Now is the time to speak to your doctor about the safety of any medications that you currently take. If you take a prescription drug for a health condition, talk to your doctor to find out if it is safe to take during your pregnancy. Your doctor may decide to change your medication or reduce the dose, or stop it altogether. You'll read more about the safety of vitamin supplements and herbal remedies in Chapter 7.

4. I work in an environment that exposes me to chemicals,
   solvents, fumes, or radiation.   TRUE   FALSE

Certain substances in the home or the workplace may make it harder for you to conceive or could harm your unborn baby. Before you plan to become pregnant, take a close look at what's around you. Think about the chemicals you use for gardening, for house cleaning, even for hobbies. Think about your workplace: are you exposed to substances such as pesticides, solvents, lead, mercury, or radiation? You may have to ask your employer these questions. Discuss your level of exposure with your doctor. While you are trying to get pregnant, it may be necessary to take precautions if you work with hazardous materials. If you are already pregnant, your doctor may advise you to avoid contact with certain chemicals.

5. My job requires strenuous physical work or long hours.   TRUE   FALSE

Very strenuous work (standing for more than four hours at a time, climbing stairs more than three times per seven- or eight-hour shift, bending over more than 10 times per shift), working shift work, and working more than 40 hours per week may slightly increase the risk of having a low-birth-weight baby, premature labour, or miscarriage. When you become pregnant, you may need to make changes to your job. Your doctor will help you determine what's safe to do and what's not.

6. I do not incorporate physical activity into my day (e.g., walking,
   climbing stairs, gardening).   TRUE   FALSE
Being healthy and energetic at any time includes being physically active. If you don't exercise now, start by adding what I call lifestyle activities to your daily routine. Short bouts of activity such as taking the stairs instead of the escalator, getting off the bus a few stops before your destination, and walking at lunch with a co-worker can make a difference to your health. And even better, they don't require a trip to the gym.

7. I do not engage in planned exercise or sports.   TRUE   FALSE

It's best to exercise regularly before you get pregnant. Being fit before you become pregnant can increase your chances of having a comfortable and active pregnancy. The type and amount of exercise you can do during your pregnancy will depend on how active you are before you become pregnant. If you want to lose a few pounds before you conceive, I recommend you add planned workouts to your weekly routine. You'll find out more about what kind of exercise you need in Chapter 3.

8. I do not get eight hours of sleep most nights.   TRUE   FALSE

Good health requires a good night's sleep. Sleep refreshes you, improves your attitude, and gives you the energy you need for exercise and to fight off fatigue and stress. It also boosts your immune system, reducing your risk of illness. It's important to establish good sleep habits now, before the nuances of pregnancy make it difficult to get a good night's sleep. See the pre-pregnancy checklist in Chapter 2 for tips on sleep.

9. My last medical checkup was more than one year ago.   TRUE   FALSE

If you have not seen your family doctor for a physical exam in the past 12 months, book an appointment today. Let your doctor know that you are planning to become pregnant in the near future. During this visit, your doctor will assess your current health status, review your medical history as well as your family's medical history, and ask questions about your lifestyle habits. Armed with this information, you and your doctor can start planning for your healthy pregnancy.

It's important that you get a clean bill of health before you become pregnant. Routine blood tests, such as hemoglobin and hematocrit, will determine if you have iron deficiency anemia. You can be iron deficient without being anemic. More sensitive blood tests, such as ferritin or total iron binding capacity (TIBC), measure your tissue iron stores and will indicate if you need to boost your iron intake before conception. If you have diabetes, blood tests will determine if your blood sugars are under control. Because high blood sugar can cause birth defects early in pregnancy, it is important for you to get your sugars well controlled before you conceive.

Your doctor will also discuss your immunity during this pre-pregnancy checkup. Diseases such as chicken pox and rubella (German measles) are harmless most of the time, but if you contract them during pregnancy, they can harm your developing baby. If you are not already, you may want to get immunized.

If you have been pregnant before, you'll be asked if you had any problems during your pregnancy, labour and delivery, and after birth. This will allow your doctor to try to prevent these problems from happening again, or plan for special care.

10. I have not discussed my sexual history with my doctor.   TRUE   FALSE

If you have had sex without using a condom, especially if you have had more than one partner, you are at risk for sexually transmitted diseases. You may have been unknowingly exposed to genital herpes, genital warts, syphilis, chlamydia, gonorrhea, or the HIV virus. Some of these diseases need to be treated so they don't infect your baby at birth. Seriously consider testing for HIV if your sexual history puts you at risk for contracting the infection. There is effective treatment for HIV-positive mothers to reduce the risk of passing on the virus to their babies. Although this may be an uncomfortable topic to broach with your doctor, it is imperative that you give your doctor an honest sexual history to reduce the risks to your baby and, if needed, to plan for special care for your baby's birth.

Now that you've completed the assessments in this chapter, let's get to work. It's time to tune up your diet, get your body moving, and give up any bad habits that can interfere with experiencing a healthy pregnancy. Perhaps you scored well on each quiz. That's great. But even the healthiest of women can make improvements. Wondering where to start? It's all spelled out in the following chapters, so keep reading.

2

———— ✺ ————

The "Training Trimester": A Pre-Pregnancy Nutrition Plan

Who would have thought that you had to follow a special diet *before* you become pregnant? The journey to motherhood begins before you conceive. While you should certainly avoid fad diets and programs before you conceive and while pregnant—indeed, at any time—making small adjustments to how you eat and keep fit can make a big difference to your unborn child, not to mention how you will feel now and during pregnancy. And it's easy. Before you know it, you'll be eating healthier than you ever thought possible.

Think of your pre-pregnancy diet as a training diet, a nutrition plan that will get your body ready for pregnancy. It's a lot like sports nutrition. In my private practice, I see many women and men who are training for a marathon. They don't wait to consult me the week before the marathon. Rather, they embark on a nutrition regime at the beginning of their training program, months before the big event. My clients understand how important it is to eat healthy throughout their training. Long before the race, they practise eating the right foods, in the right amounts, at the right times. The day before a long training run, I have those clients eat just as they would the day before the race, so that when they set out to run the marathon, their bodies are well nourished and ready to go the distance.

Think of the time before you conceive as your training trimester—three months to fine-tune your diet, build up your nutrient stores, and shape up your body. If you're not planning to become pregnant so soon, that's fine, too. Think of this as an extra-long training trimester in which to adopt healthy eating habits. Many of my clients come to see me one year before they hope to become pregnant—women who want to lose weight before they conceive, or women who feel their diet is far from optimal.

Learning how to eat properly before you become pregnant is important for many reasons:

- Your pre-pregnancy diet serves as a nutritional insurance policy. In the first days or even weeks of pregnancy, you may not even know you're pregnant. Yet from very early on, your baby is undergoing amazing transformations. In just 28 days after conception, his spinal cord and brain are completely formed. And this requires adequate amounts of folic acid, B vitamins, protein, and zinc. During this early developmental period, your unborn baby will draw on your body's stores of certain essential nutrients. A healthy diet before pregnancy ensures that these nutrients are stockpiled in your body's tissues.

- Your pre-pregnancy diet will give you the extra energy and nutrients you need during your pregnancy. A well-nourished woman will be better able to cope with the physical demands of pregnancy. And here's another bonus: learning how to eat right will help you recover quickly after your baby is born.

- Your pre-pregnancy diet will help you lose or gain weight if need be.

- Your pre-pregnancy diet can help get medical conditions, such as high blood pressure or diabetes, under control.

- Your pre-pregnancy diet will help put your mind at ease once you become pregnant. Adopting a healthy diet now means you won't have to worry about making abrupt dietary changes once you are pregnant. You'll feel confident about your nutrition choices and be well prepared for the exciting journey that lies ahead.

- Your pre-pregnancy diet will set the stage for lifelong healthy eating. You'll have the knowledge and skills you need to make healthy choices for you and your baby. The nutrition principles you follow today and throughout your pregnancy will lay the foundation for your baby's health.

As you can see, getting a head start on healthy eating means you'll be ready, both physically and emotionally, for your pregnancy. You'll have nutrients on board from the moment you become pregnant. Below, I'll tell you not only what nutrients you need and how to get them but also what to avoid. Practise these 10 nutrition strategies for three months before you plan to become pregnant.

If you are already pregnant, that's wonderful news. But don't skip to the next chapter before reading the nutrition advice below. The nutrition strategies that follow lay the foundation for a healthy pregnancy diet. These dietary modifications are important when you are expecting. No matter where you are in your pregnancy, it's not too late to make a positive impact. Here's my pre-pregnancy nutrition advice.

Fuel Up on Folate (Folic Acid): 400 Micrograms Per Day

I can't overemphasize how important it is to get enough of this B vitamin. The names "folate," "folacin," and "folic acid" are often used interchangeably. But there is a difference. Folate, or folacin, refers to the vitamin when found naturally in foods. Folic acid, on the other hand, is the synthetic form of the vitamin. Folic acid is added to vitamin supplements and enriched breads and pastas. The body absorbs folic acid much better than it does folate found in food. You'll soon see that this has great importance for women in their childbearing years.

Folate supports cell division and growth. It's used to make red blood cells and DNA, the genetic blueprint of all cells. And it's essential for the normal development of your baby's spine, brain, and skull during the early weeks of pregnancy. If the tissues that form the brain and spinal cord fail to develop properly, neural tube defects occur. These are the most serious types of birth defects. The most common neural tube defect is spina bifida, a defect in which the spinal column fails to close completely. Neural tube defects can result in stillbirth or lifelong physical and mental disabilities. Fortunately, the prevalence of neural tube defects in newborns has decreased over the past decade. Increased vitamin use as well as prenatal testing and termination of affected pregnancies have contributed to the decline.

Neural tube defects occur within the first four weeks of pregnancy, usually before a woman even knows she is pregnant. That's why Health Canada, the Canadian Paediatric Society, and the Society of Obstetricians and Gynaecologists of Canada recommend that all women of childbearing age consume 400 micrograms (0.4 milligrams) of folic acid each day to reduce the risk of neural tube defects. Folic acid has been proven to help reduce the risk of neural tube defects by more than 70 percent if taken before pregnancy.

It's recommended that you take a supplement or multivitamin, since synthetic folic acid, unlike food folate, is nearly 100 percent available to the body (folate in food is only 50 percent available). Even the best food sources won't supply all the folate you need. You need to get 400 micrograms (0.4 milligrams) of folic acid *in addition* to the folate you get from foods. Most multivitamin and mineral supplements provide 400 micrograms (0.4 milligrams) of folic acid. You might want to check your brand to see how much it contains.

Folic acid can help prevent neural tube defects only if it is taken one to three months before conception. The month prior to conception and one month after are the most critical times for getting folic acid, because the baby's neural tube (spinal column) is completely closed by four weeks after conception. So start taking a multivitamin at least three months before you plan to get pregnant, and continue taking it throughout the first trimester. (I'll discuss the use of vitamin supplements during your pregnancy in Chapter 6.)

If you've taken birth control pills recently, you must pay extra special attention to your folic acid intake. Many oral contraceptives diminish the body's folate stores (as well as stores of vitamin B6). Since it takes a while to build these stores back up, you should take a folic acid supplement or a multivitamin for three months before you try to get pregnant.

If you have had a previous pregnancy affected by a neural tube defect, or you have a family history of this problem, speak with your doctor. You have a higher than average risk of the problem recurring and you will likely be advised to take 4 milligrams of folic acid, 10 times the daily recommended dietary allowance. In this case, you will have to take a single supplement of folic acid, rather than getting it as part of a multivitamin. If you have diabetes, obesity, or epilepsy, you also may be at higher risk for having a baby with a neural tube defect. Your doctor will make folic acid recommendations to reduce your risk.

So, if you're not already taking a multivitamin, I hope you are on your way to the pharmacy now to pick one up. This doesn't mean you can stop paying attention to eating folate-rich foods. Along with taking a supplement, it's important to boost the folate content of your diet. Dietary folate can aid in building up your stores of this B vitamin. And many folate-rich foods supply other important pregnancy nutrients, such as iron, vitamin B6, and fibre. Assess how much folate you get each day from food by taking the quiz below.

Did You Get Your Folate Today?

1. I eat one serving of the following foods each day. (Place a check mark beside each food you eat on a daily basis.)

Excellent sources of folate: 55 micrograms or more per serving. One serving equals 1/2 cup (125 ml) cooked vegetable, 1 cup (250 ml) raw vegetable, 3/4 cup (175 ml) fruit juice, 1 cup (250 ml) fresh fruit, 1/2 cup (125 ml) cooked beans, 1/4 cup (50 ml) nuts or seeds, or 1/2 cup (125 ml) cooked pasta.

❑ Asparagus	❑ Lentils	❑ Romaine lettuce
❑ Avocado, 1/2	❑ Navy beans	❑ Soybeans
❑ Black beans	❑ Orange juice	❑ Soy nuts
❑ Chickpeas	❑ Peanuts	❑ Spinach, cooked
❑ Collard greens	❑ Pineapple juice	❑ Sunflower seeds
❑ Kidney beans	❑ Pinto beans	❑ Turnip greens

Good sources of folate: 33 micrograms folate or more per serving.

❑ Artichoke	❑ Endive	❑ Parsnips
❑ Almonds	❑ Green peas	❑ Raspberries
❑ Beets	❑ Hazelnuts	❑ Split peas
❑ Broccoli	❑ Honeydew melon	❑ String beans
❑ Brussels sprouts	❑ Lima beans	❑ Tomato juice
❑ Cashews	❑ Mung bean sprouts	❑ V8 juice
❑ Cauliflower	❑ Okra	❑ Walnuts
❑ Chinese cabbage	❑ Orange	❑ Wheat germ (15 ml)

2. I buy breads and pastas that are labelled "enriched."   Yes ❑   No ❑

3. I take a multivitamin or folic acid supplement each day.   Yes ❑   No ❑

By taking this quiz, you might be surprised to learn how challenging it is to eat a folate-packed diet. I'll admit, it takes careful planning to ensure you eat folate-rich foods on a daily basis. But now that you can see what foods give you the most bang for your buck, getting more folate will be a breeze . . . providing you like those foods, of course.

As of 1998, breads and pastas labelled "enriched" must be fortified with folic acid. It's estimated that adding folic acid to these products will boost the average woman's folic acid intake by approximately 0.1 milligram—one-quarter of a non-pregnant woman's daily needs. This is good news for another reason, too: researchers are learning that getting adequate folic acid may help ward off heart disease, as well as breast and colon cancer.

If you didn't check off any foods listed as excellent sources of folate, you have some work to do. To boost your folate intake, aim to include at least two servings of excellent folate foods (packing at least 55 micrograms of the vitamin per serving) in your daily diet. And take a multivitamin supplement. Here's a handy list to help you bump up your folate intake:

FOLATE CONTENT OF SELECTED FOODS (MICROGRAMS)

Legumes, Nuts, and Seeds

Beans, baked, canned, 1 cup (250 ml)	60
Black beans, cooked, 1/2 cup (125 ml)	135
Chickpeas, cooked, 1/2 cup (125 ml)	85
Kidney beans, cooked, 1/2 cup (125 ml)	120
Lentils, cooked, 1/2 cup (125 ml)	189
Navy beans, cooked, 1/2 cup (125 ml)	86
Peanuts, dry roasted, 1/4 cup (50 ml)	56
Sunflower seeds, 1/3 cup (75 ml)	96

Fruit

Orange, medium, 1	40
Orange juice, freshly squeezed, 1 cup (250 ml)	79
Orange juice, frozen, diluted, 1 cup (250 ml)	115
Pineapple juice, canned, 1 cup (250 ml)	61

FOLATE CONTENT OF SELECTED FOODS (MICROGRAMS) (continued)

Vegetables

Artichoke, medium, 1	64
Asparagus, 5 spears	110
Avocado, California, 1/2	113
Avocado, Florida, 1/2	81
Bean sprouts, 1 cup (250 ml)	91
Beets, 1/2 cup (125 ml)	72
Brussels sprouts, 1/2 cup (125 ml)	83
Corn, 1 ear or 1/2 cup (125 ml)	55

Peas, green, 1/2 cup (125 ml)	54
Pepper, sweet, yellow, 1	48
Romaine lettuce, 1 cup (250 ml)	80
Spinach, cooked, 1/2 cup (125 ml)	139
Spinach, raw, 1 cup (250 ml)	115
Turnip greens, cooked, 1/2 cup (125 ml)	90

Other Foods

Pasta, enriched, cooked, 1 cup (250 ml)	100

Nutrient Values of Some Common Foods. Health Canada (Ottawa, 1999). Adapted and Reproduced with the permission of the Minister of Public Works and Government Services Canada, 2004.

The 14-Day Meal Plan for a Healthy Pregnancy in Part Four offers plenty of recipes brimming with this superstar B vitamin. Each recipe is accompanied by a nutrient analysis so you can tell how much folate one serving provides. You'll be pleasantly surprised at how easy it is to fuel up on folate.

Can You Get Too Much Folic Acid?

Absolutely. More folic acid is not necessarily better. The daily safe upper limit of supplemental folic acid is 1 milligram (1000 micrograms). Do not take more than this without your doctor's supervision. Supplementing with doses greater than 1 milligram may cause or worsen nerve damage in people who have a vitamin B12 deficiency. If you're a strict vegetarian who eats no animal foods, you're at risk for a B12 deficiency: make sure your doctor monitors your B12 status. (You'll learn more about nutrition for vegetarian moms-to-be in Chapter 7.)

Bone Up on Calcium: 1000 Milligrams Per Day

We all know that calcium is good for strong bones and teeth. But did you also realize that this important mineral helps regulate our blood pressure, muscle contraction, and immune function? What's good for keeping our bodies strong and healthy is also good for our developing baby. Getting enough calcium can help keep your blood pressure in good control when you are pregnant. Adequate calcium during pregnancy may even reduce your risk for leg cramps and pre-eclampsia, a pregnancy complication I discuss in detail in Chapter 9.

Most women fall short of meeting the recommended dietary allowance (RDA) for this mineral. Surprisingly, your calcium requirements remain unchanged during pregnancy. That's because a woman's body amazingly adapts and uses calcium more efficiently when pregnant. Here's how much calcium you need each day.

RECOMMENDED DIETARY ALLOWANCE FOR CALCIUM (MILLIGRAMS)

	Non-Pregnant	Pregnant
Women, aged 19–50	1000	1000
Girls, aged 14–18	1300	1300
Safe upper limit	2500	2500

National Academy of Sciences, Institute of Medicine, Food and Nutrition Board. Standing Committee on the Scientific Evaluation of Dietary Reference Intakes. *Dietary Reference Intakes for Calcium, Phosphorus, Magnesium, Vitamin D, and Fluoride.* Washington, DC: The National Academy Press, 1997.

Calcium in Foods

You'll get the most calcium per serving from dairy products and calcium-fortified beverages such as soy milk or orange juice. Just 1 cup (250 ml) packs 300 milligrams of calcium. Here's how foods stack up when it comes to calcium content (notice that some of the best non-dairy calcium foods are also great sources of folate).

CALCIUM CONTENT OF SELECTED FOODS (MILLIGRAMS)

Dairy Foods

Carnation Instant Breakfast, with 1 cup (250 ml) milk	540
Cheese, cheddar, 1 1/2 oz (45 g)	300
Cheese, cottage, 1/2 cup (125 ml)	75
Cheese, mozzarella, 1 3/4 oz (50 g)	269
Cheese, ricotta, 1/2 cup (125 ml)	255
Cheese, Swiss or Gruyère, 1 1/2 oz (45 g)	480
Milk, chocolate, 1 cup (250 ml)	285
Milk, evaporated, 1/2 cup (125 ml)	350
Milk (Lactaid Milk), 1 cup (250 ml)	300
Milk (Neilson TruCalcium), 1 cup (250 ml)	420
Milk (Neilson TruTaste), 1 cup (250 ml)	360
Milk, skim powder, 3 tbsp (45 ml)	155
Sour cream, light, 1/4 cup (50 ml)	120
Yogurt, fruit, 3/4 cup (175 ml)	250
Yogurt, plain, 3/4 cup (175 ml)	300

Legumes and Soy Foods

Soybeans, cooked, 1 cup (250 ml)	175
Soybeans, roasted, 1/4 cup (50 ml)	60
Soy beverage, 1 cup (250 ml)	100
Soy beverage, fortified, 1 cup (250 ml)	300–330
Baked beans, 1 cup (250 ml)	150
Black beans, 1 cup (250 ml)	102
Kidney beans, cooked, 1 cup (250 ml)	69
Lentils, cooked, 1 cup (250 ml)	37
Tempeh, cooked, 1 cup (250 ml)	154
Tofu, raw, firm, with calcium sulphate, 4 oz (120 g)	260
Tofu, raw, regular, with calcium sulphate, 4 oz (120 g)	130

Fish

Salmon, 1/2 can (with bones)	225
Sardines, small (with bones), 8	165

Fruit

Currants, 1/2 cup (125 ml)	60
Figs, medium, 5	135
Orange, medium, 1	50

Vegetables

Broccoli, cooked, 1 cup (250 ml)	94

CALCIUM CONTENT OF SELECTED FOODS (MILLIGRAMS) (continued)

Broccoli, raw, 1 cup (250 ml)	42	**Nuts**	
Bok choy, cooked, 1 cup (250 ml)	158	Almonds, 1/4 cup (50 ml)	100
Collard greens, cooked, 1 cup (250 ml)	357	Brazil nuts, 1/4 cup (50 ml)	65
Kale, cooked, 1 cup (250 ml)	179	Hazelnuts, 1/4 cup (50 ml)	65
Okra, cooked, 1 cup (250 ml)	176	**Other Foods**	
Rutabaga, cooked, 1/2 cup (125 ml)	57	Blackstrap molasses, 2 tbsp (25 ml)	288
Swiss chard, cooked, 1 cup (250 ml)	102	Orange or grapefruit juice,	
Swiss chard, raw, 1 cup (250 ml)	21	calcium-fortified, 1 cup (250 ml)	300–360

Nutrient Values of Some Common Foods. Health Canada (Ottawa, 1999). Adapted and Reproduced with the permission of the Minister of Public Works and Government Services Canada, 2004.

Tips to Boost Calcium

Follow these tips to boost your calcium intake:

- Aim for three servings of milk or calcium-fortified beverage each day.

- Cook hot cereal, rice, and grains in low-fat milk or calcium-fortified soy beverage.

- Add milk to cream soups, puddings, and egg dishes.

- Add skim milk powder to casseroles, soups, smoothies, meatloaf, French toast, muffin batters, breads, mashed potatoes, and dips. Just 1/4 cup (50 ml) packs 210 milligrams of calcium.

- Use evaporated skim milk instead of regular milk or cream in puddings, cream soups, and pasta cream sauces. A serving of evaporated milk contains twice as much calcium as regular milk.

- Top a baked potato with 1/4 cup (50 ml) low-fat sour cream for an extra 70 milligrams of calcium.

- In a hurry? Try an instant breakfast drink with skim milk and you'll get 400 milligrams of the mighty mineral.

- Include at least one serving (1/2 cup or 125 ml cooked) of a calcium-rich vegetable in your daily diet.

Your body does not absorb calcium from all foods equally well. It's true that foods such as broccoli and almonds supply you with calcium, but natural compounds in plant foods bind some of this calcium and prevent it from being absorbed. The following strategies will help you enhance your body's absorption of calcium:

- Eat green vegetables cooked, rather than raw. Cooking releases some of the calcium that's bound to a compound called oxalic acid.

- If you are taking an iron supplement to treat a deficiency, don't take it with calcium-rich foods, since these two minerals compete with each other for absorption. Take the iron supplement two hours before or after a calcium-rich meal.

- Drink tea and coffee between meals. Natural compounds in these beverages inhibit calcium absorption.

Do You Need a Calcium Supplement?

The majority of my female clients find it challenging to meet their daily calcium requirements. They may be lactose intolerant, or they follow a vegetarian diet that excludes milk, or they have poor eating habits. Often taking a supplement is the only way they can ensure that they are meeting their calcium needs.

To help you decide if you need a calcium supplement, use my 300 Milligram Rule. Remember how I told you that one serving of dairy or calcium-fortified beverage gives you approximately 300 milligrams of calcium? Well, that means that most of you need to get three servings per day in order to meet your calcium requirements of 1000 milligrams. For every serving your diet lacks, you need to supplement with 300 milligrams of elemental calcium.

I recommend that you buy a calcium citrate supplement, for two reasons: it is absorbed more easily than other forms of calcium, and it is less likely to cause constipation and gas. Calcium citrate can be taken with meals or on an empty stomach. So if you're brushing your teeth before bed and you realize your diet was shy a glass of milk that day, you can take a calcium supplement right then. And here's another bonus: most calcium citrate pills offer 300 milligrams of elemental calcium, so it's a cinch to replace your missing dairy (or other calcium-rich food) servings. If you need 1000 milligrams of calcium each day, but you're getting only two dairy servings (600 milligrams), all you have to do is take one calcium citrate supplement.

Avoid calcium supplements made from bone meal, dolomite, coral calcium, or oyster shell calcium. Some of these products have been found to contain trace amounts of toxic contaminants such as lead and mercury, which are harmful to a developing baby—and to you, if consumed in high quantities.

Buy a brand of calcium citrate with vitamin D and magnesium added. These nutrients work in tandem with calcium to promote optimal health. For instance, vitamin D helps the body absorb calcium from foods more efficiently. If you need to take more than one calcium pill to meet your daily requirements, split large doses throughout the day. Don't take more than 500 milligrams of calcium at one time; the body absorbs larger doses less efficiently.

Include Iron-Rich Foods: 18 Milligrams Per Day

A lack of iron is the most common nutrient deficiency among women of childbearing age. Women who cut calories to lose weight, shy away from red meat and animal foods, engage in heavy exercise, or are pregnant are all at risk for missing out on this important mineral. All women of childbearing age are at risk for developing an iron deficiency because of the regular blood loss that occurs during menstruation.

Your body needs iron to make hemoglobin, the component of red blood cells that carries oxygen to all your tissues. In your muscles, oxygen is stored in a pigment called myoglobin, which is also made from iron. If your diet does not provide the amount of iron your body needs, your iron stores will become depleted. Iron deficiency eventually leads to anemia, a condition that is diagnosed when you have a low hemoglobin level in the blood.

One doesn't become anemic overnight. Iron deficiency is a progressive condition that develops in stages, but you will feel its effects along the way. Symptoms of iron deficiency include tiredness, headache, irritability, and depression. You may also look pale, lack motivation to exercise, experience breathlessness and fatigue during a workout, and have difficulty concentrating.

Treating an Iron Deficiency

As I mentioned in Chapter 1, it's important to have your iron stores tested during your pre-pregnancy medical checkup. That way, if the doctor detects a deficiency or anemia, you'll have time to build up your body's iron stores before you conceive.

Depending on the extent of your iron deficiency, you may need to take one to three iron tablets (each providing 100 milligrams of elemental iron) per day. If you are advised to take an iron pill, take it on an empty stomach to enhance absorption. Most of my clients find that taking their iron supplement before bedtime reduces stomach upset. Iron can be constipating, so you'll need to pay attention to your intake of fibre and water to prevent this side effect (more on this later). I routinely recommend the brand Palafer to my clients, and I rarely hear a client complain about uncomfortable side effects from it. You'll have to ask the pharmacist for this product, since it's kept behind the counter (as are all high-dose iron supplements). You may notice that your stools turn black while taking iron. There's no need to worry—this is a normal and harmless side effect of the treatment.

A supplementation period of 12 weeks is usually all it takes to treat an iron deficiency. However, it is sometimes necessary to supplement for up to six months to completely restore your body's iron reserves. As your iron levels improve, your symptoms will gradually disappear. Your doctor will perform occasional blood tests to ensure that your iron supply has increased to a healthy level.

When it comes to iron supplements, it is important to remember that more is *not* better. Too much iron can cause indigestion and constipation. And excessive doses of iron can be toxic, causing damage to the liver and intestines. An iron overload can even result in death. Do not take iron supplements without having a blood test to confirm that you are in fact iron deficient.

Iron and Pregnancy

It's important to make sure you have sufficient stores of iron now, since your daily iron requirements increase once you become pregnant, especially during the second and third trimesters.

RECOMMENDED DIETARY ALLOWANCE FOR IRON (MILLIGRAMS)

	Non-Pregnant Non-Vegetarians	Non-Pregnant Vegetarians	Pregnant Non-Vegetarians	Pregnant Vegetarians
Women, aged 19–50	18	32	27	48
Girls, aged 14–18	15	27	27	48
Safe upper limit	45	45	45	45

National Academy of Sciences, Institute of Medicine, Food and Nutrition Board, Standing Committee on the Scientific Evaluation of Dietary Reference Intakes. *Dietary Reference Intakes for Vitamin A, Vitamin K, Arsenic, Boron, Chromium, Copper, Iodine, Iron, Manganese, Molybdenum, Nickel, Silicon, Vanadium, and Zinc.* Washington, DC: The National Academy Press, 2002.

Pregnancy can deplete a woman's iron stores at a much faster rate than normal. That's because the growing fetus and placenta require a higher blood volume and a larger supply of iron. Pregnant women are likely to develop iron deficiency unless they take a prenatal supplement that provides extra iron (more on prenatal supplements in Chapter 7). In the meantime, here's how to get more iron from your diet.

Iron in Foods

The richest sources of iron are beef, fish, poultry, pork, and lamb. These are known as heme sources of iron, the type that can be absorbed and utilized the most efficiently by your body. Heme sources of iron contribute about 10 percent of the iron we consume each day. Even though heme iron accounts for such a small proportion of our intake, it is so well absorbed that it contributes a significant amount.

The rest of our iron comes from plant foods such as dried fruits, whole grains, leafy green vegetables, nuts, seeds, and legumes. These are called non-heme sources of iron. The body is much less efficient in absorbing and using this type of iron. Vegetarians may have difficulty maintaining healthy iron stores because their diet relies exclusively on non-heme sources. If you follow a vegetarian diet that excludes meat, poultry, or fish, your recommended dietary allowance for iron is higher than 18 milligrams. In fact, you need 1.8 times more iron than non-vegetarian women—32 milligrams per day.

Follow these tips to enhance your body's absorption of non-heme iron:

- *Add a little animal food to your diet, if you are not a vegetarian.* Meat, poultry, and fish contain MFP factor, a compound that promotes the absorption of non-heme iron from other foods eaten with them.

- *Add a source of vitamin C.* Including some vitamin C food in a plant-based meal can enhance the body's absorption of non-heme iron fourfold. The acidity of the vitamin converts iron to a form that's ready for absorption (your stomach acid enhances iron absorption in the same way). Here are winning combinations:

  - Whole-wheat pasta with tomato sauce

  - Brown rice stir-fry with broccoli and red pepper

  - Whole-grain breakfast cereal topped with strawberries

  - Whole-grain toast with a small glass of orange juice

  - Spinach salad tossed with orange or grapefruit segments

- *Don't take a calcium supplement with an iron-rich meal.* These two minerals compete with each other for absorption.

- *Drink tea and coffee between meals, not during.* These beverages contain polyphenols, compounds that bind to non-heme iron and cause it to be excreted from the gut.

- *Cook your vegetables.* Phytic acid (phytate), found in plant foods, can attach to iron and hamper its absorption. Cooking vegetables such as spinach releases some of the iron that's bound to phytates.

IRON CONTENT OF SELECTED FOODS (MILLIGRAMS)

Meat and Poultry		Legumes	
Beef, lean, cooked, 3 oz (90 g)*	3.0	Beans in tomato sauce, 1 cup (250 ml)	5.0
Chicken breast, cooked, 3 oz (90 g)	0.6	Kidney beans, 1/2 cup (125 ml)	2.5
Fish		**Fruit and Vegetables**	
Oysters, cooked, medium, 5	7.2	Apricots, dried, 6	2.8
Shrimp, cooked, large, 10	1.7	Prune juice, 1/2 cup (125 ml)	5.0
Tuna, light, canned, 1/2 cup (125 ml)	1.2	Spinach, cooked, 1 cup (250 ml)	4.0

Cereals	
All Bran, Kellogg's, 1/2 cup (125 ml)	4.7
All Bran Buds, Kellogg's, 1/2 cup (125 ml)	5.9
Bran Flakes, 3/4 cup (175 ml)	4.9
Cream of Wheat, 1/2 cup (125 ml)	8.0
Just Right, Kellogg's, 1 cup (250 ml)	6.0

Oatmeal, instant, 1 package	3.8
Raisin Bran, 3/4 cup (175 ml)	5.5
Shreddies, 3/4 cup (175 ml)	5.9

Other Foods	
Blackstrap molasses, 1 tbsp (15 ml)	3.2
Wheat germ, 1 tbsp (15 ml)	2.5

*3 oz (90 g) is the size of a deck of playing cards.

Nutrient Values of Some Common Foods. Health Canada (Ottawa, 1999). Adapted and Reproduced with the permission of the Minister of Public Works and Government Services, 2004.

Getting 18 milligrams of iron each day can be challenging, especially if you seldom eat red meat. That's why I recommend that all menstruating women take a multivitamin and mineral supplement each day. Not only will a multivitamin supply your daily share of folic acid, it will also provide 10 to 18 milligrams of iron, depending on the brand. Women's one-a-day formulas usually have 18 milligrams of iron, a good choice if you're a vegetarian. Be sure to check the label to determine how much iron you're getting.

Get Enough Protein: 50 Grams Per Day

Protein-rich foods such as lean meat, poultry, fish, legumes, and dairy products supply your body with amino acids, the building blocks for tissue growth and repair. Cells cannot be formed without protein in your diet. The amino acids in protein foods are used to form muscle tissues, connective tissues, skin, hair, and nails. They are also used to make hormones, enzymes, and important immune compounds that keep you healthy.

Protein and Pregnancy

As you'll read in the next few chapters, your protein requirements increase during pregnancy. That makes sense, since protein supports cell growth and division, activities that are continually occurring in your developing baby. If your diet is too low in protein during pregnancy, the placenta may not function efficiently to prevent harmful substances passing from you to your baby's bloodstream. Many protein-rich foods supply a fair amount of vitamin B6, iron, and zinc, nutrients that play important roles in the development of your baby. As you'll see below, your daily protein requirements are based on your body weight.

RECOMMENDED DIETARY PROTEIN INTAKES FOR HEALTHY WOMEN

Sedentary (no regular exercise)	0.36 grams per pound body weight (0.8 grams per kilogram)
Recreational exercise	0.5–0.7 grams per pound body weight (1.1–1.5 grams per kilogram)
Endurance athlete	0.5–0.6 grams per pound body weight (1.2–1.4 grams per kilogram)
Maximum for healthy adults	0.9 grams per pound body weight (2.0 grams per kilogram)

Position of the American Dietetic Association, Dietitians of Canada, and the American College of Sports Medicine: Nutrition and athletic performance. *Journal of the American Dietetic Association* 2000, 100(12):1543–1556; *Manual of Clinical Dietetics*, 6th ed. Chicago: American Dietetic Association, 2000.

To find out how much protein you need to eat each day, multiply your recommended dietary allowance for protein by your body weight. For example:

- A 135-pound woman, no exercise: $135 \times 0.36 = 48$ grams protein

- A 135-pound woman, three workouts per week: $135 \times 0.5 = 67$ grams protein

- A 135-pound woman, training for a marathon: $135 \times 0.6 = 81$ grams protein

The average non-pregnant woman needs to consume roughly 50 grams of protein each day. As you can see, if you exercise, you need a little more. Here's a look at some of the best sources of protein, and how much protein a serving of each supplies.

PROTEIN CONTENT OF SELECTED FOODS (GRAMS)

Meat, Poultry, and Fish

Meat, 3 oz (90 g)*	21–25
Chicken, 3 oz (90 g)	21
Salmon, 3 oz (90 g)	25
Sole, 3 oz (90 g)	17
Tuna, canned, 1/2 cup (125 ml)	30

Eggs

Egg, white, large, 1	3
Egg, whole, large, 1	6

Milk and Milk Alternates

Cheese, cheddar, 1 oz (30 g)	10
Milk, 1 cup (250 ml)	8
Soy milk, 1 cup (250 ml)	9
Yogurt, fruit-bottom, 3/4 cup (175 ml)	8

Legumes and Soy Foods

Beans, baked, cooked, 1 cup (250 ml)	13
Black beans, cooked, 1 cup (250 ml)	16
Kidney beans, cooked, 1 cup (250 ml)	16
Lentils, cooked, 1 cup (250 ml)	19
Soybeans, cooked, 1 cup (250 ml)	30
Soy ground round, cooked, 1/3 cup (55 g)	11
Tofu, firm, 6 cm × 4 cm × 4 cm piece (80 g)	13
Veggie dog, small, 1 (46 g)	11
Veggie burger (soy protein based), 1 patty (71 g)	12–14

Nuts and Seeds

Almonds, 1/2 cup (125 ml)	12

Mixed nuts, 1/2 cup (125 ml)	13	Energy Bars, high-carbohydrate (PowerBar, Clif Bar)	7
Peanuts, 1/2 cup (125 ml)	18		
Peanut butter, 2 tbsp (25 ml)	9	Energy Bars, high-protein (Pure Protein, ProMax)	21–35
Sunflower seeds, 1/3 cup (75 ml)	8	Soy protein powder, flavoured, 1 scoop (28 g)	14–16
Tahini (sesame butter), 2 tbsp (25 ml)	2		

Protein Supplements

		Soy protein powder, plain, 1 scoop (28 g)	25
Energy Bars, 40/30/30 (Balance Bar, Zone Bar)	14–18	Whey protein powder, 1 scoop (32 g)	22–25

*3 oz (90 g) is the size of a deck of cards.

Nutrient Values of Some Common Foods. Health Canada (Ottawa, 1999). Adapted and Reproduced with the permission of the Minister of Public Works and Government Services Canada, 2004.

Here's a handy way to ensure you're getting enough protein before you become pregnant:

Breakfast	Include 8 to 15 grams (e.g., 1 cup [250 ml] milk or yogurt, 1 egg, or 1/2 cup [125 ml] cottage cheese)
Lunch	Include 15 to 20 grams (e.g., three slices of chicken breast, 1 cup [250 ml] bean salad, or 1/2 can of salmon)
Dinner	Include 20 grams

You can also make sure your snacks contain protein. Snack foods such as yogurt, milk, soy milk, and nuts will help you meet your daily protein requirements and keep you feeling full longer. That's because protein slows down the rate of digestion, giving your meal or snack staying power. You won't feel hungry soon after eating.

Don't forget that whole grains (e.g., whole-wheat bread, brown rice, oatmeal) and vegetables add a little protein to your diet, too. For instance, 1/2 cup (125 ml) of cooked vegetables supplies about 2 grams of protein, a whole-wheat pita pocket provides 6 grams.

It's fairly easy to get enough protein in your diet each day. In fact, most women I meet with do not lack protein in their diet, nor do they need to add protein powders to boost their intake. But if you're a vegetarian, you may be at risk for under-eating protein. Be sure you add a serving of beans or soy to both lunch and dinner.

Leslie's Pre-Pregnancy Meal Plans and Protein

The pre-pregnancy meal plans below provide enough protein for a healthy woman who exercises regularly, at a moderate pace. Whether you're running, power walking, taking aerobics classes, or using weights, you can rest assured you're getting enough protein. If you aren't active right now, I recommend you add exercise to your weekly routine. You'll find plenty of ideas for doing so in Chapter 10.

If you honestly can't see yourself starting to exercise on a regular basis, then you can cut back your portion size of meat, poultry, fish, tofu, or beans. Drop two protein food servings from the meal plan you choose (weight loss, weight maintenance, or weight gain). But, you must add back the calories with something else—either with one fruit serving or one grain food serving.

Another note: I have designed each plan to provide 1000 milligrams of calcium, to cover your daily requirement.

Eat the Right Kind of Fish:
Two to Three Times Per Week

Fish is a great source of protein that's low in cholesterol-raising saturated fat. If fish is not part of your weekly menu, I encourage you to include it. Fish, in particular fatty fish, contains omega-3 fatty acids, fats that help ward off heart disease and may even boost your mood. While these fats are good for your heart, they're also important for a healthy pregnancy. If fish isn't a part of your weekly menu, I suggest you try the delicious fish recipes featured in my 14-Day Meal Plan for a Healthy Pregnancy. Here are a few more reasons why you need to get more omega-3s in your diet.

Fish contains two omega-3 fats: docosahexaenoic acid (DHA) and eicosapentaenoic acid (EPA). DHA appears to be the most important omega-3 fatty acid when it comes to fetal health and your baby's brain and eye development, especially during the third trimester. DHA accumulates in a developing baby's brain, increasing three to five times during the final trimester.

How much DHA reaches your baby's brain depends on your diet during pregnancy. Animal studies suggest that offspring born to mothers who had DHA-deficient diets have behavioural problems and abnormal vision. Although DHA accumulates in the later part of pregnancy, it's important to consume omega-3 fats before and during your pregnancy.

Although the evidence is not conclusive, eating fish and seafood during pregnancy might ward off postpartum depression. Studies suggest that mothers with low DHA levels in their blood cells have a higher risk of postpartum blues. Observational studies show that countries such as Japan, Hong Kong, and Sweden, where fish intake is high, have the lowest rates of postpartum depression.[1]

For the best sources of omega-3 fats, choose oilier fish—salmon, lake trout, sardines, anchovies, herring, and mackerel are good choices. Include these types of fish in your diet two to three times per week.

Mercury and Fish

Now, about the types of fish to limit or avoid in your diet. In 2001, Health Canada and the US Federal Drug Administration (FDA) issued advisories recommending that people limit their intake of swordfish, shark, king mackerel, and fresh and frozen tuna. That's because these species of fish can accumulate high levels of methyl mercury. Mercury is a naturally occurring metal found in very low levels in the air, soil, lakes, streams, and oceans. But it can also make its way into the environment from industry: pulp and paper processing, mining operations, and burning garbage and fossil fuels all release mercury. Mercury is converted to methyl mercury by bacteria in water. In fish, these levels of methyl mercury can be toxic.

Methyl mercury can accumulate in the body and affect the nervous system. If women consume too much before and during their pregnancy, it can be harmful to the developing fetus and could cause birth defects and learning disabilities in their children. Even a relatively small amount can cause subtle changes to the developing brain. Women of childbearing years, pregnant and nursing women, and children under the age of 15 are particularly at risk from methyl mercury exposure. These people must limit their intake of these kinds of fish to once a month. Other people should not eat these types of fish more than once a week. And the portion should be no larger than 6 ounces, 2 ounces for children.

While *Health Canada advises pregnant and nursing women, other women of child-bearing age, and young children to eat swordfish, shark, king mackerel, and fresh and frozen tuna no more than once a month,* the US FDA goes one step farther and advises women to avoid these fish altogether during their pregnancies. So what about that tuna sandwich? Well, according to Health Canada, canned tuna is safe to eat, since the species of tuna used for canning are small and don't live long enough to accumulate harmful levels of mercury. Tests have revealed canned tuna to have mercury levels below Health Canada's upper safe limit. However, at the time of writing, the US FDA was preparing an advisory, warning consumers that some types of canned tuna fish may contain higher levels of mercury. New testing data revealed that levels of mercury in some US brands of albacore (white) tuna were three times as high as the mercury in "light" tuna, which is made from smaller fish. The testing found that mercury levels in white canned tuna averaged above the FDA's safe intake limit of 0.5 parts per million (ppm). (Health Canada's guideline level is also 0.5 ppm.)

If you're a lover of tuna sandwiches, I advise you choose "light" tuna instead of albacore. And don't eat tuna every day—add a variety of protein foods to your diet to limit your exposure to mercury.

Some experts say the US government's list of mercury-contaminated fish falls short and should be expanded to protect pregnant women from mercury exposure. In April 2001, the US Environmental Working Group issued the following recommendations to women considering pregnancy, who are pregnant, and who are breastfeeding:

Avoid	Once Per Month	Safe/Low Mercury
Halibut	Blue crab (Gulf of Mexico)	Blue crab (mid-Atlantic)
King Mackerel	Blue mussels	Catfish (farmed)
Largemouth bass	Catfish (wild)	Croaker
Marlin	Cod	Fish sticks
Oysters (Gulf Coast)	Eastern oysters	Flounder
Sea bass	Lake whitefish	Haddock
Shark	Mahi mahi	Perch
Swordfish	Pollock	Salmon (wild Pacific)
Tilefish	Salmon (Great Lakes)	Shrimp
Tuna, canned		Talapia
Tuna steaks		Trout (farmed)
Walleye		
White croaker		

US Environmental Working Group (EWG) and the US Public Interest Research Group (US PIRG), 2001. *Brain Food: What Women Should Know About Mercury Contamination in Fish.* Available at: www.ewg.org/reports/brainfood/execsumm.html.

Other fish low in mercury and high in omega-3 fats include sardines, herring, and rainbow trout.

Farmed Salmon and PCBs

In January 2004, an American study raised concern about eating farmed salmon too often.[2] The researchers tested levels of toxic chemicals, such as polychlorinated biphenyls (PCBs) and organic pesticides, in 700 salmon purchased from around the world, including Vancouver and Toronto, and found that farm-raised salmon contains higher levels of these contaminants than wild salmon. The average PCB level was 36.6 parts per billion (ppb) in farm-raised salmon and 4.75 ppb in wild salmon. While it's true that farmed salmon contain more PCBs, these levels are still incredibly low. In fact they are only a fraction of the limit of 2,000 ppb set by the Canadian and American governments.

PCBs were used widely for industrial purposes from the 1930s to the 1970s. They have been banned in North America since 1977, but they are persistent chemicals and don't break down easily, remaining in the environment for years. PCBs are present in soil, water, and even animal fat. Because these chemicals are stored in body fat, eating contaminated foods can cause PCBs to build up in your body over time.

PCBs enter the bodies of fish from water, sediment, and eating prey that have PCBs in their bodies. PCBs build up in fish and can reach levels hundreds of thousands of times higher than the levels in water. Farmed salmon are raised in ocean pens, where they are given feed and antibiotics to make them grow quickly. Farmed salmon are fed from a global supply of fish meal and fish oil manufactured from small open-sea fish, which studies show are the source of PCBs in most farmed salmon.

Excessive exposure to PCBs may cause a wide variety of adverse health effects. Our knowledge about the effects of PCBs comes from studies of people exposed in the workplace or who ate contaminated food, and from experimental studies with animals. Of particular concern are the effects on development in infants whose mothers have been exposed before and during pregnancy. PCBs are known to increase the risk of cancer, depress the immune system, and cause learning disabilities in children.

Over the past decade, a growing body of research suggests that infants and children with higher PCB exposures during development score lower on many measures of neurological function, ranging from decreased IQ scores to reduced hearing sensitivity. Some of these effects have even been observed at low levels of PCB exposure. PCB exposure also appears to impair the immune system. Exposure early in life may make people more susceptible to chicken pox or infections of the inner ear and respiratory tract.

PCBs are found throughout the environment, not just in farmed salmon. What's more, a report by the US Environmental Working Group clearly shows that we get far more PCBs from beef than we do from salmon. Even milk, poultry, and pork contribute more PCBs to our diet than does farmed salmon.

So, what should you do? For starters, don't give up on salmon. The benefits of eating fish rich in omega-3 fats are more clearly proven and far outweigh the potential risk of PCB exposure. And you might be reassured to hear that the Canadian Food Inspection Agency and Health Canada recently completed a survey of fish, both farmed and wild, that involved gathering a large number of samples and analyzing for PCBs. The results indicate that the levels of PCBs are well below Health Canada's current guidelines for both farmed and wild salmon. But to minimize your exposure, here are a few recommendations:

- Choose wild salmon over farmed salmon when it's in season (late spring to early summer). Types of wild salmon include sockeye, chum, coho, chinook, pink, and canned salmon. Farmed salmon includes Atlantic salmon and "fresh" salmon. Some salmon pâtés also use farmed salmon. Canned salmon is always wild.

- Trim fat (which contains the PCBs) from fish before cooking.

- Choose broiling, baking, or grilling over frying, as these cooking methods allow the fat to cook off the fish.

- If you eat salmon often, include a mix of wild and farmed. Wild salmon is in season only four months of the year, from midspring to midsummer.

Omega-3 Supplements

What if you just don't like fish but still want to get your omega-3 fats? Fish oil supplements are a good way to get a concentrated source of DHA and EPA. These capsules generally contain oil from cod, salmon, tuna, sardines, mackerel, and anchovies—none of which is listed in Health Canada's or the US FDA's warning lists. Methyl mercury is stored in the muscle (protein) of fish, not in the fat. This significantly reduces the amount of methyl mercury in fish oil supplements as compared with fish. Avoid fish *liver* oil supplements, which have concentrated amounts of vitamins A and D. As you'll read in Chapter 7, too much vitamin A during pregnancy is linked to birth defects. Buy a fish oil supplement that provides both DHA and EPA. Most fish oil supplements contain 12 percent DHA and 18 percent EPA by weight. That means that one 1000-milligram (1 gram) capsule supplies 120 mg of DHA and 180 mg of EPA for a total of 300 milligrams of omega-3 fats. But check the label to be sure of what you're getting.

You need 1.1 grams of omega-3 fatty acids each day, 1.4 grams if you're pregnant. Fatty fish, fish oils, and foods containing alpha-linolenic acid (ALA) all contribute to your daily omega-3 intake. ALA is another omega-3 fatty acid, found in flax oil, canola oil, walnuts, omega-3 eggs, and soy beans. When consumed through diet, the body converts some ALA to DHA, but not a lot. Flax oil supplements usually are sold as 1000-milligram capsules, providing 500 milligrams of ALA.

Limit Your Intake of Trans Fat

In addition to boosting your intake of the healthy omega-3 fats, it's important to limit your intake of the bad fats. Chances are you're already a pro at eating a diet that's low in saturated fat—the type of fat in animal foods that's linked to a higher risk of heart disease and certain cancers. Choosing lower-fat dairy products, lean meats, and skinless poultry breast are important ways to help you keep your saturated fat intake low.

But there's another type of fat that may be the most heart-unhealthy fat of them all— *trans fat*. It's a fat that lurks in many foods, and what's more, it's not easy to detect. Faced with new nutrition labelling laws and the threat of obesity lawsuits, large food makers are promising to reduce trans fat levels in many products. In the meantime, it's important to learn how to sleuth out trans fat.

Trans Fat 101

When a liquid vegetable oil is hydrogenated, trans fat is created. Essentially, the chemical process of hydrogenation turns a healthy vegetable oil into an unhealthy one. For food manufacturers, partially hydrogenated vegetable oils are cheap, and foods made with them have a longer shelf life—they don't turn rancid as quickly as foods made with pure vegetable oils and animal fats.

But what's good for the bottom line isn't so good for your health. Trans fat raises your LDL (bad cholesterol) and lowers your HDL (good cholesterol) levels, thereby increasing your risk for heart disease, and it's been shown to damage artery walls. Studies have even linked a diet high in trans fat to a greater risk of type 2 diabetes.

Consuming too much trans fat during pregnancy can also interfere with the metabolism of omega-3 fats. There is evidence to suggest that a high intake of these unhealthy fats may impair the growth and development of infants.[3] It's important to cut out sources of trans fat in your diet before you become pregnant, during pregnancy, and when nursing. The level of trans fat in breast milk relates directly to how much a nursing mother consumes in her diet. The bottom line—trans fat is to be avoided as often as possible.

How Much Trans Fat Is Safe to Eat?

In July 2002, the National Academy of Sciences issued a report that stated there is *no safe level of trans fat*. In other words: avoid this type of fat as much as possible! But that doesn't mean that trans fat–free foods that are high in saturated fat (e.g. cheeseburgers) are okay to eat. In fact, Canadians consume far more artery clogging saturated fat than trans fat. Limit both fats in your diet.

Where's the Trans Fat?

Roughly 70 percent of the trans fat in our diet comes from commercial baked goods, snack foods, and fried fast food and 20 percent comes from margarines. The remainder comes from meat and dairy products, where trans fat occurs naturally. Here's a look at how much trans fat is hiding in some common foods.

TRANS FAT IN COMMON FOODS (GRAMS)

Fast Food

Burger King Chicken Tenders, 6	3.0
Burger King French Fries, large	6.0
Harvey's Veggie Burger	1.0
McDonalds' Chicken McNuggets, 6	6.0
McDonald's Fries, large	4.3
McDonald's McVeggie Burger	2.0
Wendy's Biggie Fries	1.0
Wendy's Crispy Chicken Nuggets, 6	0.3

Commercial Baked Goods

Dunkin Donuts Glazed Donut	4.0
Dad's Cookies, 3	0.9
Kellogg's Eggo Waffles, 2	1.5
Krispy Kreme Glazed Donut	4.2
Nabisco Animal Crackers, 8	1.0
Nabisco Snackwell's Chocolate Chip Bite Size, 13	1.0
Oreo Cookies, 3	1.5
Quaker Chewy Granola Bar Chocolate Chip	0.5
Quaker Chewy Granola Bar, Low Fat	0.5

Crackers & Snack Foods

Microwave Popcorn, regular, 2 cups	3.5
Nabisco Wheat Thins, 8	1.0
Potato Chips, plain, 14 chips (28 g)	0.7
Ritz Crackers, 7	2.0

Don't be fooled by "low fat" labels. Even foods marketed as low fat can harbour trans fat. For example, almost one-third of the fat in a serving of Snackwell's low fat cookies comes from trans. The same goes for Nabisco Graham Crackers labelled 40 percent less fat.

Detecting Trans Fat

To eat less trans fat, read ingredient lists. Words such as "partially hydrogenated vegetable oils," "shortening," or "vegetable shortening" mean that trans fat is present. Eat foods that list these on the label less often. As much as 50 percent of the fat in foods like French fries, fast food, doughnuts, pastries, snack foods, and store bought cookies and crackers is trans fat.

If you use margarine, choose one that's made with "non-hydrogenated" fat. Many brands state this right on the label. If you can't find "non-hydrogenated" printed on your tub of margarine, use the nutrition information panel to add the values for polyunsaturated and monounsaturated fats. For a 10 gram (2 teaspoon/10 ml) serving, these fats should add up to at least 6 grams for a regular margarine and 3 grams for a light margarine. If the values don't add up to these numbers, this means there are more saturated and trans fats present.

Soon we will be able to see the grams of trans fat listed on the nutrition label of packaged foods. In January 2003, Health Canada legislated mandatory nutrition labels on pre-packaged foods. In other words, food manufacturers must disclose the nutrient content per serving of food, including the amount of trans fat and saturated fat. Large food companies have been given three years to comply with this new law. Over the next two years, you'll see more and more packaged foods bearing new and improved nutrition labels.

The new nutrition label will display the "% daily value" for saturated fat and trans fat combined. Restrict your intake of these combined bad fats to less than 10 percent of daily calories (or no more than 20 grams per day.).

If you see an old nutrition label that gives the breakdown of saturated, polyunsaturated, and monounsaturated fat grams, here's a trick for learning how much trans fat is present: add up the values for these three types of fat and if the number is less than the total grams of fat that means the unaccounted-for fat is trans fat!

Boost Your Fibre Intake: 25 Grams Per Day

The average Canadian consumes about 14 grams of fibre each day, about half of the daily recommended intake. Dietary fibre has many health benefits. By absorbing water and adding bulk, fibre helps move food through the digestive tract faster. Not only does this bulking action keep you regular, but it can also reduce the exposure of cells in your colon to cancer-causing substances. Fibre may also inactivate these harmful compounds before they can do harm to your colon. And certain types of fibre can act to help keep your heart healthy, too.

Foods are made up of two types of fibre: soluble and insoluble. Both are present in varying proportions in plant foods, but some foods will be rich in one or the other. For instance, dried peas, beans and lentils, oats, barley, psyllium husks, apples, and citrus fruits are good sources of soluble fibre. Soluble fibre forms a gel in your stomach and slows the rate of digestion and absorption. As soluble fibre passes through the digestive tract, its gel-like property can trap substances related to high cholesterol. Indeed, there's plenty of evidence that supports the cholesterol-lowering effect of oats, beans, and psyllium.

Diets rich in soluble fibre may also be helpful for people with diabetes. By delaying the rate at which food empties from the stomach into the intestine, the rise in blood sugar after a meal is blunted. Not only does this put less wear and tear on your pancreas but insulin requirements also may be reduced in people with type 1 diabetes.

Foods such as wheat bran, whole grains, and certain vegetables contain mainly insoluble fibre. This fibre has a significant capacity for retaining water and acts to increase stool bulk and promote regularity. By reducing constipation, a diet high in fibre may also prevent a condition called diverticulosis. Since high-fibre diets are usually lower in fat and calories, they may help people achieve and maintain a healthy weight.

Fibre and Pregnancy

Pregnant or not, you need to get 25 grams of fibre every day from your diet. Once you become pregnant, your need for fibre will become more obvious. That's because during pregnancy, food moves slower through the bowel and—you guessed it—constipation can result. To make matters worse, the iron in prenatal multivitamins can also lead to constipation. You'll learn more about treating pregnancy-related constipation in Chapter 9. In the meantime, you need to establish a diet that's high in fibre so you can reduce your chances of suffering this discomfort.

Fibre in Foods

Boosting your fibre intake means more than making a sandwich on whole-grain bread. And eating a green salad for dinner won't make a big difference either. You'll need to ensure you eat high-fibre foods at least once during the day. As you will see from the list below, 100 percent bran cereals and cooked legumes are winners when it comes to fibre.

FIBRE CONTENT OF SELECTED FOODS (GRAMS)

Legumes

Beans and tomato sauce, canned, 1 cup (250 ml)	20.7
Black beans, cooked, 1 cup (250 ml)	13.0
Chickpeas, cooked, 1 cup (250 ml)	6.1
Kidney beans, cooked, 1 cup (250 ml)	6.7
Lentils, cooked, 1 cup (250 ml)	9.0

Nuts

Almonds, 1/2 cup (125 ml)	8.2
Peanuts, dry roasted, 1/2 cup (125 ml)	6.9

Cereals

100% bran cereal, 1/2 cup (125 ml)	10.0
Bran Flakes, 3/4 cup (175 ml)	6.3
Grape Nuts, 1/2 cup (125 ml)	6.0
Kellogg's All-Bran Buds, 1/3 cup (75 ml)	13.0
Oat bran, cooked, 1 cup (250 ml)	4.5
Oatmeal, cooked, 1 cup (250 ml)	3.6
Quaker Corn Bran, 1 cup (250 ml)	6.3
Red River Cereal, cooked, 1 cup (250 ml)	4.8
Shreddies, 3/4 cup (175 ml)	4.4

Bread and Other Grain Foods

Flaxseed, ground, 2 tbsp (25 ml)	4.5
Pita pocket, whole-wheat, 1	4.8
Rice, brown, cooked, 1 cup (250 ml)	3.1
Spaghetti, whole-wheat, cooked, 1 cup (250 ml)	4.8
Wheat bran, 2 tbsp (25 ml)	2.4
Whole-wheat (100%) bread, 2 slices	4.0

Fruit

Apple, medium with skin, 1	2.6
Apricots, dried, 1/4 cup (50 ml)	2.6
Banana, medium, 1	1.9
Blueberries, 1/2 cup (125 ml)	2.0
Figs, dried, 5	8.5
Orange, medium, 1	2.4
Pear, medium with skin, 1	5.1
Prunes, dried, 3	3.0
Raisins, seedless, 1/2 cup (125 ml)	2.8
Strawberries, 1 cup (250 ml)	3.8

Vegetables

Broccoli, 1/2 cup (125 ml)	2.0
Brussels sprouts, 1/2 cup (125 ml)	2.6
Carrots, 1/2 cup (125 ml)	2.2
Corn niblets, 1/2 cup (125 ml)	2.3
Green peas, 1/2 cup (125 ml)	3.7
Lima beans, 1/2 cup (125 ml)	3.8
Potato, medium, baked with skin, 1	5.0
Sweet potato, mashed, 1/2 cup (125 ml)	3.9

Nutrient Values of Some Common Foods. Health Canada (Ottawa, 1999). Adapted and Reproduced with the permission of the Minister of Public Works and Government Services Canada, 2004.

Tips to Boost Fibre

Follow these tips to boost your fibre intake:

- Strive to eat at least five servings of fruits and vegetables each day.

- Leave the peel on fruits and vegetables whenever possible (but wash thoroughly).

- Eat at least three servings of whole-grain foods each day.

- Buy high-fibre breakfast cereals. Aim for a minimum of 4 to 5 grams of fibre per serving (check the nutrition information panel). Better yet, choose a 100 percent bran cereal that packs 10 to 13 grams of fibre per 1/2 cup (125 ml) serving.

- Top breakfast cereal with berries, dried cranberries, or raisins.

- Add 1 to 2 tablespoons (15 to 25 ml) of natural wheat bran, oat bran, or ground flaxseed to cereals, yogurt, applesauce, casseroles, and soup.

- Eat legumes more often; add white kidney beans to pasta sauce, black beans to tacos, chickpeas to salads, lentils to soup (these are also excellent sources of folate).

- Add a handful of seeds, nuts, or raisins to salads.

- Add nuts to a vegetable stir-fry.

- Reach for high-fibre snacks such as popcorn, dried apricots, and dates.

Drink Plenty of Fluids: 9 Cups (2.2 Litres) Per Day

Guess what dietary fibre needs to do its job? That's right—fluid. But there are other important reasons to be sure you are drinking enough fluid each day. Water lives inside and around every single cell in the body. In fact, there's not one system in your body that does not rely on a steady supply of water. Every biochemical reaction that takes place in your body does so with the help of water. Water in saliva and digestive juices help break down the food you eat into smaller nutrients that can be absorbed into your bloodstream. These nutrients are then transported to your cells and tissues via water in the blood. And your cells would not get the oxygen they need to survive if it weren't for water in your bloodstream. Fluid in your blood, urine, and stool also helps remove toxic waste products from your body.

Even your body's ability to regulate its temperature is dependent on water. The fluid in your sweat allows your muscles to release heat that builds up during exercise. The amount of water in your bloodstream also regulates your blood pressure and heart function. And finally, water acts as your body's central lubricant. It cushions your joints, moistens your eyes, and protects your brain and spinal cord.

The average women needs to drink 9 cups (2.2 litres) of non-caffeinated, non-alcoholic fluid each day to meet her needs. Of course, fluid needs vary depending on your size, activity level, and the weather—high temperatures and low humidity increase your fluid needs.

Plain water, juice, milk, soy milk, soup, herbal tea, and foods containing high amounts of water, such as fruit and vegetables, will all help you meet your daily fluid requirements (notice that soft drinks are not on this list). Depending on your diet, solid foods can actually provide about 4 cups (1 litre) of fluid each day. And the water generated by your body's metabolic reactions contributes another 1 cup (250 ml). The rest you have to make up by drinking fluids, preferably plain water.

Water and Pregnancy

Once you become pregnant, you need to drink more fluid than the 9 cups (2.2 litres) recommended above. During pregnancy, the fluid spaces between your cells enlarge, demanding more water. The growing fetus and the amniotic fluid surrounding your baby also require more fluid. When you're pregnant, you need to drink an additional 1 cup (250 ml) of water each day. In Chapter 7, you'll read how your fluid needs increase even more.

If you drink water from the tap, I strongly recommend that you filter it first. Most public drinking water supplies are disinfected with chlorine to remove disease-causing viruses and bacteria. Some cities use ozone to disinfect the water. But because ozone breaks down quickly, small amounts of chlorine must still be added.

Chlorination is a good thing; it keeps our drinking water safe. Yet there remain concerns about the potential harmful effects of chlorine by-products in tap water. When chlorine is added to water, it reacts with organic matter such as decaying leaves. This chemical reaction forms a group of chemicals known as disinfection by-products, the most common ones being trihalomethanes (e.g., chloroform). Recent scientific data suggests that these by-products may be harmful during pregnancy.

It's not possible to remove all disinfection by-products from tap water, but you can minimize your exposure to them by using a water-treatment device at home. Not only will such devices remove a fair amount of chlorine and its by-products from drinking water, they will also improve the water's taste and smell. Pitcher-type products use activated carbon filters, and some may include an ion-exchange resin to remove inorganic chemicals responsible for the hardness of water.

You may prefer to drink bottled water during your pregnancy. Many companies will deliver a month's supply right to your door. Bottled water differs from tap water in two ways. One main difference is the source of the water. While tap water comes from the surface of lakes and rivers, bottled spring waters originate from a protected underground source. Another difference is in how these waters are distributed. Municipal water is pumped through miles of piping, whereas bottled water is produced in food plants and packaged in clean, sealed containers. And finally, bottled waters do not contain chlorine or chlorine by-products.

Give Up Alcohol

Most women are aware that heavy drinking during pregnancy can cause birth defects. You probably know that heavy drinking or binge drinking during pregnancy can cause fetal alcohol syndrome (FAS), one of the most common causes of mental retardation. Babies born with FAS are smaller than normal at birth, have smaller eyes, a short nose, and flat cheeks. Many babies with FAS exhibit some degree of mental disability and behavioural problems as a result of being born with an abnormally formed brain. Sadly, the effects of FAS last a lifetime.

Keep in mind that fetal alcohol syndrome is more likely to occur in babies born to women who drink continuously and heavily during their pregnancies. At this time, it remains unclear what amount of alcohol can be considered safe during pregnancy. The evidence suggests that an *occasional* drink during pregnancy is unlikely to cause any harm to a developing fetus. So if you are concerned about an occasional drink, rest assured.

However, because no safe level of alcohol during pregnancy has been established, I recommend that you abstain from drinking when you pregnant. This usually isn't a problem, since many women are turned off alcoholic beverages when they are expecting.

What if you had a few drinks at a party before you realized you were pregnant? This is a common concern, since many pregnancies are a surprise. There is no need to worry or stress about what has happened in the past. It is unlikely that having an occasional drink or two, before you realized you are pregnant, will harm your baby. What's most important is that you abstain from alcoholic beverages as soon as you learn you are pregnant. Stop drinking even if you suspect you could be pregnant.

I also recommend that you abstain from alcohol while you are trying to get pregnant. For starters, you may not know you are pregnant until well into the first trimester, a critical time for your baby's brain development. Second, some studies suggest that even a moderate alcohol intake can delay conception. In a study of 430 Danish couples, women who consumed 1 to 5 drinks per week were 40 percent less likely to get pregnant over six months compared with non-drinkers. And the more a woman imbibed, the lower her odds of conceiving. Women in the study who had more than 10 drinks each week were 65 percent less likely to become pregnant.[4]

Women with endometriosis may have a harder time getting pregnant if they drink alcohol. Researchers from the Harvard School of Public Health studied women who drink alcohol and determined that those who drank a moderate amount (one or two drinks a day) had a 60 percent higher risk of infertility compared with non-drinkers.[5]

Drinking can affect men's fertility, too. Researchers are learning that alcohol can lower sperm count, change the sperm's ability to move, and damage sperm, which could lead to miscarriage.

If you're looking for an alternative to an alcoholic cocktail, try a virgin Caesar, tomato juice, or a glass of soda water with a splash of cranberry juice.

Cut Back on Caffeine: No More than 250 Milligrams Per Day

If you're a java junkie, it's time to cut down on caffeine. Many studies have shown that consuming more than 300 milligrams of caffeine each day (the amount in three small cups of coffee) delays a woman's ability to conceive.[6] A study by CK Stanton and RH Gray found that women whose daily diet included at least 300 milligrams of caffeine were more than twice as likely to have conception delayed for longer than one year.[7]

There's also evidence to suggest that consuming similar amounts of caffeine when you are pregnant increases the risk of miscarriage.[8] What's more, it seems that the more caffeine consumed, the higher the risk. Canadian researchers in Montreal found that an intake of as little as 48 milligrams of caffeine per day was linked with a slightly greater risk of miscarriage.[9] In fact, scientists at the University of Toronto analyzed 32 studies and concluded that there is a small increase in risk for miscarriage and low-birth-weight babies in pregnant women who consume more than 150 milligrams of caffeine per day.[10]

Caffeine enters your central nervous system within 15 minutes after consumption. Here, it acts as a stimulant, increasing blood pressure and heart rate. Caffeine also acts as a diuretic, causing your body to lose fluid. As you will read later, when you are pregnant, your body needs more fluid, not less.

If you consume caffeine during your pregnancy, keep in mind that your developing baby is consuming it too. That's because caffeine easily passes from you to your unborn baby through the placenta. And because a developing baby has an immature metabolism, caffeine may stay in his system longer. Some research suggests that caffeine does affect fetal heart rate and breathing.

So how much caffeine can you safely consume? It's hard to say. An intake of less than 300 milligrams does not appear to harm your ability to become pregnant. Based on this, I recommend that you keep your daily caffeine intake to a maximum of 250 milligrams while trying to conceive. Cut back your caffeine intake further once you become pregnant. If you want to go cold turkey now, that's even better.

Don't forget that caffeine is found in other products besides coffee. Use the table below to estimate your daily caffeine intake. (The averages listed below for coffee and tea will be affected by brewing time, brewing method, and water temperature, all of which influence the amount of caffeine that gets transferred to your brew.)

CAFFEINE CONTENT OF SELECTED FOODS (MILLIGRAMS)

Beverage or Food		Beverage or Food	
Coffee, decaffeinated, 8 oz (250 ml)	4	Espresso, 2 oz (60 g)	90–100
Coffee, filter drip, 8 oz (250 ml)	110–180	Tea, black, 8 oz (250 ml)	46
Coffee, filter, Starbucks, 8 oz (250 ml)	200	Tea, green, 8 oz (250 ml)	33
		Cola, diet, 12 oz (355 ml)	46
Coffee, filter, Starbucks, 16 oz (500 ml)	400	Cola, regular, 12 oz (350 ml)	35
		Root Beer, Barq's, 12 oz (355 ml)	15
Coffee, instant, 8 oz (250 ml)	80–120	Chocolate cake, 1 slice	20–30
		Chocolate, dark, 1 oz (30 g)	20

Chocolate milk, 1 oz (30 g)	6
Chocolate milk, 1 cup (250 ml)	8
Coffee-flavoured ice cream, Haagen-Dazs, 1 cup (250 ml)	48

Medication (2 tablets)	
Anacin	64
Excedrin	130
Midol	64

If you find you need to reduce your caffeine intake, do so gradually over a period of three weeks to minimize withdrawal symptoms such as headache, muscle pain, and fatigue. To help you start your caffeine countdown, choose a cut-off time for drinking caffeine-containing beverages. For instance, I tell my clients to cut out all sources of caffeine after lunchtime. It helps them gradually cut back, and they sleep better, too. Switch to caffeine-free or low-caffeine beverages such as low-fat milk, soy milk, vegetable juice, unsweetened fruit juice, water, herbal tea, decaffeinated tea and coffee, weak tea, hot chocolate, and cereal coffee (e.g., grain-based hot beverages such as Ovaltine).

Minimize Exposure to Pesticide Residues

Approximately 6000 types of pesticides are used in Canada. These products are used in agriculture, on lawns, and on golf courses to combat weeds, insects, and fungi that destroy plant life. The use of pesticides in fruit and vegetable farming allows us to enjoy a wide variety of foods at a relatively low cost.

Health Canada's Pest Management Regulatory Agency (PMRA) monitors pesticide residues on food. The PMRA sets maximum residue limits for all pesticides. These limits have built-in safety margins that set the final level at a minimum of 100 times below the limit that could cause health problems. The PMRA and the Canadian Food Inspection Agency test thousands of produce samples each year to ensure that maximum residue limits are not exceeded.

Despite this, many Canadians are worried about the possible ill effects of pesticide residues that linger on the surface of fruit and vegetables. Some pesticides disrupt hormone function, some cause nerve damage, and others are carcinogenic. Certain pesticides don't break down in the environment and can accumulate in fatty tissues.

Some scientists and watchdog groups worry that some people may be more vulnerable to the effects of toxic pesticide residues than others. Pregnant women, breastfeeding moms, and children may be at higher risk. From conception to puberty, children's bodies are developing and are more sensitive to disruption.

To play it safe, practise these simple measures at home to minimize your exposure:

- Rinse produce with running water to remove most trace residues. Special produce washes are unnecessary.

- Avoid using detergents to wash produce, since these may leave trace residues of chemicals that have not been tested for human consumption.

- Remove and discard outer leaves of lettuce and cabbage.

- Scrub thick-skinned produce such as potatoes, carrots, and parsnips.

Consider Organic

Many people are turning to organically grown fruit and vegetables to minimize their intake of pesticide residues. Finding organic produce has become increasingly easy. No longer available only in health food stores, these fruits and vegetables are found in the produce section of most grocery stores, next to their non-organic counterparts.

Organic fruit and vegetables are grown and processed without the use of genetic engineering, synthetic or artificial fertilizers, pesticides, growth regulators, antibiotics, preservatives, dyes, or additives. However, most processed organic foods (e.g., organic frozen food meals, canned chili con carne) are allowed to contain a small percentage of non-organic ingredients.

Organic produce is more expensive but not because it's more nutritious than non-organic fruit and vegetables. Organic produce costs more because organic farmers produce smaller amounts—insects and weeds compete with the crops more effectively. Many people say that organic produce tastes better. For some, this is worth the extra cost. And organic agriculture is better for the environment.

Third-party certification bodies have been established to assure consumers that the produce they're buying is indeed organic. However, because there are about 45 certifiers in Canada, it is not as easy as looking for just one logo when shopping for organic foods. Certification logos come in all shapes and sizes. "Certified organic" logos to look for include those of the Organic Crop Improvement Association (OCIA), Demeter, Organic Crop Producers and Processors, Quality Assurance International, and Canadian Organic Producers Association.

While there are many certification bodies, they all use similar national standards. And organic farms have to reapply for certification each year. It is anticipated that one day there will be a common "Canada Organic" seal. Such a national organic standard has been developed but awaits support of the federal government.

Putting It All Together: Pre-Pregnancy Meal Plans

Now that you know what you need to eat to prepare your body for pregnancy, it's time to map these foods onto a meal plan. I recommend that you start by planning three meals and two snacks each day. To get the calories and nutrients you need before and during pregnancy, you will need to eat more than three square meals each day. Eating snacks might seem foreign to you, but once you enter the second trimester, you'll probably notice an increased appetite that drives you to eat more often. (Your goal later in your pregnancy is to not overeat and gain too much weight.) Now is a good time to learn how to spread nutrients and calories out over the course of the day.

Eating more often is an important strategy to boost your energy level and prevent hunger during the day. Planning for healthful snacks means you won't grab that chocolate bar when late-afternoon fatigue hits. Once you review the meal plans below, you'll notice that the midday snacks include milk and fruit, a great combination for protein, fibre, calcium, and antioxidants such as vitamins A and C. Eating these types of snacks will result in you spending your calories wisely, rather than wasting them on refined starchy foods full of white flour and sugar.

Using the Right Meal Plan for Your Weight Goal

So how much do you need to eat? No two women are alike. How much food you need to eat depends on your weight and activity level. The meal plans below are for three calorie levels. Which is right for you depends on your goal: 1600, 1900, or 2200 calories per day? The average woman needs roughly 1900 calories to maintain her weight. If your body mass index (BMI) falls within the healthy zone, start at this level and adjust only if your weight changes. If you want to lose a few pounds before you become pregnant, start at the 1600-calorie level. Don't attempt to lose more than 1 to 2 pounds (0.5 to 1 kilogram) per week. Losing weight more quickly than this can rob your body of important nutrients. And don't go lower than 1200 calories per day. If your doctor has advised that you gain weight to help prepare for pregnancy, start by following the 2200-calorie plan.

You'll probably have to experiment to learn which calorie level works for you. For instance, if you find that you gain weight on the maintenance level of 1900 calories, drop your daily calorie intake by 100. Same thing goes for the weight-loss plan: if you don't lose weight after two weeks, take away 100 calories (and be sure you exercise). I suggest you cut 100 calories by removing one grain serving from your plan. That way, you'll be sure to get the protein, vitamins, and minerals you need each day. But no matter which calorie level you're following, be sure to take a daily multivitamin and mineral supplement for folic acid.

MEAL PLAN FOR WEIGHT LOSS: 1600 CALORIES

Breakfast:

Protein servings: 1 (optional)

Starch servings: 1

Fruit servings: 1

Milk servings: 1

Water: 2 cups (500 ml)

Morning Snack:

Fruit servings: 1

OR

Milk servings: 1

Water: 1 to 2 cups (250 to 500 ml)

Lunch:

Protein servings: 3

Starch servings: 2

Vegetable servings: 1 to 2

Fat servings: 2

Water: 2 cups (500 ml)

Afternoon Snack:

Fruit servings: 1

Milk servings: 1

Water: 2 cups (500 ml)

Dinner:

Protein servings: 3

Starch servings: 2

Vegetable servings: 2 to 3

Fat servings: 2

Water: 2 cups (500 ml)

MEAL PLAN FOR WEIGHT MAINTENANCE: 1900 CALORIES

Breakfast:

Protein servings: 1 (optional)

Starch servings: 2

Fruit servings: 1

Milk servings: 1

Water: 2 cups (500 ml)

Morning Snack:

Fruit servings: 1

Milk servings: 1

Water: 1 to 2 cups (250 to 500 ml)

Lunch:

Protein servings: 3

Starch servings: 2

Vegetable servings: 1 or 2

Fat servings: 2

Water: 2 cups (500 ml)

Afternoon Snack:

Fruit servings: 1

Milk servings: 1

Fat servings: 1

Water: 2 cups (500 ml)

Dinner:

Protein servings: 4

Starch servings: 2

Vegetable servings: 2 to 3

Fat servings: 2

Water: 2 cups (500 ml)

MEAL PLAN FOR WEIGHT GAIN: 2200 CALORIES

Breakfast:

Protein servings: 1 (optional)

Starch servings: 2

Fruit servings: 2

Milk servings: 1

Water: 2 cups (500 ml)

Morning Snack:

Fruit servings: 1

Milk servings: 1

Water: 1 to 2 cups (250 to 500 ml)

Lunch:

Protein servings: 3

Starch servings: 2

Vegetable servings: 1 to 2

Fat servings: 2

Water: 2 cups (500 ml)

Afternoon Snack:

Fruit servings: 1

Fat servings: 1

Water: 2 cups (500 ml)

Dinner:

Protein servings: 4

Starch servings: 3

Vegetable servings: 2 to 3

Fat servings: 2

Water: 2 cups (500 ml)

Bedtime Snack:

Grain servings: 1

Milk servings: 1

To learn what a serving size is, see A Guide to Serving Sizes on page 303.

Using the 14-Day Meal Plan from
The Canadian Living Test Kitchen

I encourage you to use the recipes outlined in Part Four. If you don't have time to plan menus, think of this meal plan as a starter kit. All you need to do is prepare a list and head to the grocery store. But don't feel you have to use the meal plan exactly as it's presented. You might not want to adhere to a two-week schedule. Perhaps you'd rather pick and choose recipes to add to your own repertoire of healthy meals. If that's the case, you'll find plenty to choose from. In addition to the 14 breakfasts, lunches, and dinners planned, I've provided extra recipes for vegetables, grain side dishes, snacks, and desserts.

To achieve your calorie goals, you will have to add in your own snacks, be it fruit and yogurt or one of the 10 snack recipes, such as Fig and Orange Bars or Spa Trail Mix. Depending on the recipe, you may have to add side dishes to your meal; for example, milk and fruit at breakfast, or vegetables and whole grains to lunch and dinner.

You might find that you don't need one of your midday snacks. For instance, if you eat breakfast at 8 A.M. and lunch at noon, you might not be hungry for something in between. To maintain your calorie intake, I recommend you snack on a serving of (healthy) dessert, such as Chocolate Banana Pudding or Pure and Simple Vanilla Pudding with Fruit, with lunch or dinner.

Your Pre-Pregnancy Nutrition Checklist

Use this checklist to ensure your pre-pregnancy nutrition plan is in place, so that you are nourishing your body in preparation for pregnancy.

- Take a daily multivitamin and mineral supplement to ensure you get 400 micrograms of folic acid each day.

- Aim to include three servings of milk, yogurt, or calcium-enriched beverage in your daily diet to get 1000 milligrams of calcium. If you fall short, take a calcium citrate supplement with vitamin D added.

- Add good sources of iron to your meals. Lean red meat, legumes, dried fruit, and nuts are foods that will help you meet your daily requirement of 18 milligrams. Your multivitamin and mineral supplement should supply 10 to 18 milligrams of iron.

- Include protein-rich foods such as lean meat, poultry, fish, legumes, nuts, and dairy products in meals.

- Choose fish wisely. Include fish that's rich in omega-3 fats and low in mercury in your diet twice a week. If you don't like fish, consider adding one 1000-milligram fish oil capsule to your daily nutrition regime. If you're a vegetarian, take one 1000-milligram flax oil capsule.

- Limit your intake of saturated and trans fats. Choose lower-fat dairy products, lean meats, and skinless chicken breasts. Read ingredient lists and avoid foods that list "partially hydrogenated oil," "vegetable shortening," and "shortening"—all sources of trans fat.

- Boost your intake of fibre-rich foods to achieve a daily intake of 25 grams.

- Ensure you get 9 cups (2.2 litres) of fluid each day from non-caffeinated, non-alcoholic beverages. If you drink tap water, use a filter to reduce chlorine by-products.

- Consume no more than 250 milligrams of caffeine each day. This is the equivalent of two small cups of coffee.

- Avoid all alcoholic beverages while you are trying to get pregnant and after you have conceived.

- Minimize your exposure to pesticide residues by washing produce under running water. Consider buying organic fruit and vegetables.

3

---⌘---

Your Pre-Pregnancy Checklist: Gearing Up

Taking the plunge into parenthood is an incredibly exciting time, and a time to contemplate this new chapter in your life. It will be both exhilarating and exhausting. If you're planning for your first pregnancy, you might be feeling a little anxious. I would be surprised if you weren't. After all, there are a lot of things to think about and plan for: getting your body healthy, prenatal care, and child care arrangements, not to mention career and financial considerations. You've probably spent many moments wondering what you need to do to get ready to bring a baby into the world.

If you are just considering pregnancy, you are one step ahead of the game. You have time to get your body and your lifestyle habits into top-notch shape. If you haven't done so already, I strongly recommend that you assess your diet and lifestyle by taking the quizzes in Chapter 1. If you have taken stock of your habits, then you are aware of what you need to do before becoming pregnant. On the nutrition front, I've already given you plenty of diet advice to put into action.

You'll also need to think through other aspects of pregnancy and parenthood. Take the next three months to get a few things done—important things you should do *before* conceiving to get your body and your lifestyle ready for pregnancy.

Make a Pre-Conception Visit to Your Health Care Provider

Schedule a checkup with your doctor before you get pregnant. The objective of this visit is to prevent any problems that may occur during your pregnancy. Your doctor will ask about medications you take, as well as about your medical history, family medical history, diet, activity level, and past pregnancies. Be completely honest about your health and lifestyle practices.

If you need to learn about your medical roots, start asking questions. Has anyone in you or the baby's father's family had genetic disorders such as Down syndrome, sickle-cell anemia, cerebral palsy, muscular dystrophy, cystic fibrosis, or bleeding disorders? Your doctor may suggest you are a good candidate for genetic counselling, depending on your family medical history. Find out if any of your relatives were born with a heart defect or a neural tube defect. Your doctor needs to know the whole picture in order to help you deliver the healthiest baby possible.

Get Immunized

Undoubtedly, you'll cover this topic during your pre-conception visit. Your doctor will determine if your vaccines are up to date. Although some vaccines are safe to get when you are pregnant, it's best to have any necessary immunizations before you become pregnant. Here's what is recommended:

Three months before pregnancy:

- Rubella (German measles) vaccine. During your pre-conception visit, your doctor will do a rubella test to determine if you are immune to the disease. If you are not, you will need to get this vaccine.

- Varicella (chicken pox) vaccine (if not immune)

Safe during pregnancy:

- Tetanus (diphtheria) booster (once every 10 years)

- Hepatitis A and B vaccines

- Influenza vaccine (if you will be in your second or third trimester during flu season)

Visit Your Dentist

If it's been more than six months since your last trip to the dentist's office, make an appointment for a checkup and cleaning. You might not realize it, but your oral health can have a significant effect on your pregnancy. Many studies have revealed that pregnant women with periodontal disease (a bacterial infection that affects your gums and bones supporting your teeth) have babies too early and at low birth weights (less than 88 ounces or 2500 grams).[1] Researchers have found that pregnant women with periodontitis were up to seven and a half times more likely to have a preterm low-birth-weight infant than were women with healthy gums.[2] In fact, it's widely believed that periodontal disease is an independent risk factor for preterm low-birth-weight babies.

Gum Disease 101

Gum disease in the early stages is commonly referred to as gingivitis. Gingivitis develops when plaque builds up on the teeth and irritates the gums. Plaque actually begins to form within minutes after you brush. If left on the teeth for more than 72 hours, plaque hardens into tartar or calculus, a tough, discoloured deposit that cannot be completely removed by brushing or flossing. As bacteria accumulate on your teeth, they release toxins that irritate the oral tissues. Swollen, tender gums that bleed easily are common signs of gingivitis.

The advanced stage of gum disease is known as periodontitis or periodontal disease. Untreated gingivitis leads to a buildup of plaque and tartar along the gum line at the base of your teeth. Gradually, tartar extends below the gum line, causing the gums to pull away from the teeth. In the airless environment below the gums, bacteria flourish and pockets of infection form, slowly deepening as the disease progresses. Eventually, periodontitis can destroy the tissue and bone that keep your teeth in an upright position, causing them to loosen and fall out.

Oral bacteria can enter your bloodstream whenever you brush, floss, or chew. It's thought that these microbes make their way to the placenta, where they can influence pregnancy. Researchers have learned that women who have periodontal disease *and* receive oral care during their pregnancy are much less likely to have preterm (born before 37 completed weeks of pregnancy) low-birth-weight babies.[3]

Even if you have healthy gums right now, the hormonal shifts during pregnancy make you more susceptible to gingivitis. It's estimated that 60 to 75 percent of pregnant women get gingivitis.[4] Increased estrogen and progesterone levels together with vascular changes can cause the gums to react differently to oral bacteria, resulting in swollen, bleeding, tender gums. The bottom line: if you take care of your oral health before and during pregnancy, you'll be much less likely to experience pregnancy complications.

Quit Smoking

If you are a smoker, no doubt you already know that the habit is bad for your health. But if you are unaware of the effects of cigarette smoke on your pregnancy, here are the sobering facts:

- Women who smoke are at greater risk for infertility. Research suggests that, compared with non-smoking women, it takes longer for women who smoke to conceive.

- Women who smoke may have a higher risk for ectopic pregnancy and spontaneous abortion. In an ectopic pregnancy, the embryo becomes implanted in a fallopian tube or other abnormal site instead of the uterus. These pregnancies do not result in the birth of a baby. Instead, they must be removed surgically or with drugs to protect the woman's life.

- Smoking nearly doubles a woman's risk of having a low-birth-weight baby. The longer a woman smokes during pregnancy, the greater the effect on her baby's weight. Low-birth-weight babies, who weigh less than 5.5 pounds (2.5 kg), face a higher risk of health problems during the newborn period, chronic disabilities, and even death. A baby may be born too small if she did not grow properly in the womb, was born too early, or a combination of both.

- Smoking can increase a woman's chance of giving birth prematurely by roughly 30 percent. If a woman stops smoking by her 16th week of pregnancy, she is no more likely to have a low-birth-weight baby than a woman who never smoked.

- Babies who are exposed to smoke before they are born may have a higher risk of asthma as well as learning and behavioural problems.

If you are considering pregnancy, quit smoking now, before you conceive. If you are already pregnant and smoke, it's not too late to quit. It's also important to stay smoke-free after your baby is born. Make your home a smoke-free environment: babies exposed to second-hand smoke suffer more health problems than other babies. And according to the March of Dimes, babies of mothers who smoke are twice as likely to die from sudden infant death syndrome (SIDS) as babies of non-smokers.[5] While exposure to cigarette smoke after birth poses a risk, it seems that exposure to smoke while still in the womb is a bigger risk for SIDS.

Understanding the harmful effects of smoking can make it easier to quit. It's also important to get support from friends and family. Discuss your smoking habit with your doctor. He or she can refer you to a smoking cessation program that's right for you.

Plan for Your Pregnancy (Prenatal) Care

It's also time to think about who you want to care for you during your pregnancy and to be at the birth of your baby. You also need to decide where you want to have your baby—in the hospital or at home? The majority of women rely on their family physician or obstetrician for medical care during pregnancy. But a growing number of women are turning to midwives to guide them through the many stages of pregnancy, delivery, and postpartum care.

In addition to offering a personalized and professional level of service, using a midwife allows you to deliver your baby at home, an option that has tremendous appeal for many women. If you're wondering whether a midwife is the right choice for you, take time to learn about the services midwives offer. Ask friends and colleagues, too; chances are good that someone you know has used one. Ask for recommendations.

The Role of a Midwife

A midwife is a registered health professional, trained to provide "primary care to low-risk women throughout their pregnancy, labour and birth."[6] The "low-risk" part of this statement is important. If you have a history of medical problems or are at risk of complications during your pregnancy or delivery, a midwife is not the right heath care provider for you: a doctor or an obstetrician must monitor high-risk pregnancies. However, if you're healthy and your pregnancy is normal, a midwife can offer many of the same services as your family doctor.

Midwives usually work in small group practices and share responsibility for your care. The prenatal routine is similar to the one followed by your family doctor. You will have regularly scheduled visits with the midwives, and they will provide you with clinical examinations, counselling, advice, and education. If you choose a midwife as your heath care provider, you will not see a doctor during your pregnancy and delivery unless you run into a problem or complication requiring medical attention.

Midwives also provide care and support for you and your baby during the first six weeks after delivery. They will check in on you regularly during those critical early weeks to make sure everything is progressing as it should. Because they are available 24 hours a day, seven days a week, midwives are wonderful resources for new mothers, helping you deal with many of those "new baby" issues that often seem so overwhelming and worrisome at first.

To give you an example of the level of service that midwives offer, let me share with you a story my friend Jennifer told me. It was the day after delivery and both Jen and her little bundle of joy were having difficulty getting the hang of breastfeeding. By one o'clock in the morning, the baby was hysterical with hunger and Jen was frantic with worry—no wonder the breastfeeding wasn't working. Jen's husband, at his wit's end trying to cope with his crying females, decided to call their midwife. Undeterred by the early hour, the midwife came to their house immediately, calmed Jen down, and gave her a few tips to get the milk flowing. She then helped the baby latch on properly and guided the entire feeding process. Within an hour, the crisis was over and everyone was able to settle down and catch up on greatly needed sleep. It's that type of commitment and support that has won midwives a strong following in the centres where their services are available.

Many of my clients tell me that the best part of using a midwife is the highly personalized care they offer. Midwives tend to establish close relationships with their clients and offer a woman-to-woman connection that you won't often find in a doctor's office. One of my friends describes her association with her midwife as more like a friendship than a doctor–patient relationship. Because of this personal connection, you may feel that you can ask a midwife questions about pregnancy and childbirth that you would feel too silly or embarrassed to ask someone else. Women tell me that having a midwife is like having a trusted friend to mentor and guide you through your pregnancy.

If you have a hospital phobia, the prospect of a home birth can be reassuring. Midwives attend and support home births and will give you a number of options for delivery, including water births. Many women prefer midwives because they offer a greater degree of control over their pregnancy and delivery. Although midwives are not the right choice for everyone, many women value the level of service and support they provide.

Professional Training of Midwives

Until recently, midwifery was an unregulated profession. Anyone could claim the title of midwife and it was up to the consumer to decide whether the midwife's qualifications were valid. But as the number of family doctors continues to decline across the country, provincial governments are now looking much more seriously at the advantages midwives can bring to the health care system. When properly trained and qualified, midwives can significantly reduce the pressures on overburdened medical doctors by providing high-quality, cost-efficient care for pregnant women. In many cases, midwives have the authority to order all the prenatal testing you will need during your pregnancy. In Ontario, for example, midwives can order laboratory and diagnostic tests, as well as ultrasounds and genetic screening.

A number of provinces have developed regulations to govern midwives, and others are in the process of considering new legislation. Most provinces require midwives to meet specific training requirements, both clinical and academic, before they can register as heath care professionals. In late 1993, Ontario was the first province to integrate midwives into the heath care system and now fully funds all midwife services through the Ontario Ministry of Health.[7] Other provinces are following Ontario's lead. The Canadian Association of Midwives is the national organization of the midwifery profession; its website (see the Resources section at the back of this book) is an excellent source of information about the current status of legislation across the country.

For most women, the biggest concern about using a midwife is what will happen if something goes wrong with the pregnancy or delivery. Because midwives are an accepted part of the heath care team, they are closely associated with medical professionals and local hospitals. Whenever necessary, midwives will consult with doctors or specialists about your care. If there is any risk of complications with your pregnancy, your midwife can transfer you to the care of an obstetrician or your baby to the care of a pediatrician. If that does happen, and you end up in the care of another heath care professional, your midwife will continue to take an active role in supporting you until your baby is born.

Improve Your Diet

It's critical that you make dietary changes to get your body ready for pregnancy. What changes are those? Well, chances are, you got a few strong hints after answering the questions in Chapter 1 about your current diet. Take a close look at your "No" responses. These indicate areas for improvement. Determine your body mass index and make any necessary changes to get your weight in check. In Chapter 2, you'll find all the advice you'll need to improve your diet and feel confident that you are eating well for both you and your future baby.

Get Your Partner Eating Healthy

More and more women today are choosing to have children on their own or with their female partners. However, if the father is part of the pregnancy process, he too should be following many of the tips I present in this book. Have him read through Chapters 1 and 2 and take the nutrition quiz in Chapter 1. Think of the pre-pregnancy diet as a "before baby" diet for both of you. Since sperm develops over a three-month period, it's vital that daddy-to-be eats well for healthy sperm production. As you read in Chapter 2, men also should abstain from alcohol and get adequate amounts of certain vitamins and minerals to enhance their fertility.

Consult a Qualified Nutrition Expert

Although this book offers plenty of nutrition advice for before, during, and after your pregnancy, if you have a specific concern about your health or your diet, it makes good sense to seek one-on-one help. If you're overweight, a dietitian can design a safe weight-loss plan that fits your lifestyle. Conversely, if you're underweight and need to add a little padding, a dietitian can prescribe an eating plan that promotes healthy weight gain. Or perhaps you have a health condition that you'd like to learn to manage through diet before you become pregnant.

Over the years, I've helped hundreds of women get ready for their pregnancies by revamping their diets. Many have wanted to lose those extra 10 pounds, others have wanted to boost their energy level during the day, and some have had a specific health problem, such as reflux (heartburn) or anemia. See the Resources section (page 304) for help in finding a registered dietitian in your community.

Create an Exercise Program—and Stick with It

Women who exercise before and during pregnancy are better able to handle the stress pregnancy puts on the body; they have fewer backaches, and less ankle swelling, fatigue, and excess weight gain. If you start a fitness program now, you'll be rewarded with a healthy body that's ready for pregnancy. According to experts, we need to accumulate 60 minutes of physical activity every day to stay healthy or improve our health. That can include lifestyle activities, such as walking, climbing stairs, and gardening, as I mentioned in Chapter 1. Ways to activate your day include:

- Walk whenever you can—park at the back of the lot, walk partway to work, take the dog for an extra walk.

- Ride a bike instead of driving to a friend's house.

- Walk rather than using moving sidewalks at airports (unless you're late for a flight!).

- Use the stairs instead of the elevator, even if only partway.

- Walk to visit a co-worker instead of sending an email.

- Play actively with your kids.

- Get up off the couch and stretch for a few minutes each hour.

- Ride a stationary bicycle while watching TV.

The time you need to spend being active depends on the amount of effort the activity takes. As you progress to moderate intensity activities, you can cut down to 30 minutes, four days a week. In other words, the higher the exercise intensity, the shorter the duration of exercise.

An ideal fitness program includes the following components:

- *Cardiovascular exercise four to seven days per week.* These exercises get your heart and lungs in shape. Brisk walking, jogging, swimming, stair climbing, cycling, cross-country skiing, boxing, and aerobics classes are all great ways to enjoy a cardio workout. Depending on the amount of effort you're expending, exercise for 20 to 60 minutes continuously.

- *Flexibility exercise four to seven days per week.* Gentle reaching, bending, and stretching your muscles keep your joints flexible and your muscles relaxed. The more flexible you are, the less likely you'll be to injure yourself during exercise. If you're not sure what to do, get help from a fitness expert at your health club or gym. Or pick up a book on stretching at the local bookstore.

- *Strength exercise two to four days per week.* Muscular strength, tone, and endurance are important to your overall health and physical fitness. Strength training (also called resistance training) improves your posture, prevents injuries, gives you definition, reshapes problem areas, increases your metabolism, and helps prevent osteoporosis. Getting your muscles in shape doesn't mean you have to pump iron at the gym. You can do push-ups, sit-ups, lunges, and squats at home. Or consider taking yoga or Pilates classes to tone up. If you already work out at a gym, ask a personal trainer to demonstrate the weight machines.

If you're used to sitting on the couch, I strongly recommend that you consult with a certified personal trainer before you jump into an exercise program. A fitness expert can set up a program that's right for you, and, most importantly, he or she can show you how to exercise safely. If you belong to a health club, there are bound to be personal trainers on staff. If you work out at home and would like the help of a personal trainer, contact the Canadian Personal Trainers Network (see Resources, page 304). Tell them your goals, where you live, and whether you prefer a male or female trainer, and they'll offer you a referral. Some trainers even specialize in prenatal exercise.

Most healthy people can safely start an exercise program. However, consult with your doctor if you have two or more of the following risk factors:

- High blood pressure

- High blood cholesterol

- Diabetes

- You're a smoker

- You have a family history of early onset heart disease (father before the age of 55 or mother before the age of 65)

Once you become pregnant, it's okay (and recommended) to continue exercising. Of course, as your pregnancy progresses, you won't be able to work out at the same intensity. And certain exercises should be avoided. You'll learn all about fitness for moms-to-be in Chapter 10.

Practise Healthful Sleep Habits

If you have difficulty sleeping, the following tips may help improve your sleep. Consult with your doctor if you find that none of these strategies helps. He or she will work with you to investigate the cause of your sleep disturbances and find possible solutions.

- *Stick to a schedule.* Try to go to bed at the same time each night and get up at the same time each morning. This goes for Saturday and Sunday nights, too; if you sleep in late on the weekend, you might have trouble falling asleep on Sunday night.

- *Establish a regular bedtime routine.* Following a regular evening routine of brushing your teeth, washing your face, and setting your alarm will help set the mood for sleep. Avoid daytime naps that might interfere with nighttime sleep.

- *Control your sleep environment.* Keep your bedroom dark and quiet, and make sure it is not too warm or cold. Use your bedroom as a place to sleep; don't use it for watching television, eating, exercising, working, or other activities associated with wakefulness.

- *Don't eat heavy meals close to bedtime.* Plan to finish dinner at least three hours before retiring for the night. Avoid spicy and fatty foods that could cause heartburn and keep you up at night.

- *Avoid alcoholic beverages and caffeine.* These interfere with your ability to sleep soundly.

- *Get regular exercise.* Physical activity not only helps you get to sleep but helps you sleep better. But don't exercise in the evening, since this can rev you up and make it difficult to fall asleep. For a sound sleep, the best time to exercise is in the late afternoon.

- *Relax.* Stress and worry can trigger insomnia. Relax at bedtime by taking a warm bath, enjoying a cup of herbal tea, or reading until sleepy. Try to avoid worrying about daytime problems. Some people find that alternative therapies, such as biofeedback, muscle relaxation, behavioural therapy, or psychotherapy, help them achieve a more restful sleep.

Learn to Manage Stress

We all live with stress. In fact, a certain amount of stress serves to motivate and energize us. But too much stress, day after day, can lead to health problems, including high blood pressure, irritable bowel, and increased susceptibility to colds and flu. Extreme stress is believed to affect fertility, reducing your chances of conceiving. And stress may also play a role in a baby's low birth weight.

If you feel you have too much stress in your life, now, more than ever, is the time to learn to manage it. You may not be able to get rid of all your stressors, but you can change how you react to them. Learning how to relax and put things in perspective will prove invaluable skills once you become pregnant. You'll be in a better mental and physical state to prepare for the arrival of your baby. I am not a stress management expert, but I do have a few tips that can help:

- *Set realistic goals.* If you're like me, you set out to accomplish too many things. One of the most important things I have done to manage my stress was learning how to say no. It took years of feeling stressed and unfulfilled to realize I was trying to do too much. I started managing stress by reducing my commitments and giving up responsibilities that were not rewarding or positive. Over the years, I've learned my limits and how to prioritize my goals, as well as my daily tasks. Learn how to set priorities: do only those things you feel are truly important.

My girlfriend Sandra, a mother of two and a successful businesswoman, has a motto she lives by to manage work stress. As she looks over her overwhelming list of memos, reports, emails, and phone calls to get done in between meetings, she asks herself, "If it doesn't get done, who's going to notice?" In other words, if no one will notice, it's not a priority.

- *Learn to recognize stressful situations*. Avoid situations you know will generate stress, or try to alter the circumstances in some way to create a more positive result.

- *Learn to put yourself first*. This is a tough one, especially if you already have children. But it's important to make time to go for a walk, go to the gym, get more sleep, and prepare healthy meals. And if that means not getting the laundry done on time, so be it. Shave a few things from your hectic schedule if necessary. Once you become pregnant, you might not have the physical energy to do all the things you do now.

- *Discuss problems and frustrations with friends, colleagues, or close relatives*. Make a regular date with your friends and family to share, have fun, and relax. If you already have kids, you probably know how challenging it can be to make "couple time" with your partner. If you make "dating" a priority now, there's a good chance you'll keep up this ritual once the baby is born, whether it's once a week or once a month.

- *Learn relaxation techniques*. Deep breathing or meditation can help you cope with stressful situations. There are many audio- and videotapes available in music and bookstores, with relaxing music and scenery. They can really help you unwind.

- *Consider getting professional help*. This is important if you find you can't cope with the stressors in your life.

Consult a Financial Advisor

Frequent shopping sprees at Baby Gap are only the start. Don't forget about formula, baby food, child care, school supplies, even college. Some of these milestones may sound like they're a long way off, but if you don't plan for them, they will catch you off guard. By investing just a little bit of money each month now, you will build a nest egg for your child's education. A financial advisor can tell you how to start saving for your child's near and distant future.

Part Two

———— ⦸⦸⦸ ————

During Your Pregnancy

4

———— ∞∞∞ ————

The First Trimester: Weeks 1 to 12

Over the next nine months, you'll ride a roller coaster of emotional and physical change. Joy, anticipation, fear, and worry—pregnancy is often accompanied by a whirlwind of emotions. And physically, something new is happening to your body every day. At first, the changes will be subtle and almost unnoticeable. But it won't take long before you'll see and feel undeniable signs of the precious new life you're nurturing.

As you set off down the road to motherhood, it's comforting to think about the countless numbers of women who've travelled this path before you. But it's equally important to remember that every woman experiences pregnancy in her own way. Your pregnancy will be different from your mother's or your best friend's. And if you've already had a baby, this pregnancy will undoubtedly be different from your first.

During your pregnancy, take time to listen to your body. Understand that your normal routine will change. If you're feeling tired, rest. If you're hungry, eat something nutritious. And don't be afraid to ask questions. The more you learn about pregnancy, the more you'll understand how to give your baby a safe and healthy start in life.

Over the years, scientists have learned a great deal about pregnancy. We know that these next nine months are crucial to your baby's development. There's a mountain of evidence to prove that you can profoundly influence your baby's future simply by taking care of yourself. If you eat a healthy diet, keep fit, and avoid harmful substances, such as cigarette smoke and alcohol, you'll protect your baby from many health problems. And as an added bonus, you'll recover faster after delivery—your body will snap back into shape with much less effort.

There's no question that pregnancy comes with plenty of responsibility. At times, you may feel overwhelmed by all the decisions that lie ahead. In the next few chapters, I'll try to make your life a little easier by helping you make good choices for yourself and your baby. I'll explain the physical changes that both you and your developing baby will experience in each trimester. In Part One of this book, I offered advice and suggestions to help you get your diet and lifestyle ready for pregnancy. Now it's time to show you how to get the extra nutrients and calories you need as your unborn baby grows. In the chapters that follow, you'll find nutrition advice for every stage of your pregnancy. I'll share with you the strategies that have helped my clients enjoy a happy, healthy journey to motherhood. And I'll also offer plenty of tips to help you deal with common discomforts of pregnancy.

A Nine-Month Odyssey

A normal pregnancy lasts approximately 40 weeks. Yet, how often do you hear women talk about their pregnancy in terms of weeks? Almost never. Ask any woman and she'll tell you that it takes nine months to grow a baby. If she's pregnant, she'll be happy to tell you exactly how many of those months she's already ticked off on the calendar.

If you're doing the math, you've already figured out that 40 weeks is closer to 10 months than to 9. The reason for this discrepancy is that it can be difficult to determine the exact date you conceived. To simplify the process of establishing your baby's gestational age, your due date is calculated from the beginning of your last menstrual period. So, officially, you aren't pregnant for the first few weeks of the 40-week calculation. It can be a bit confusing to hear your doctor refer to your pregnancy in terms of weeks, while everyone else wants to know what month you're in. You may have to do some mental gymnastics to keep the months and weeks straight, but, ultimately, the calculation that will matter most to you is your due date.

Mathematics aside, a nine-month pregnancy is divided into three parts, called trimesters. Each trimester is approximately three months. The first trimester covers weeks 1 to 12, the second trimester covers weeks 13 to 27, and the third trimester covers weeks 28 to 40.

One of the most interesting things about pregnancy is that it seems to usher you into a vast and global sisterhood of mothers. As soon as you announce your pregnancy, it will seem as though every woman you know feels compelled to share the intimate details of her own pregnancy, labour, and delivery. And you, oscillating daily between fear and anticipation, will be equally compelled to listen, often with fascinated horror. While most women genuinely share your joy and are well intentioned, some of their war stories may make you nervous, worried, or even frightened about what lies ahead.

One of the purposes of this book is to set the story straight, to clear up any confusion about what you might expect over the next nine months. My goal is to help you have a safe, healthy, and happy pregnancy, and to usher you gently into that wonderful sisterhood of mothers. So let's get started.

During the first three months of pregnancy, your body is hard at work, creating an ideal environment for nurturing your baby. From the moment of conception, extraordinary events are taking place in the hidden reaches of your womb. Yet despite all this internal activity, the earliest signs of pregnancy are minor and usually go unnoticed. You may not even know you're pregnant for several weeks after you've conceived.

You may meet women who claim to know the exact moment they became pregnant. While I'm not disputing their stories, this level of physical intuition is rare. If you don't have a mystical experience at the moment of conception, don't worry; you're not alone. The vast majority of women are unaware of their pregnancy until they miss their period, and many still aren't convinced until they confirm it with a pregnancy test.

What you should keep in mind, though, is that these first three months are critical to the development of your baby. While you're going about things, oblivious to the fact that you're pregnant, your tiny fetus is busily laying the foundation for major organs, such as the heart, lungs, and brain. At this stage, your baby is extremely vulnerable. The food you eat, the drugs you take, the diseases you catch, even the air you breathe can significantly impact the future health of your child.

Your Changing Body

Your body undergoes many changes, even before you may realize you are pregnant.

Hormonal Changes

Most of the symptoms you'll experience during pregnancy are triggered by changes in your normal hormonal balance. Hormones are highly versatile architects of change. Within a few days of conception, they're already working their magic, preparing your body to accommodate the demanding needs of your growing baby.

Hormonal changes occur as soon as the fertilized egg enters your uterus. The minuscule ball of cells immediately attaches itself to the wall of the uterus, where it begins to form a placenta. The placenta produces several hormones that play a major role in maintaining your pregnancy. Placental hormones prevent your ovaries from releasing more eggs for the duration of your pregnancy. They also sustain the development of your fetus by stimulating increased production of estrogen and progesterone. Essentially, these important hormones ensure that your body will support a healthy pregnancy.

As those pregnancy hormones surge through your bloodstream, your body responds by altering its rhythms and functions of its major organs. These changes are normal and necessary to help you nourish and protect your baby. In most cases, your body will quickly return to its pre-pregnancy state after delivery.

Breasts

The good news is that you'll soon have those big, beautiful breasts you've always dreamed of (or not). The bad news is that they'll be so tender and sore for the first few weeks that you won't want your partner, or your nightgown, or the water in the shower, or anything else for that matter, to come near them. A number of my friends have told me that their suddenly sensitive breasts gave them the first clue that they were pregnant. But don't worry; the sensitivity settles down after the second or third month and you can really enjoy your lush new figure—at least until your stomach starts demanding all the attention.

Breast tenderness develops because your body is getting ready for breastfeeding. The fat layer in your breasts is growing and milk glands are developing. As the blood supply gradually increases, your breast veins will become larger and more noticeable. And all the while, your breasts keep getting bigger. This is a good time to pack away the lacy lingerie and invest in a sturdy support bra. You'll be glad you did, because a little extra support right now will save your breasts from a lot of stretching and sagging later on.

Heart and Circulatory System

In the first trimester, your heart starts to work overtime, keeping up this accelerated pace until you deliver your baby. Over the course of the pregnancy, your hard-working heart will pump between 30 and 50 percent more blood than usual. Nutrients are carried to the fetus through your bloodstream, so your body needs all that extra blood to meet the ever increasing demands of your growing baby. Your blood supply gradually begins to increase by the 6th week of pregnancy and peaks somewhere around the 24th week. Naturally, your heart has to pump harder to move all that blood through your system. As your pregnancy progresses, you may notice that your pulse rate quickens by as much as 10 to 15 beats per minute.

Kidneys

Like your heart, your kidneys work much harder during pregnancy. The kidneys are responsible for filtering impurities out of your bloodstream and eliminating them as urine. As soon as your heart begins pumping a larger-than-usual blood supply, your kidneys kick into overdrive to keep up with the increased volume. Which means that your body produces lots of extra urine and you spend plenty of time hunting for bathrooms.

Lungs

Pregnancy also has an impact on your lungs and respiratory system. Your body needs more oxygen to nourish both you and your baby, so you'll find yourself breathing faster and more deeply. As your pregnancy progresses, the blood supply to your lungs and respiratory tract increases. Vital oxygen molecules are transferred from your lungs into your bloodstream and carried to the fetus. You may notice that the circumference of your chest actually increases slightly to accommodate the changes in your respiratory activity.

Digestive System

Until now, you've probably taken your digestive system for granted, never really giving it much thought. But during pregnancy, your digestion is always top-of-mind. Unfortunately, the high levels of progesterone you need to sustain a healthy pregnancy can play havoc with your stomach and intestines. Progesterone relaxes the muscles in your esophagus and rectum, slowing down the intestinal contractions that move food through your digestive tract. So food stays in your stomach and intestines longer than usual.

Food that lingers in your intestine is easy prey for the bacteria residing there. These tiny organisms will work overtime to ferment undigested food particles. This means you'll experience plenty of unwanted gas in the form of burping, bloating, and flatulence. Indeed, pregnancy can bring with it a whole range of digestive complaints, from constipation and heartburn to stomach ulcers and gallbladder disease. While none of these conditions adds to the joy of pregnancy, most are easily managed through diet and exercise.

Signs and Symptoms

Now that you know a little more about what's going on in your body, let's talk about what all this internal activity means to you. These physical changes may look fairly minor on paper, but they can have a dramatic effect on how you look and feel. It's highly unlikely that you'll have to cope with all the classic symptoms of pregnancy, but you are certain to encounter a few. The list below will give you some idea of what to expect. It will help you prepare for the adjustments you'll have to make as your body tackles the complex task of growing a baby.

Bleeding

Everybody knows that the one surefire sign of pregnancy is a missed period. Or is it? Many women don't have a regular menstrual cycle and often don't keep track of their shifting schedule. If your period fluctuates from month to month and you're not on a consistent

28-day cycle, you may not even notice that you've missed your period by a week or two. So don't count on a missed period to alert you that you're pregnant. However, whether you notice it or not, your period does come to a halt when you're pregnant. The placenta produces a hormone, called human chorionic gonadotropin (hCG), which prevents your ovaries from releasing any more eggs once a fertilized egg reaches your uterus.

Even though your period has stopped, you may experience sporadic bleeding, especially during the first trimester. Every woman worries about bleeding during pregnancy, so it's only natural to feel a little panicky if you find blood on your underwear. Although it doesn't necessarily mean you're heading for a miscarriage, it's wise to report all bleeding to your doctor. If the bleeding is light and the blood is brown with no clots in it, your doctor will likely recommend that you take it easy and spend time lying down with your feet up. If the blood is bright red or has clots in it, there's no need to get overly alarmed, but you should call your doctor immediately. He or she may want to monitor your pregnancy more closely and may suggest an ultrasound to check the health of your baby.

Fatigue

In the early stages of pregnancy, you can expect to feel tired most of the time. Fatigue can completely overwhelm you, making it difficult to work, concentrate, or even think. Don't be surprised if you fall asleep everywhere and anywhere—in a staff meeting, in the passenger seat of a car, or watching TV. When you do give in to your sleep cravings, you'll sleep like a log. Unfortunately, the chances are good that you won't feel refreshed when you wake up, just groggy and still tired. Your body is working hard to grow this tiny, new human being, and you're burning up a lot of energy just sitting still. So don't fight your urge to sleep. Listen to your body and rest whenever you can. After all, once your little angel arrives, sleep will be nothing more than a distant memory.

Morning Sickness

I hate to tell you this, but "morning sickness" is the wrong name for this particularly unpleasant pregnancy symptom. It should really be called "any time, anywhere sickness." In the first trimester, as many as 70 percent of all pregnant women suffer some degree of nausea.[1] If you manage to get through your pregnancy without streaking to the bathroom with a horrible churning sensation in your stomach, consider yourself lucky. I'll go into more detail about morning sickness in Chapter 9, but, for now, suffice it to say that nausea is the bane of the pregnant woman's existence.

Most women are particularly prone to nausea in the first trimester, when pregnancy hormones are high. For some women, mornings really are the worst time of day. When my researcher, Anne, was pregnant with her first child, she lived in Toronto and worked in

Hamilton. Her morning drive to the office included several carefully organized vomit stops. After a number of urgent bathroom visits en route, she'd get to work and feel fine for the rest of the day. Other women feel sick all day long. One of my clients, Andrea, was so easily nauseated that she couldn't walk into a grocery store without throwing up. Her husband had to do all the food shopping until she was well into her second trimester.

Morning sickness is often accompanied by an incredibly strong aversion to certain smells, due to the hormonal changes going on in your body. My friend Lisa's husband would only have to walk through the door with a cup of coffee in his hand and she'd be charging for the bathroom. Anne once threw up in a garbage bin when she became overwhelmed by the exhaust smells in an underground parking lot. There's no way of knowing exactly what will set your stomach off, as your food and smell aversions can change from day to day.

Plan on taking it one day at a time, and experiment with a variety of foods to find the ones your body can tolerate. The goal is to try to eat a balanced diet and incorporate at least some foods from the four major food groups into your daily diet. But don't be too hard on yourself if you can't always manage it for the first little while. Though you may not have much of an appetite now, you'll want to eat everything in sight by the time the second trimester rolls around.

Frequent Urination

Remember those kidneys in overdrive I mentioned earlier? Well, they're the culprits behind your sudden need to pee every few seconds. Even when you know you've just been to the bathroom and you couldn't possibly have another ounce of urine in your bladder, you'll still feel an urge to urinate. That's because your kidneys are busily cleaning the waste products out of your bloodstream and making urine to flush them out of your body. As your uterus enlarges, the additional pressure on your bladder can also aggravate that sense of urination urgency.

In the second trimester, some of these pressures ease off and your bladder settles down. But the peeing problem will return to plague you in the third trimester. By the end of her pregnancy, my friend Sheila swore that she could get out of bed, use the bathroom, and get back into bed without even waking up. Now that's a skill worth cultivating!

Dizziness

As your blood volume increases and your heart starts working harder, your blood pressure changes. This can lead to episodes of dizziness and light-headedness. Bending over or standing up too quickly can leave you swooning like a Southern belle. Because more blood is flowing through the respiratory tract, you may also feel a little congested and short of breath. Respiratory and circulatory changes, as well as nausea and fatigue, can all contribute to that light-headedness. There's not much you can do about any of this except to move a little more slowly so your heart and lungs can adjust to their new workload. Take it easy when you get up after sitting or lying down, drink plenty of fluids, and avoid driving when you feel faint or dizzy.

Weight Gain

If your pre-pregnancy body mass index was between 20 and 27, you need to gain between 25 and 35 pounds (11 and 16 kilograms) over the duration of your pregnancy. This amount of weight gain will result in the healthiest pregnancy outcome for you and your baby. But you'll gain little of this weight in the first trimester. Weight maintenance, even slight weight losses, are normal during the first trimester. Despite this, most women gain between 2 and 8 pounds (1 and 3.5 kilograms) during the first trimester. You'll read more about weight gain in the first trimester in Chapter 7.

Your Changing Emotions

When you were planning your pregnancy, you may have thought you'd drift through the entire nine months in a lovely state of tranquility. But now that your pregnancy is a reality, I'm willing to bet that you aren't feeling the least bit tranquil. Those pesky pregnancy hormones, estrogen and progesterone, are playing havoc with your emotions, causing you to feel up one minute and down the next.

Mood Swings

Mood swings are a fact of life in pregnancy, especially during the first trimester. You'll be amazed at how quickly you career from one end of the emotional spectrum to the other. Swinging wildly from deep despair to great joy will soon become a normal state of affairs for you. The littlest thing can bring you to tears, and you may become completely irrational without even realizing it. One of my clients told me that she became hysterical when her husband, a low-key man, reacted with less than overwhelming excitement to the news of her pregnancy. Once her husband managed to convince her that he was indeed thrilled with her news, she started crying all over again. As she rather shame-facedly confessed later, she launched into a tirade, accusing her by now completely confused husband of ruining her career by getting her pregnant. The poor man couldn't win for losing! This to say that your husband, family, and friends may find you a little difficult to live with over the next few months.

It's only natural to struggle with a mixed bag of emotions as you face the enormity of the demands and responsibilities that lie ahead. So don't be too hard on yourself when you indulge in a crying jag or two. If you have a partner, do try to spare a thought for him or her now and then. He or she is going through serious emotional changes, too. Just like you, your partner may be feeling uncertain and anxious about the future, and is probably sharing your concerns about financial stresses, lifestyle change, and shifting priorities. He or she may also be feeling a little neglected as you become increasingly focused on your changing body and the imminent arrival of the baby. As the pregnancy slowly begins to dominate your life, it's important to be mutually supportive and to keep the lines of communication open. Take time to talk about your feelings and concerns, and try to resolve issues before they become too big to handle.

Your Developing Baby

The development of a baby, from the moment of conception to the moment of birth, is a complex and miraculous process. Thousands of steps are involved, each seemingly more intricate than the previous one. When you think about the precise orchestration necessary to create the countless building blocks of human life, it seems incredible that it all comes together so reliably. Of course, birth defects do occur, and it would be naïve to overlook the possibility of inherited genetic abnormalities. But, many birth defects are not inherited and can be avoided by following a healthy lifestyle during pregnancy.

Researchers have found that birth defects can often be traced back to external factors that have influenced or interrupted the normal genetic program. After all, babies don't grow in a vacuum. The environment surrounding your baby in the womb profoundly shapes the development process. By ensuring that your baby is supplied with essential nutrients and protected from damaging toxins, you can reduce the risk of birth defects and long-term health problems. Let's take a look at what's happening with your baby in the first three months of life.

Implantation

The first trimester is the most important in your baby's development. This is the stage when all major body organs and systems are formed. The process starts almost as soon as your egg is fertilized. The fertilized egg, known as a zygote, travels down the fallopian tubes to the uterus, dividing repeatedly as it moves. Three to five days after conception, it enters the uterus. The hollow ball of cells, now referred to as a blastocyst, implants itself near the top of the uterus wall. The inner cells of the blastocyst develop into the embryo, and the outer cells attach to the uterine wall to form the placenta. An umbilical cord begins to form, containing blood vessels that allow vital nutrients to pass from your bloodstream into the embryo. The umbilical cord and placenta provide an essential exchange of nourishment, oxygen, and waste products between you and your baby. The embryo floats in a fluid-filled amniotic sac, which expands as the baby grows. The amniotic sac protects the embryo from bumps, pressure, and unexpected blows.

The First Month

By the time the embryo is four weeks old, the spinal cord and brain are completely formed. The embryo soon develops a head and trunk and starts sprouting arm and leg buds. Internal organs, such as the heart, lungs, and brain, are developing rapidly at this stage. The heart begins to beat approximately 18 days after conception, just about the same time as the circulatory system takes shape. At four weeks, the embryo is about 1/8 inch (3 millimetres) long, approximately the length of a grain of rice. By six weeks, it has already grown to 1/2 inch (12 millimetres), with the head and brain making up nearly one-third of the baby's total body length. This is a critical stage for the development of healthy brain tissue and internal organs. Your diet and physical condition in these first few weeks will directly affect the health of the embryo.

The Second Month

During the second month of pregnancy, all the major organs and systems of the embryo are developed and growing rapidly. The liver, stomach, and skin have all taken shape and other essential systems, such as blood vessels, intestines, and the urinary tract, are well underway. The inner ear is forming and eyelids start to grow, although they still cannot open and close. In an orderly pattern, the tiny arm buds begin to sprout hand buds, and then finger buds. The leg buds follow suit by sprouting feet buds and toe buds. By the end of the 8th week, the embryo's cartilage tissue starts to change into bone tissue. At this stage, the sex organs also begin to form. If your baby is a boy, high levels of the hormone testosterone will be released in the embryo and a tiny penis will appear. After eight weeks, the embryo is referred to as a fetus. It is now about 1 inch (2.5 centimetres) long and weighs less than 1 ounce (28 grams).

The Third Month

As the third month progresses, your baby begins to look more like a human and less like a tadpole. The head is still oversized compared with the rest of the body and may be covered with the beginnings of hair. Soft nails form on the fingers and toes, and 20 tooth buds appear in the mouth. Body organs are maturing and will soon be fully developed. Reflexes have started to fire, and nerves and muscles are working. Your baby may start to make small movements and to open and close her mouth. But, despite all the activity, the movements are still too tiny for you to feel. The baby's heart beats at 120 to 160 beats per minute and is pumping 50 pints (140 litres) of blood a day through her circulatory system. Even the tiny kidneys are working, sending urine into her bladder. The umbilical cord, now fully developed, removes these waste products and exchanges them for nutrients to help your baby grow. At the end of the 12th week, the fetus is about 4 inches (10 centimetres) long and weighs a little more than 1 ounce (28 grams).

Health Care Needs in the First Trimester

Prenatal checkups begin in the first trimester. Now is also the time to find a suitable health care provider.

Pregnancy Tests

The first thing you need to do if you think you may be pregnant is to take a pregnancy test. The sooner you confirm your pregnancy, the sooner you can start taking proper care of your developing baby. If you're like most women, you'll probably rush out and buy a home pregnancy kit as soon as you suspect you're pregnant. It used to be that you had to wait several weeks after you missed your period to get an accurate confirmation of your pregnancy. But now, the testing process is very sensitive, so you can find out whether you're pregnant within 8 to 10 days after conception—often as soon as one day after you miss your period.

The home pregnancy test measures the level of hCG (human chorionic gonadotropin) that is floating in your urine. I mentioned earlier that hCG is a placental hormone that plays a major role in maintaining your pregnancy. This hormone enters your bloodstream shortly after conception and can be accurately detected in a urine test. For best results, test your urine first thing in the morning, when hCG levels are highest. While the modern home pregnancy kits are usually accurate, testing too soon after conception may lead to a false negative. That's because the hormone levels are still too low to register on the testing tool. Every woman's hormone levels are different, so don't give up hope if you get a negative result the first time. Wait a few days and try it again to be sure. This type of test can also produce a false positive, though that doesn't happen often.

If you get a positive result with a home pregnancy test, make an appointment with your doctor right away. He or she will send you for a blood test, which is the most accurate way to confirm your pregnancy. Pregnancy blood tests work the same way as pregnancy urine tests, measuring the level of hCG in the bloodstream. However, the measurement process used in the blood test is more precise than the one used in the home pregnancy kit. If you get a positive on this test, it's definite: you're pregnant.

Finding a Health Care Provider

If you don't have a family doctor, try to get one right away. (If you planned the pregnancy and completed the pre-pregnancy to-do list in Chapter 3, then you've already been for a checkup.) Your health care provider will oversee your pregnancy and monitor your progress on a regular basis. Many women are comfortable using their family doctor, though more and more women are turning to a midwife for their routine prenatal care. If your pregnancy is normal and you have no history of high-risk pregnancy, a midwife is an option worth considering (see Chapter 3 for more information on midwives). If you have a complicated or high-risk pregnancy, you may be referred to an obstetrician for specialized care.

In Part One, I encouraged you to think ahead and choose your health care provider before you became pregnant. You may or may not have had time to do this. If not, now is the time. When selecting your caregiver, keep in mind that your doctor is a crucial member of the project team, with a vital role to play in ensuring a successful outcome of your pregnancy. You're going to be spending a lot of time together in the next little while, so choose carefully.

Look for someone who is patient and understanding. He or she should be willing to make time for the hundreds of questions you'll want to ask. You should have confidence in your practitioner's skills and experience, and feel comfortable when you're in his or her office. Most importantly, your concerns should be treated with respect. Though your doctor or midwife may have been through this complicated process many times, this may be your first time. You deserve to be taken seriously, even when you fuss and worry about little problems and issues. Of course, I'm not suggesting that you rush to the doctor for every ache and pain. However, reasonable questions deserve reasonable responses.

One of the best ways to find a suitable health care provider is to ask for recommendations from friends or family. If you know someone who's had a good pregnancy and successful delivery, get her doctor's or midwife's name. If you ask around a little, you'll soon find out who's good and who's not, in your area. You could also ask other health care providers for a referral or contact your regional health authority for a list of doctors taking on maternity patients.

Your First Prenatal Visit

This visit can be quite long, especially if you didn't have a medical checkup before you became pregnant. Expect to spend time discussing your health history and having tests to rule out existing medical conditions. The tests you receive will vary, depending on your health and family medical history. Your first visit could include:

- An internal pelvic exam to check your uterus and cervix
- A Pap smear to detect cancer in your cervix (the opening of your uterus)

- Blood tests to determine your blood type and Rh factor (see below), and to check for conditions such as anemia, diabetes, and hepatitis B. If you haven't been tested previously, blood tests will be done to determine if your body is protected against rubella, the virus responsible for German measles.

- Inquiry about your exposure to chicken pox

- A urine test to check for infections or kidney problems

- Tests to determine whether you've been exposed to sexually transmitted diseases, such as syphilis

- An HIV test, which you can refuse if you wish. However, many people don't know they have the virus simply because they haven't been tested. I strongly recommend that you be tested for HIV. Today there is treatment available to prevent passing the virus to your unborn child or to your newborn through breast milk.

- A breast exam to identify changes in your breasts

- Weight measurements to assess your health and your baby's growth

Rh factor is a protein that can sometimes attach to blood cells (A, B, AB, O). If your blood has this protein, it is Rh-positive. If it does not, it's Rh-negative. If you are Rh-negative and your baby's father is Rh-positive, your child might inherit his Rh factor rather than yours. If an Rh-positive baby is growing inside an Rh-negative mother, the two blood types are incompatible. If the mother's blood mixes with the baby's blood at birth, or if bleeding occurs during pregnancy, the mother can react as if she were allergic, forming antibodies to her baby. This can lead to serious illness or even death for the baby. Today, this incompatibility is preventable and therefore rarely seen. If your blood test reveals potential for an incompatibility, you will be given Rh-immune globulin when you are at 28 to 32 weeks. Details about other conditions you will be tested for on this visit are provided in Chapter 6.

To be sure that you and your doctor are on the same wavelength about your pregnancy, the first visit is a good time to ask a few important questions, including:

- *Where will my baby be born?* Doctors have medical privileges at specific hospitals only, and it's important to know which hospital he or she will be sending you to for labour and delivery.

- *Will you be attending the birth of my baby?* Because of the demanding, unpredictable hours associated with maternity patients, many doctors belong to medical groups and rotate their on-call responsibilities with other physicians. If your doctor belongs to this type of medical group, there is no guarantee that he or she will be available to deliver your baby when you go into labour.

- *What are my choices for labour and delivery?* It's important to know how your doctor prefers to handle the labour and delivery process. Ask questions about birth positions, labour support (midwives and family members), labour induction, medications and anesthesia, episiotomies (a small incision in the skin and the perinatal muscle at the time of delivery to enlarge the vaginal opening, making it easier for the baby's head or body to emerge or to insert birthing instruments), and induction of labour. You will eliminate a great deal of anxiety and stress if you know how your delivery will be handled before you arrive at the hospital in full labour.

Other Prenatal Checkups

If your pregnancy is normal, you can expect to see your doctor on a monthly basis, from the second month right up to the seventh month. After the seventh month, your doctor will want to monitor your progression more closely and visits will gradually increase. Most prenatal appointments are routine and brief. Your doctor will check your weight, blood pressure, and urine. He or she will also check your baby's heartbeat and the size of your uterus. This helps ensure that everything's still on track and that your baby is growing normally. If you and your baby are healthy and you have no pressing issues to discuss, you will be in and out of the doctor's office with the minimum of fuss. But if you have any questions, ask. That's what your doctor is there for.

Prenatal Tests and Chorionic Villus Sampling

It used to be that the baby's sex was a complete surprise; the excited parents anxiously awaited the announcement in the delivery room. The same thing applied to your baby's health. If there was a problem, you didn't find out about it until you delivered the baby. In recent years, all that has changed. Now prenatal tests can reliably determine the sex of your baby well ahead of your due date. There are also a number of tests that will help your doctor assess your baby's health and identify birth defects or genetic abnormalities. This testing allows you to make informed decisions about continuing with the pregnancy.

Most of these prenatal tests are conducted in the second trimester; I'll tell you more about the various testing processes in Chapter 5. However, chorionic villus sampling, or CVS, is a prenatal test that takes place when you are between 9 and 11 weeks pregnant. CVS tests your baby's genetic information to identify specific problems. This test is used to screen for chromosome abnormalities, such as Down syndrome, and genetic disorders, such as cystic fibrosis. Because it does not sample amniotic fluid, it does not detect neural tube defects, such as spina bifida. And it cannot identify all causes of mental retardation. There is also a 1 in 100 risk of miscarriage with this procedure. The CVS test is not part of a routine prenatal checkup. Rather, it may be performed for certain high-risk pregnancies.

The process involves taking samples of chorionic villi, the cells lining the placenta. These cells contain the same genetic information as the cells in your baby. Usually, the placenta can be easily reached through your vagina and samples can be taken with minimum discomfort.

Using an ultrasound to guide progress, the doctor will collect a sample of the chorionic villi by inserting a thin tube through the cervix into the uterus. The procedure feels a bit like a Pap smear and takes about 45 minutes (most of that time is spent preparing for the procedure; the actual sampling takes only five minutes). Occasionally, the placenta may not be accessible and samples will be taken by inserting a long needle into the uterus through your abdomen. You may experience slight bleeding, which you should report to your doctor, but usually that is not cause for alarm.

The advantage of CVS over other genetic screening tests is that you get the results within a few days, instead of having to wait a few weeks. Preliminary results are available in two days and final results are ready in a week. CVS is 98 percent accurate in detecting chromosomal problems. While many women are anxious to get results about the health of their baby as early as possible, amniocenteses (discussed in Chapter 5), which are performed at 16 weeks, have a better safety record. To determine what's best for you, consult with your doctor.

Sex During Pregnancy

In a normal pregnancy, sex is safe right up to the final weeks of your third trimester. The strong muscles of your uterus and a thick cushion of amniotic fluid keep your baby safely protected, so even a night of vigorous lovemaking won't harm the fetus. You have to limit sexual intercourse only if you're at high risk of pregnancy complications, preterm labour, or miscarriage.

Now that you know it's okay to have sex during pregnancy, let's consider the real question. Are you *interested* in sex during pregnancy? If you're like many women, the answer is probably not, or at least not often. Many women find that their sex drive goes into a decline during pregnancy. In the early weeks, nausea and fatigue might keep you from thinking of your bed as anything other than a place to sleep. And as your belly becomes bigger, you may start to feel unattractive and ungainly. To be honest, pregnancy may not be the most sexually fulfilling time of your life. It can be hard to feel sexy when your breasts hurt, your back aches, and you have to pee every five minutes.

For each woman who is uninterested in sex during pregnancy, there's another who says her sex drive surges instead of declines. This often happens to women during their first trimester. The increased blood flow to your sexual organs coupled with the high hormone levels of pregnancy make your breasts and vulva more sensitive. As a result, lovemaking can be more appealing than ever. You may find yourself more easily aroused and more sexually responsive—even your dreams may become dramatically sexual.

As your pregnancy continues and your uterus expands, lovemaking becomes more challenging. You and your partner may have to experiment to find a position that comfortably accommodates your beach ball–like stomach. Be aware, however, that sexual stimulation may cause your breasts to leak and orgasms may trigger uncomfortable uterine contractions. These responses are normal and not in the least bit harmful to your pregnancy.

There's no way to predict how your sex life will fare during pregnancy. A lot depends on how you and your partner communicate. This is a time to express yourself openly and to discuss your feelings honestly. Be creative—explore your sexual options. Experiment until you find the positions that give you the greatest comfort and pleasure. If penetration becomes too uncomfortable, consider alternatives, such as mutual masturbation and oral sex. Sometimes, just gentle touching and cuddling is enough to maintain a feeling of closeness with your partner. Take time to talk about what feels right for you; it will help you and your partner to share the experience of pregnancy in a positive and fulfilling way.

The Risk of Miscarriage

No doubt about it, the first trimester is an exciting stage of pregnancy. Your body is nurturing, your baby is growing, and your life is changing dramatically. At a time when so much joy abounds, it's tempting to ignore the frightening prospect of losing your baby through miscarriage. But the risks of miscarriage are very real, particularly during the first three months of pregnancy. Nearly 15 percent of all confirmed pregnancies end in the loss of the baby. Factor in the number of miscarriages that occur very early in pregnancy—before women even realize they're pregnant—and that figure is estimated to be as high as 50 percent.[2]

Miscarriage is still a bit of a taboo subject in our society. No one wants to upset a newly pregnant woman by talking about the loss of her baby, so the topic is usually ignored or avoided. As a result, many women are unaware of the potential for miscarriage and are overwhelmed with shock when it happens to them. Yet, you would probably be surprised at how many of your friends and family have lost a baby. My researcher, Anne, miscarried her first pregnancy at 12 weeks and was astonished at the number of women who comforted her by sharing their own stories. Miscarriage tends to be a private grief, one a woman keeps close to her heart. If Anne hadn't lost her baby, she would never have known that so many of her friends and acquaintances had lost one, too. Fortunately, most of the women went on to have healthy babies from subsequent pregnancies, so Anne found a great deal of hope and support in these personal tales of loss and renewal.

My point is that miscarriage is a reality of pregnancy, and you should be aware of it. Some women are so fearful of miscarriage that they spend the entire nine months in a state of high anxiety. But there's simply no point in spending so much energy on need-less worrying. If you're going to miscarry, there's not a lot you can do to prevent it. However, for your peace of mind, it is a good idea to understand the risks and recognize the warning signs.

What Causes a Miscarriage?

Although a miscarriage is defined as the loss of a baby before the 20th week of pregnancy, most miscarriages occur during the first 12 weeks.[3] Women who have miscarried once will often keep the news of their next pregnancy a secret until they've passed the critical 12-week period, just in case it happens again. While some women do have repeated miscarriages, the good news is that approximately 85 percent of women go on to have normal pregnancies after their first miscarriage.[4] Anne, for example, gave birth to three healthy children after she lost her first pregnancy.

Miscarriages that occur in the first trimester are usually the result of chromosomal or genetic abnormalities. This means that something is developmentally wrong with the fetus and it will not survive outside the womb. Sometimes the placenta does not implant prop-erly in your uterus and, as a result, it isn't capable of nurturing the growing fetus. Hormonal problems, abnormalities in your uterus or cervix, medical conditions such as diabetes, and certain illnesses or infections may also trigger a miscarriage.

The important thing to note here is that miscarriages are usually caused by circum-stances that you can't control. In most cases, they are nature's way of ending a pregnancy that would not produce a healthy baby. If your pregnancy is destined to miscarry, there is nothing that you or your doctor can do to prevent it.

Now, that's easy enough to say, but it's difficult for a grieving woman to accept. When you've lost a baby, the overwhelming urge is to look for someone or something to blame. Many women burden themselves with guilt, blaming themselves for doing something that harmed their baby. One woman I know was convinced that she lost her baby because she had played soccer the day before. Another told me that she miscarried because she was having too much sex. And some of my clients ask me whether it was something they did or didn't eat that caused their loss.

Let me reassure you that there is nothing in your normal daily activities that would cause the loss of your baby. The fetus is well protected by the amniotic sac, so exercise, sex, even minor falls, will not injure your baby. I always recommend a healthy diet dur-ing pregnancy, but your nutrition—or lack of it—will not trigger a miscarriage. Difficult as it is to accept, miscarriages are a fact of life. Blaming yourself or your partner will not make the loss any easier to bear and will only cloud future pregnancies with unhealthy worry and fear.

Warning Signs

The signs of a miscarriage are usually clear. You will experience light to heavy vaginal bleeding and may pass large blood clots. You may also have cramping, chills, or a fever and may notice a foul-smelling vaginal discharge. If you have any of these symptoms, notify your doctor immediately. While these warning signs accompany most miscarriages, some women have no symptoms at all when they lose their pregnancy. These are known as silent miscarriages and are discovered only through an ultrasound. A silent miscarriage can be particularly distressing because the news of the loss comes as a complete shock.

Not all spotting or bleeding means you will miscarry. Women frequently have bleeding in the early stages of pregnancy and go on to have a successful pregnancy. Notify your doctor of your symptoms; he or she will explain the possible causes of the bleeding and perform an internal examination. You might also have an ultrasound to determine if the fetus is still alive. The pregnancy could continue successfully or could progress into a miscarriage: again, there are no guarantees and no known ways to stop a miscarriage. Bedrest may help ease the bleeding and cramping symptoms of an impending miscarriage but will not likely change the outcome.

If the fetus is not alive, your doctor will check to see if all the tissue and blood have been expelled from the uterus. If there is still material left in the womb, you may need to have a medical procedure to remove the remaining contents. This procedure is necessary to prevent infection and is usually quick and painless.

After the Miscarriage

After your miscarriage, rest for a day or two. However, it is often helpful to get back to your usual routine as soon as possible. While your body will recover quickly, your emotions may take longer to heal. The pain of your loss may affect you in many ways, and you need to give yourself time to grieve. Everyone experiences grief in her own way. Because the pregnancy and the feelings for your baby were more real to you than to anyone else, others may not understand the extent of your grief and may expect you to bounce back faster than you do. Although you may find it difficult to share your loss with those around you, talk to your partner, friends, and family. It's important that you get emotional support at this difficult time, so ask for the help you need and consider grief counselling if you feel that you're not coping well with your loss.

If you want to try to get pregnant again, it's recommended that you wait until you've had at least one normal menstrual period. This will help give your body and uterus time to heal.

5

The Second Trimester:
Weeks 13 to 27

Ask any woman to describe the best part of her pregnancy and chances are, she'll talk about the second trimester. This is the time in your nine-month odyssey when you look and feel your best. You're over the worst of your morning sickness, your energy is picking up again, and all that extra blood circulating in your system is giving you a rosy glow of good health. Your belly is getting round, and you'll soon feel the baby kicking. Family, friends, even strangers, will start complimenting you on how terrific you look. Take advantage of the extra attention and enjoy this wonderful stage in your pregnancy.

Your Changing Body

In the second trimester, your body continues to undergo tremendous change.

Uterus

Your uterus is an amazing organ. Before pregnancy, it's about the size and shape of a pear. It sits, nicely tucked away, at the top of your vagina. Once you get pregnant, though, your uterus starts behaving like the Incredible Hulk, stretching and growing and busting right out of its normal pelvic confines. It's not long before your waistline is nothing more than a dim memory. While it may take time to get used to your new, rounder silhouette, keep in mind that this steady expansion is necessary to accommodate your growing baby.

By the time you're 12 weeks pregnant, your uterus has expanded beyond the pelvis and extends into the abdomen. At 20 weeks, the uterus has grown as high as your belly button and has started to compress your stomach and bladder. All that extra pressure makes you feel as if your bladder is the size of a pea (no pun intended) and your stomach is shrinking daily. As the uterus grows, it eventually displaces your entire digestive tract. Toward the end of your pregnancy, the uterus will have expanded right up under your lungs—and your baby will be drumming a tattoo on your rib cage. At each prenatal visit, your doctor will check the size of your uterus to be sure that the baby is growing normally.

Breasts

Your breasts are probably still feeling tingly and a little bit sore, but the extreme sensitivity that plagued you in the first trimester is easing off. You may feel lumpiness in your breasts, but that's a normal part of the milk production process and shouldn't be cause for concern. In the second trimester, you will probably notice enlarged veins appearing under your skin. These veins have always been there but are much more noticeable now because of the increased blood supply to your breasts.

As your cleavage continues to increase dramatically, you'll notice that your nipples are becoming much darker. If you examine your body carefully, you may be surprised to find that moles, freckles, and other pigmented areas are becoming darker, too. You can thank those hyperactive placental hormones for your new look. They stimulate increased production of melanin, a dark brown skin pigment, which deepens your skin tone in specific areas.

Skin

Many women sail through pregnancy without any skin problems. Their skin takes on a rosy luminescence, glowing with good health. Other women, unfortunately, find that their skin is very temperamental at this time and needs a lot of extra attention. Women who have never had a pimple in their lives suddenly find themselves coping with acne. Stretch marks, dry skin, rashes—you name it and pregnant women get it. Your skin takes a lot of abuse during the journey to motherhood.

One of the most commonly reported skin problems in pregnancy is melasma, or "the mask" of pregnancy. A pregnancy mask can develop as early as the fourth month and is caused by a combination of pregnancy hormones and exposure to the sun's ultraviolet rays. The mask will appear as blotchy, brown spots on your forehead and cheeks. These spots will become steadily darker if you go out in the sunshine without proper protection. If you start to see brownish spots developing on your face, avoid going out in the sun without a sunscreen that's SPF15 or higher. Unfortunately, there's not much else you can do to prevent the discolouration. The mask usually fades after pregnancy and may disappear completely. If it's still visible after your baby is born, Retinol-A creams and lightening agents may help reduce the pigmentation.

You must be careful with acne treatments during pregnancy. If your skin starts breaking out, check with your doctor before starting any new skin-care programs. Some acne treatments have been known to cause birth defects in fetuses.[1] Your skin is delicate, so treat it gently at every stage of your pregnancy. Avoid brushes, exfoliants, facial scrubs, and harsh cleansers, and use only the mildest products for cleaning your face.

Ironically, while the oil glands in your face are working overtime, the skin on the rest of your body is probably extremely dry and itchy. Several of my clients have complained that the itchiness is the worst part of pregnancy. I know a number of women who've been driven to distraction by itchy skin and have scratched their bellies and breasts so hard that they've left welts. During pregnancy, your skin is being stretched in every direction, so some dryness and itchiness is to be expected. Right from the beginning of your pregnancy, try to keep your skin well moisturized. Regular applications of lotions and creams will protect its natural elasticity.

You may want to save the long soaks in the bathtub until after the baby's born. Hot showers and bubble baths can remove the natural, protective oils of the skin, which will only aggravate a dry skin problem. If the itchiness is too much to bear, ask your doctor for medicated creams or antihistamines to keep the worst of it under control.

You will probably notice other small changes in your skin during these next few weeks. Almost every pregnant woman develops a dark line (linea nigra) on the skin of her belly, running from the top of the pubic bone to just below the belly button. Some women also develop tiny skin tags in unexpected places, such as under their breasts, on their eyelids, or along their panty line. Skin tags are little flaps of loose tissue that are caused by clothing or skin rubbing on skin. Skin tags won't go away once they've developed, but they are easily removed after the baby's born. You may also notice little red marks on your skin or broken capillaries. Again, these are permanent, so if they bother you, you can have them removed after pregnancy.

Stretch Marks

Most women hate stretch marks, but I think of them as the battle scars of pregnancy. They identify you as one of the initiated—a mother. Even if you dread the thought of stretch marks, you might as well get used to it, because almost every pregnant woman gets them. Stretch marks are red or purple lines that usually appear on your breasts, abdomen, thighs, and buttocks. They're caused by all the stretching and pulling that's going on under the surface of your skin. Stretch marks tend to be obvious at first but gradually fade to a soft silvery colour.

There is some indication that stretch marks may be hereditary. If your mother got them, chances are, so will you. If you developed stretch marks during your teenage growth spurt, you're almost sure to get them. Many cosmetic firms promote creams and lotions for preventing or eliminating stretch marks. Some doctors recommend laser surgery as a means of removing them. But no treatment has been proven to prevent or remove stretch marks. So, wear your battle scars proudly and don't waste energy worrying about something you likely can't change.

Teeth and Gums

When you think about pregnancy, I'll bet that teeth and gums are the last things that come to mind. But, as I mentioned in Chapter 3, your oral health is very much affected by your changing hormonal state. And the condition of your teeth and gums may have a significant impact on the health of your baby. During pregnancy, 60 to 75 percent of all women develop gingivitis or later stages gum (periodontal) disease.

Gum disease is caused by plaque, which is the bacteria that naturally builds up on your teeth when you eat. If you floss and brush your teeth regularly, most of this plaque is removed before it can cause health problems. However, when you don't keep your teeth clean, the bacteria quickly accumulate in the spaces between your teeth and gums. Your body normally treats this type of bacteria as an irritant and reacts by causing your gums to become inflamed and infected. During pregnancy, hormonal activity and changes in your circulatory system exaggerate your body's inflammatory response to plaque, making the situation much worse. As a result, pregnant women develop gingivitis easily.

Studies have shown that women with gingivitis in their second trimester have a four-and-a-half to seven times greater risk of delivering preterm, low-birth-weight babies.[2] While gum disease is not yet clearly identified as a cause of preterm birth, all the signs indicate that it may be a contributing factor.

You take care of the rest of your body during pregnancy; it's just as important to take care of your oral health. Why take a chance on a preterm delivery, when the simple act of brushing and flossing your teeth could protect you and your baby from a serious health risk? You might recall that in Chapter 3 I encouraged you to visit your dentist before you became pregnant. If you haven't had a chance to do so, make an appointment to have your teeth properly cleaned today. Make sure you get treatment immediately for any problems with your teeth or gums.

Heart and Circulatory System

Throughout the second trimester, your heart continues to pump an ever increasing supply of blood. By about 24 weeks, the amount of blood your heart pumps into your system reaches its peak. Your resting heart rate will increase from a normal rate of 70 beats per minute to 80 or 90 beats per minute. You may experience a slight drop in blood pressure during the second trimester, but that usually returns to normal during the third trimester.

Lungs

As the increased blood supply circulates through your body, it can affect the lining of your respiratory tract, making you feel a little congested and short of breath. You may find that your nose is stuffy all the time and your throat feels thick and phlegmy. Your ears may become plugged and even the tone of your voice may change. Don't worry; all these symptoms go away once you've delivered your baby and your blood supply returns to normal.

Digestive System

As I mentioned earlier, your rapidly expanding uterus has started to encroach on the space usually occupied by your stomach. The pressure from the uterus pushes it higher and higher into your abdomen. Pregnancy hormones have also slowed down the action of your intestines. Food stays longer in your stomach to give your body more time to absorb the nutrients and send them on to the fetus. If you didn't encounter any digestive problems in the first trimester, consider yourself lucky. During the second trimester, digestion definitely becomes an issue, and you may start to experience heartburn, constipation, bloating, and gas. In Chapter 9, I'll tell you how good nutrition can help minimize these irritating conditions.

Signs and Symptoms

During the second trimester, you'll notice more signs and symptoms of your pregnancy as your body continues to change.

Appetite

By the time you reach the second trimester, your morning sickness should be gone, or at least easing off, and your appetite returning with a vengeance. When a pregnant woman is hungry, she's *hungry!* During pregnancy, you will periodically find yourself in the grip of overwhelming forces of nature that leave you helpless and unable to resist or ignore the demands of your body (labour contractions being the most obvious).

The need to eat—what you want, when you want—is one of the most powerful of these out-of-your-control forces. My friend Ashley was six months pregnant when she was invited to a formal New Year's Eve dinner at a posh downtown hotel. After she arrived, she discovered to her horror that food would not be served until after an hour-long floorshow.

Frantic with hunger, she marched into the hotel's kitchen and pleaded with the chef for food. Never one to deny a pregnant lady, he made a lovely presentation of soup and salad for her right there and then. Hunger temporarily appeased, Ashley went on to enjoy the floorshow—and to eat the four-course dinner that followed. Believe me, you stand between a pregnant woman and her food at your peril.

Food Cravings

Food cravings have always been part of the folklore surrounding pregnancy. There are more myths and jokes about pregnant women and food cravings than there are about almost any other aspect of pregnancy. To all those men and non-pregnant women who scoff at food cravings as self-indulgent claptrap, let me state, unequivocally, that food cravings are a very real part of the pregnancy process.

Researchers don't really know what causes food cravings, but so many women report having them that we can't deny their existence. Some people believe they're related to hormonal changes; others think they're caused by nutritional deficiencies. The most common cravings are for sweet, salty, or spicy foods. Some women crave a combination of unusual foods, which has given rise to the popular notion of pregnant women demanding pickles and ice cream.

Surprisingly, a lot of women crave foods that you usually couldn't pay them to eat. Much to my despair, my researcher, Anne, has never been a fruit eater. Apples and the occasional bowl of strawberries were the full extent of her fruit repertoire. But during her pregnancy, Anne astonished friends and family by becoming addicted to oranges. She bought bags of them and kept them at her desk, in her car, and by her bed. You could always tell when a pregnant Anne was coming your way—the tangy smell of oranges preceded her by half a block.

Of course, I have a number of clients who have indulged in daily cravings for chocolate bars or potato chips, instead of healthy foods such as fruit. Many months after their pregnancies, these women are still struggling to lose their unwanted pregnancy pounds. So don't use food cravings as an excuse to overeat foods you know aren't good for you. Indulge healthy food cravings as much as you want, but try to keep the chocolate and chips to a minimum. If you find yourself craving a big bowl of ice cream, change your focus by going for a brisk walk or eating something nutritious, such as a peach or pear. If you just can't resist the urge, reach for low-fat frozen yogurt instead of high-fat ice cream. I'll give you more advice on managing food cravings in Chapter 9.

Food Aversions

The flip side of food cravings is food aversions. Some women become so sensitive to certain foods that they can't stand the smell of them. Most food aversions are just an aggravated response to foods that you didn't like anyway. One of my clients always hated the taste and smell of cheese. When she was pregnant, her dislike of cheese became a thousand times worse. Even a Kraft Dinner commercial on TV was enough to make her feel nauseated.

I'm sorry to be the one to tell you, but you can also develop an aversion to foods you adore. Before she became pregnant, a friend of mine was a cereal addict, eating two or three bowls of cereal each day. Sometime during the second trimester, she developed such an aversion to cereal that she couldn't be in the kitchen when the rest of her family was eating breakfast.

Food aversions can make it difficult for women to get healthy foods in their diet. Often I counsel pregnant women who are completely turned off eating fish. Even the thought of fish turns their stomachs. Vegetables and eggs are other common food aversions during pregnancy. You'll find nutrition strategies for managing food aversions in Chapter 9.

Back Pain

Approximately half of all pregnant women experience some type of low-back pain. Part of the problem is caused by the extra weight you're carrying in your uterus. Throughout the second trimester, your growing baby is steadily gaining weight, which changes your centre of gravity. Gradually, you'll find that you start leaning backwards slightly to balance the forward pull of your heavy uterus. This type of posture adjustment helps accommodate the strain on your abdominal muscles, but it can cause problems with your back. Your abdominal muscles are now stretched far beyond their normal capacity, so they can no longer effectively support the spine or help maintain good body posture. The lower back is then forced to handle the bulk of your body weight and your back muscles are recruited to stabilize your spine.

As if this wasn't enough wear and tear on your back, those pregnancy hormones are causing trouble again. During pregnancy, the hormone relaxin circulates through the body in high concentrations. Relaxin does just what its name suggests; it relaxes and loosens the joints in the pelvis, so the baby can pass easily through the birth canal. But it also loosens many other joints in your body, causing inflammation and pain, particularly in your back.

In combination, these two factors can easily lead to chronic back pain that will plague you throughout your pregnancy. Most back pain clears up within a few months of delivery as the hormonal effects of pregnancy recede. But you can expect to encounter a whole new set of stresses and strains on your back as soon as you start lifting and carrying the baby.

In Chapter 10, you'll find exercises and stretches for strengthening your back muscles. In the meantime, here are tips to help prevent back problems:

- Lose the spike heels and high platform shoes; they only accentuate the misalignment of your spine. Buy low-heeled shoes with a good support to reduce the strain on your back.

- Avoid lifting heavy objects. If you have to lift something, don't bend over at the waist to pick up the object. Bend at the knees, keeping your back straight, and use your leg muscles to push your body upright.

- Sit in chairs with good low-back support and put a pillow at your back to help keep your spine straight.

- Don't stand for long periods. When you're sitting or standing, take some of the pressure off your back by resting one foot on a small stool.

- Sleep on a firm mattress.

- When you sleep, lie on your left side to improve the flow of blood and nutrients to the placenta. Doing so will also help your kidneys efficiently eliminate waste products from your body. Tuck a pillow between your legs. As your uterus grows, you can add a second pillow under your abdomen to take the strain off your abdominal muscles. Bedding down with a fortress of pillows takes getting used to, but it will help keep your spine in alignment and prevent additional strain on your back muscles. Anne has always been plagued with back problems, and she found the pillows eased her back so much that she continues to this day to sleep with a leg pillow. Avoid sleeping on your back, as this position puts the full weight of your uterus on the spine, back muscles, intestines, and inferior vena cava (the vein that transports blood from your lower body to the heart).

- If you do experience low-back pain, use a combination of heat and ice to soothe the aching muscles. Massages also can provide short-term pain relief. Anti-inflammatory drugs are not recommended during pregnancy. Don't take any medication without consulting with your doctor.

Abdominal and Leg Pain

All the stretching and pressure from your expanding uterus may result in other mysterious aches and pains. A lot of women report sharp pains in their abdomen or groin area. This is usually caused by the stretching of ligaments and muscles around your uterus. Leg cramps are another common problem at this stage of pregnancy. Sometimes, leg pain is caused by the pressure of the uterus on the nerves in your legs, or it might be caused by fatigue. As you'll read in Chapter 9, a lack of calcium in your diet may trigger leg cramps. Are you getting 1000 milligrams of calcium each day? It might be time to review the calcium information provided in Chapter 2.

Vaginal Discharge

As your pregnancy progresses, you will find that your vagina becomes much more drippy. Vaginal discharges, or leukorrhea, increase during pregnancy because of the increased blood supply to the vaginal area. A normal discharge is white or creamy yellow. If the amount of discharge increases significantly during your second or third trimester, make sure you mention it to your doctor; it could be a sign of preterm labour. If the discharge is greenish in colour, has a strong odour, or if your vaginal area itches and burns, you could be suffering from a vaginal infection. Again, tell your doctor so that the problem can be cleared up safely with medications that won't harm your baby.

Weight Gain

In the second trimester, women with a healthy pre-pregnancy body mass index should expect to gain about 1 pound (0.5 kilogram) per week. Your weight gain may fluctuate slightly; some weeks you'll gain only 1/2 pound (0.2 kilogram) and other weeks you might gain 2 or 3 pounds (0.9 to 1.4 kilograms). It will all even out in the end. As long as your weight gain is steady, there's no cause for concern.

And don't worry when you see the scale start to creep up during your monthly check-ups. Only 20 percent of your total weight gain is stored as body fat, and much of this is used for breastfeeding. Almost half of your weight gain is related to the placenta, your baby, and the amniotic fluid. The rest is caused by your increased blood supply, extra body fluids, additional breast tissue, and expanded uterus.

In the second trimester, your waistline disappears and your clothes start stretching at the seams. It won't be long before you'll feel the urge to add maternity clothes to your wardrobe. If you read the fashion magazines, the current trend is to stay in regular clothes for as long as you're comfortable. My girlfriend Lisa shopped at The Gap for the first half of her pregnancy, buying her pants one size larger than usual.

Many of my friends couldn't wait to put on their first maternity outfit. They really are so much more comfortable than squeezing into too-tight pants and skirts that will no longer button up. When my friend Sandra was pregnant with her first child, I helped her choose outfits at a trendy maternity shop. The maternity clothes I saw that day were a lot more fashionable than most of my wardrobe—I started to get excited about the prospect of my own pregnancy someday. Yet, while they might be fun to wear early on, many women are heartily sick of their maternity clothes by the end of their pregnancy.

Your Changing Emotions

The second trimester marks a turning point in your pregnancy. This is the time when your pregnancy begins to feel "real." Your stomach is getting round and full, and you're starting to really look pregnant. Don't be surprised if strangers come up to you and ask questions about your due date, name choices, and gender preferences—people often want to share in your experience. All this extra attention can be disconcerting, but it goes with the territory.

Sometime during the fourth and fifth months, you'll start to feel slight flutterings and bubblings in your belly. This perception of fetal movement, known as "quickening," is a clear sign that your baby is alive and active in your womb. The first time you feel him move is an exciting, long-awaited moment in your pregnancy and you'll probably want to share every little bump and bubble with those close to you. Unfortunately, because the baby is still so small, others won't be able to feel much at this stage.

As I mentioned earlier, during these next few months, you'll start to feel more like your pre-pregnant self. You'll have more energy and won't be as fatigued, which will help keep you in a positive frame of mind. Mood swings are still a reality, though, and you might find yourself easily irritated or somewhat scatterbrained and forgetful. As your pregnancy becomes more "real," so, too, will some of your worries and concerns. Instead of focusing on the negatives, put your energy to good use by learning more about child care, investigating local prenatal classes, discussing baby names, and shopping for baby furniture. This is generally a happy, optimistic stage of your pregnancy and is a good time to concentrate on preparing for the future of your new family.

Your Developing Baby

Let's take a look at what's happening with your baby in the first four to six months of life.

The Fourth Month

Those little flutters you're feeling in your stomach are signs that your baby is sleeping, kicking, swallowing, and waving his arms and legs. As neck and back muscles get stronger, the fetus starts to stretch out, lifting the head off the chest. By now, your baby's skin is pink and slightly transparent. Eyelids and eyelashes are beginning to appear, and tiny ear buds are developing on the side of the head. Even your baby's face is starting to take on a defined shape now. At this stage, the fetus is 8 to 10 inches (20 to 25 centimetres) long and weighs about 6 ounces (170 grams).

The Fifth Month

The fifth month is a period of rapid growth for your baby. You'll start to feel a definite increase in activity inside your womb, as the tiny fetus rolls from side to side, does somersaults, and sucks his thumb. By now, your baby's heartbeat can be heard with a stethoscope. At your five-month checkup, most doctors will let you listen in and hear that thrilling sound.

A white, cheese-like coating, called vernix, develops at this stage, covering the baby from head to toe. Vernix protects your baby's skin from chapping during his long swim in the amniotic fluid. The miniature gallbladder has started to produce bile for the digestive system. Body hair, including eyebrows and eyelashes, is beginning to grow. By the end of the fifth month, your baby is about 10 to 12 inches (25 to 30 centimetres) long and weighs almost 1 pound (0.5 kilogram).

The Sixth Month

A vital layer of fat is now beginning to develop beneath your baby's skin, and a soft, fine layer of body hair, called lanugo, appears all over the body. A special type of brown fat that keeps your baby warm at birth is also forming. Bones are becoming solid, and finger and toenails are strengthening. Muscles are growing, and your baby is starting to exhibit a startle reflex. The skin is wrinkled and red, and the eyelids are finally starting to open.

Your fetus, almost fully formed now, is recognizable as a human baby. By the time it is 24 weeks old, the fetus is considered viable. If your baby is born at this stage, there is a slight chance that he could survive with highly specialized care. But the lungs are not yet well developed, so babies born in the sixth month are at high risk. As you enter the third trimester, your baby is 11 to 14 inches (28 to 35 centimetres) long and weighs 1.5 to 2 pounds (0.7 to 1 kilogram).

Health Care Needs in the Second Trimester

Routine health care visits continue on a monthly basis throughout the second trimester. At each visit, your doctor will check your:

- Weight
- Blood pressure
- Urine
- Fetal heartbeat
- Uterus size
- Physical symptoms, such as swelling of the hands and feet, vaginal discharge, or problems with your digestive system

Prenatal Screening and Diagnostic Testing

In Chapter 4, I mentioned the possibility of undergoing prenatal diagnostic testing during your pregnancy. A few of these diagnostic tests, particularly ultrasounds, are prescribed so often that they are now considered an integral part of a healthy pregnancy workup. But most prenatal testing is reserved for women who have a significant risk of pregnancy complications or genetic abnormalities.

Approximately 2 to 3 percent of babies are born with a major birth defect.[3] The risk of giving birth to a baby with a genetic abnormality, such as Down syndrome, also increases with age. Women who are most likely to be candidates for prenatal testing include those who:

- Are 35 years of age or older on the due date
- Have a family history of birth defects or genetic abnormalities
- Are known carriers of genetic conditions that can be determined by diagnostic testing
- Were exposed to toxic chemicals, such as chemotherapy or radiation, during pregnancy
- Have abnormal results on routine maternal screening tests[4]

If the baby's father was 45 years of age or older at the time of conception, or a known carrier of certain genetic conditions, this also makes you a candidate for prenatal testing.

While prenatal testing can determine genetic and other potential health problems, these tests pose some degree of risk to your pregnancy. The risk of miscarriage, for example, increases with almost all types of diagnostic testing. Before going ahead with testing, it is important to consider the moral, ethical, and religious implications of the testing process. It's difficult to predict what effect the test results will have; they may change the way you prepare for your baby's birth or they may cause you to consider terminating the pregnancy. These are difficult decisions for anyone to make, and it's important to spend time discussing the "what-ifs" before proceeding with any recommended tests. If necessary, get counselling or professional advice to help you resolve the most challenging issues.

Prenatal tests fall into two categories: screening and diagnostic. Screening tests provide a great deal of information to your doctor and are the first step in evaluating the health of your pregnancy. This type of test is usually performed on women who have no apparent risk factors for birth defects. They are used to determine if there are hidden risk factors that may affect the health of your baby. The two main screening tests are ultrasounds and maternal blood tests. Screening tests can't be used to diagnose a medical condition, but they can determine if you might benefit from a more advanced, diagnostic test.

Prenatal Ultrasound

Almost all women are offered a prenatal ultrasound in their 18th week of pregnancy. An ultrasound is a screening test that helps determine the health and condition of your baby. Ultrasounds use sound waves to create a picture of your baby on a screen. The sound waves pass through your abdomen, reflect off bones and tissue, and are then converted into black-and-white images. These images create a sonogram, a picture that provides valuable information about your pregnancy. Through a prenatal ultrasound, your doctor can:

- Assess the size, structure, and movement of your fetus
- Check for major birth defects and abnormalities
- Confirm your due date and estimate the baby's gestational age
- Determine whether you are having more than one baby
- Establish the location of the placenta and check the amniotic fluid around the fetus
- Assess your uterus and ovaries

If the sonogram shows clear evidence of a penis, your doctor may be able to determine the baby's gender. But it is not a reliable test for gender identification, and the Society of Obstetricians and Gynecologists of Canada doesn't recommend it for this purpose.

Ultrasounds have been used in diagnostic testing for more than 35 years and pose no known risk to your pregnancy. The process is painless and takes less than an hour. Approximately one and a half hours before the procedure, you will be asked to drink a large quantity of water. You may feel a strong urge to urinate after drinking all that liquid, but you won't be allowed to empty your bladder, even if you feel uncomfortable. A gel will be put on your stomach to conduct sound waves, and the technician will scan your belly with a hand-held scanner. The sonogram will be reviewed by a specialist, and the results will be reported to your doctor, usually within two weeks.

The ultrasound is an exciting test because you will have an opportunity to see your baby on the screen. This can be a thrilling moment for you as you see the little arms and legs, the tiny head, and round body floating in your womb. Some facilities will let your partner or someone else of your choosing, such as a friend or family member, join you for the ultra-sound and may give you a videotape of the sonogram for your collection of baby mementoes.

Maternal Serum Screen (MSS)

The maternal serum screen (MSS), or single screen test, is usually done at 15 to 16 weeks of pregnancy. It is a blood test that identifies the level of alpha fetoprotein (AFP) in your bloodstream. AFP is a protein produced by the fetus. Normally, a small amount of this protein passes through the placenta to enter your bloodstream. If the AFP level in your bloodstream is higher than normal, it could indicate that the baby has spina bifida. A low level of AFP may mean that the baby has Down syndrome. The single screen test identifies approximately 30 percent of babies with Down syndrome.

Only 2 or 3 out of 100 women with an abnormal MSS will have a child with a birth defect.[5] An incorrectly estimated due date will make your hormone levels appear abnormal, producing a misleading MSS result. This is a common cause of false results.

Double, Triple, and Quadruple Screen Tests

Like the single screen test, these tests require a sample of your blood for analysis. The double screen test will identify approximately 60 percent of all babies with Down syndrome. The testing process involves measuring both the AFP level and the level of hCG hormones in your blood.

The triple test adds one more measurement to the mix and increases the detection rate for Down syndrome to 62 percent. This test looks for the presence of estriol, an estrogen produced by both the placenta and the fetus. Abnormal levels of hCG and estriol may indicate chromosomal abnormalities.

The quadruple test measures diametric inhibin A, a protein produced by the placenta and which is increased in the presence of Down syndrome. When this test is integrated with the triple screen, it significantly improves the detection rate of Down syndrome to 70 percent. In southwestern Ontario, the quadruple screen has replaced the triple screen method for the detection of Down syndrome in the second trimester.

All these screening tests produce the most accurate results when they are performed between the 15th and 20th weeks of pregnancy. Results are available within one to two weeks. All provinces currently cover the cost of the single screen (AFP). The double screen is covered in some provinces, and if not, costs approximately $40. The triple screen is covered in some provinces, and if not, costs approximately $80.

If the results of your screening tests are not within normal ranges or there is a concern about the health of your fetus, you may be sent for advanced diagnostic testing. Diagnostic testing is used to identify chromosomal or genetic abnormalities that may affect your baby. If there is a history of birth defects in your family, or you have previously had a child with an inherited disorder, you can expect to be sent for diagnostic testing at the earliest possible stage of your pregnancy.

Amniocentesis

Amniocentesis is the test used most often to diagnose prenatal chromosome problems. It can detect genetic abnormalities (e.g., Down syndrome), genetic disorders (e.g., cystic fibrosis), and neural tube defects (e.g., spina bifida). At a later stage of pregnancy, amniocentesis can be used to determine if the baby's lungs are developed enough for her to breathe on her own.

During the amniocentesis, a small sample of the amniotic fluid that surrounds the baby is removed from your uterus. Before the sampling process begins, an ultrasound is used to determine the location of the placenta and the baby. A long, thin needle is inserted through your abdomen into the amniotic sac to gather the fluid. The fluid sample contains cells that the baby has shed from her skin and bladder, which are then analyzed in a laboratory. The procedure may seem frightening, but I've heard from many of my clients that, although it can be slightly uncomfortable, it isn't as bad as it sounds. After the amniocentesis you may have slight cramping or spotting, so it's a good idea to go home to rest for a few hours before returning to your usual activities.

According to the Society of Obstetricians and Gynaecologists of Canada, an amniocentesis increases the risk of miscarriage to 1 in 200, or by approximately 0.5 percent. It is usually conducted between the 15th and 16th week of pregnancy. Results are available two to three weeks later.

An amniocentesis can be used to accurately determine the sex of your baby, although that, alone, is not a reason to have it. The test must be conducted in the second trimester; by the time you get the results, you'll be five months along in your pregnancy. You'll have felt the baby kick, heard the tiny heartbeat—the bonding process will be well underway. This makes it even more difficult to deal with any bad news or to consider making the challenging decision of terminating the pregnancy. These are things to consider as you weigh the advantages and disadvantages of proceeding with this test.

Glucose Test

Gestational diabetes is a pregnancy-related condition affecting approximately 3 percent of pregnant women. Gestational diabetes does not always cause obvious symptoms, so it may be difficult to detect. As a result, the Canadian Medical Association recommends that all pregnant women be screened for the condition with a random blood-glucose test. Your doctor will usually suggest that you have it done between the 26th and 28th week of pregnancy, near the end of the second trimester. If you are at greater risk for gestational diabetes, your doctor may have sent you for testing earlier, at 16 weeks.

Approximately 15 percent of women tested have high blood-glucose levels, but only a few will develop gestational diabetes during pregnancy. If your glucose levels are elevated, your doctor will recommend a glucose-load screening test to determine whether you do indeed have gestational diabetes. To prepare for this test, you will drink a sugary solution that contains a specified amount of glucose. Your blood-glucose level is then tested twice: one hour and then two hours after drinking the solution. High sugar readings indicate you have a problem with glucose control.

If you do have gestational diabetes, you will need special diet advice from a registered dietitian, and possibly medication, such as insulin. You'll find more information about gestational diabetes in Chapter 9. Gestational diabetes usually disappears quickly after pregnancy. However, about half of all women who develop gestational diabetes will develop type 2 diabetes later in life.

6

―∞∞∞―

The Third Trimester:
Weeks 28 to Birth

This trimester is filled with both excitement and trepidation. Your baby will be arriving soon and impending parenthood is but a few weeks away. Baby names, nursery furniture, prenatal classes, and maternity leave are only a few of the details that will dominate your thinking during these next few months. As your due date inches closer, anticipation builds. But so, too, do the fears, worries, and insecurities. How will you handle labour pains? Will you be a good mother? Will you know how to care for this long-awaited child? It's only natural to have thoughts like these swirling around in your mind. Whether this is your first child or your fourth, there is always some upheaval in your life when a new baby arrives.

Your Changing Body

The final months of pregnancy are often the most uncomfortable, too. All your internal organs have been shifted out of place, causing more than a few aches and pains. Some people speculate that the many discomforts of the final trimester are nature's way of conditioning you for labour and delivery. The theory goes that, by the ninth month, you're so thoroughly tired of being pregnant that you'll endure anything to get the baby out! Scared, worried, excited—no matter how you're feeling in these last few weeks, the countdown has started and your new life is about to begin.

Uterus

In Chapter 4, I told you that a uterus is normally about the size of a pear. Well, by the end of the third trimester, your uterus has been transformed from a pear to a watermelon. It now weighs almost 2.5 pounds (1 kilogram) and has expanded to accommodate a full-term baby, nearly 4 cups (1 litre) of amniotic fluid, and a bulky placenta. No mean feat for such a tiny organ.

The uterus is now pushing on your diaphragm and lungs, making the simple act of breathing a real chore. All that extra pressure, plus the chronic congestion of your over-stimulated respiratory tract, may make you feel as if you're slowly suffocating. Don't worry, just breathe deeply and relax. Everything will return to normal in a few weeks.

Breasts

Each of your breasts contains 15 to 20 groups of milk-secreting glands, which are connected to the nipple by milk ducts. Two major pregnancy hormones, estrogen and progesterone, stimulate these glands to produce a thin, milky fluid, called colostrum. Your breasts produce colostrum in the last weeks of pregnancy and in the first few days after birth. Colostrum is high in minerals and proteins and contains maternal antibodies that protect your baby from infection. As you approach the end of your pregnancy, your breasts are intensively preparing for milk production, and you may find that they leak some of this precious fluid every now and then.

Your breasts are also very heavy and full at this stage, so a maternity bra is essential. Maternity bras offer the support you need to avoid stretching the ligaments underlying your breasts. They also have wider straps and bands for greater comfort. Maternity bras ease back and shoulder strain so much that you might consider wearing one to bed.

Heart and Circulatory System

Fluid buildup in your body can cause mild swelling, or edema, in the last months of pregnancy. Most pregnant women complain of swollen ankles and feet, but swelling can also develop in your face, hands, and wrists. One of my clients had such swollen feet and ankles that she couldn't wear shoes for the last two weeks of her pregnancy. She accessorized her maternity outfits with a lovely pair of her husband's sheepskin slippers. If you're suffering from swollen feet and ankles, your heavy uterus is usually the culprit. All the extra weight you're carrying in your abdomen compresses your veins and reduces circulation to your legs. You may also develop varicose veins in your legs (I discuss these in detail in Chapter 9).

You can ease the pressure on your circulatory system by putting your feet up whenever you sit or lie down. Add to your pillow fortress by putting a pillow under your legs when you sleep. If you keep your legs elevated as much as possible when you sleep, you'll probably find that most swelling disappears overnight. If swelling does not disappear with rest or seems to develop suddenly, it may be a sign of pre-eclampsia. Pre-eclampsia is a life-threatening condition that affects your blood pressure and is characterized by rapid swelling of the hands, feet, and face. You'll read more about it in Chapter 9.

Lungs

Shortness of breath is a real problem for women in the third trimester. At this stage, any amount of exertion can leave you huffing and puffing. The baby is crowding your lungs and the effort of lugging around 20 to 30 pounds (9 to 13.5 kilograms) of baby weight puts a lot of strain on your overburdened respiratory tract.

The good news is that a few weeks or days before delivery, the baby will push away from your lungs and drop deep into your pelvis. This is called engagement or lightening, and means that the baby is assuming the proper position for birth. Once the baby has dropped, you can be confident that the end of your pregnancy is drawing near. You'll also welcome the feeling of being able to breathe more easily again; as the baby engages, more space opens up between the uterus and the lungs.

The bad news is that the baby's head puts tremendous pressure on your bladder. Expect to spend a lot of time running—or rather, waddling—to the bathroom. As the baby's head moves deeper into your pelvis, you may find that walking becomes increasingly awkward or uncomfortable. A number of my friends have said that it feels as if they're walking with a football between their legs.

Digestive System

Constipation and hemorrhoids plague many women in the third trimester. Regularity is a thing of the past, as bowel movements become increasingly unpredictable. It takes a lot more effort to have a bowel movement, too—hence the high incidence of hemorrhoids in the final stages of pregnancy. A client once confided that she thought all the extra pushing and straining during a bowel movement strengthened her muscles for pushing the baby out during delivery! There are some things, though, that you can do to keep the risk of constipation and hemorrhoids to a minimum. I'll tell you more in Chapter 9.

By now, your rapidly growing baby has steamrollered your stomach to the size of a pancake, so you'll find it hard to eat more than a small amount of food at each meal. You won't starve over the next few weeks, but you may find that eating several small meals during the day, instead of three larger meals, makes you feel more comfortable.

Signs and Symptoms

The third trimester brings with it certain signs and symptoms as you near the end of your pregnancy.

Braxton-Hicks Contractions

Braxton-Hicks contractions often cause women to mistakenly think they are in labour. These mini-contractions, usually painless, are common in pregnancy. They typically start around the middle of pregnancy, though sometimes earlier. Braxton-Hicks contractions are caused by a tightening of the muscles in the uterus and are a normal part of pregnancy. They are usually irregular, weak, and relatively painless—women tell me that these contractions feel more like menstrual cramps than labour pains.

Sometimes, Braxton-Hicks can masquerade as true labour, causing painful contractions that can last about 30 seconds. This is referred to as false labour. Many women have made hair-raising trips to the hospital, only to discover that they were driven out of bed in the middle of the night by nothing more than extra-strong Braxton-Hicks.

If you aren't sure whether you're in labour, rest for a while and see if the contractions settle down. False labour will often subside or stop altogether if you rest or change position. True labour normally continues and progresses, no matter what you do. When in doubt, call your doctor. It's far better to go to your doctor in false labour than to ignore or overlook the risk that you might be going into preterm labour.

Fetal Activity

You may feel as if you're going 10 rounds with a world-class boxer in the final stages of your pregnancy. As your baby gets more and more cramped for space, you'll feel him kick strongly, stretch, and roll around as he exercises his tiny limbs. You may even be able to see the bump of a small hand or foot, as the baby pummels away at your insides.

Fatigue

Along with discomfort, fatigue has returned in the third trimester. It's hard to find a comfortable position in bed, and lying down can trigger heartburn. Even though you're feeling exhausted, you'll find sleeping a challenge. Doctors recommend that you sleep or lie on your left side during the last months of pregnancy, as it takes pressure off the large vein that carries blood from your legs and feet to your heart. It will also relieve the pressure on your lower back. Use your newly acquired pillow collection to prop up everything that needs support, from your head to your abdomen to your feet. Rest when you can, even if it means taking catnaps during the day.

Although you may feel incredible fatigue during your final trimester, don't be surprised if you get a sudden burst of energy in the last few days or weeks before you go into labour. As your body readies for the marathon of birth, your adrenalin levels pick up and you may feel unusually energetic. Some women find that this unexpected energy surge inspires a powerful nesting instinct.

It's not unusual to hear of women spending their ninth month cleaning their houses from top to bottom, completely redecorating the baby's room, and tackling other monumental tasks. On the day my researcher, Anne, went into labour, her husband snapped a great photograph of her with her torso stuck under the sink, scouring away the last specks of dirt hiding away there. When you think of the logistics of a heavily pregnant woman squeezing under a kitchen sink, you'll know how powerful her cleaning urge was that day. So, if you get that burst of energy, be grateful, but try not to wear yourself out with household chores. You'll need to conserve your strength for the bigger effort that lies ahead.

Leaking and Discharge

Leaking and dripping is a fact of life in pregnancy, and the situation only gets worse toward the end. Your leukorrhea, or vaginal discharge, will become heavier and may be tinged with brown or pink streaks of blood after intercourse or a pelvic exam. The pressure of your uterus on your internal organs is probably playing havoc with your bladder control, too. A laugh, cough, or sneeze can easily start you peeing. To avoid this embarrassing problem, make a point of going to the bathroom often. An overly full bladder is a major cause of bladder leakage. Wear pantyliners to keep you dry, and practise Kegel exercises (discussed in Chapter 10) to strengthen the muscles that control urination.

Aches and Pains

In the third trimester everything aches. Your back, your hips, your hands, even your vagina, hurts. In Chapter 5, I discussed back pain and told you how to protect your back from unnecessary stresses and strains. During the last weeks of pregnancy, many women suffer from sciatica, a painful and debilitating type of back pain. The sciatic nerve runs from the lower back down through the buttocks and legs, all the way to the feet. The heavy weight of the uterus can press on this nerve, causing numbness, tingling, or pain anywhere along the nerve pathway.

Anyone who has suffered from sciatica can tell you horror stories. One very pregnant client of mine told me she was walking down a corridor, talking to her boss, when the baby shifted just enough to press on her sciatic nerve. The pain was so intense that she couldn't move. As her boss looked on in astonishment, this normally cool and composed professional abruptly stopped walking and started pushing frantically at the side of her belly.

She was trying to shift the baby off her tortured nerve but, for a moment, her boss thought she'd completely taken leave of her senses. Although my client and her boss were able to laugh about the incident afterward, the excruciating pain of sciatica is nothing to joke about. Fortunately, sciatica tends to ease up after the baby drops into the pelvis and usually clears up completely after delivery.

Hip pain develops during late pregnancy because hormones are loosening the ligaments and joints. Your bones seem to wobble in their sockets, and you'll feel clumsy and awkward as you try to do even the simplest tasks. Your ribs are also expanding to make more room for the rapidly growing fetus, so you may feel pain or crampiness in your chest area. Warm baths and heating pads may make you feel more comfortable and soothe the aching. Try gentle stretches to relieve rib pain. Pelvic tilts may help ease the pain in your hips. Chapter 10 describes lots of easy stretches.

Surprisingly, as many as 25 percent of all pregnant women suffer from carpal tunnel syndrome during pregnancy.[1] Pregnancy hormones, swelling, weight gain, and heavy breast tissue can put pressure on the median nerve that travels down the arm into the hand. As the nerve passes through the narrow opening or tunnel at the wrist, it can be squeezed too tight, causing the fingers to feel painfully numb or tingly. Wearing a wrist splint when you're driving, working on the computer, or sleeping may help relieve the discomfort. Carpal tunnel is another pregnancy-related ailment that usually disappears after the baby is born.

Last but not least, you can expect some vaginal pain in the third trimester. Many women complain about sharp stabbing pains in their vagina during late pregnancy. This is usually associated with the important changes that are now taking place in your cervix. Sometime after the 36th week, your cervix will start to efface, becoming thinner and shorter. It will also begin to gradually open, or dilate, in preparation for birth.

The process of effacement (thinning) and dilation (opening) proceeds quite slowly during this stage of pregnancy. However, once you go into labour, the cervix effaces and dilates rapidly. During labour, powerful uterine contractions force the cervix to dilate from a fraction of an inch to 4 inches (1 centimetre to 10 centimetres) in a matter of hours. While some vaginal pain is normal during the last trimester, report any severe abdominal pain to your doctor immediately.

Weight Gain

In the second trimester, your expanding tissues—the placenta, your body fat, your breasts—caused most of your weight gain. But now, during the last few months of pregnancy, it's your growing baby that accounts for most of your weight gain. During the third trimester, the baby will double in size. The fact that your breasts are gearing up for nursing is also behind some of your third trimester weight gain.

Just as in the second trimester, women who had a healthy pre-pregnancy weight can expect to gain about 1 pound (0.5 kilogram) each week. If you were overweight before pregnancy, aim for 1/2 pound (0.25 kilogram) per week. Conversely, if you were underweight and had a body mass index below 20, aim for a weekly weight gain of 1.5 pounds (0.7 kilogram).

Healthy weight gain is critical during the third trimester. Evidence suggests that maternal weight during the third trimester is the most important indicator of the baby's birth weight. No matter how heavy you feel, now is *not* the time to cut back on your calories to limit weight gain. But remember, healthy weight gain does not give you the license to gorge on all your favourite foods.

Your Changing Emotions

As the end of your pregnancy approaches, you're bound to feel a bit apprehensive about becoming a mother and taking responsibility for the new life you're bringing into the world. It's only natural for lurking fears about labour and delivery to start surfacing at this point, as well. Prenatal classes are informative, but, no matter how many rehearsals you have, they're not the same as actually giving birth. As the big day draws ever closer, you may feel increasingly anxious and nervous about what lies ahead. To add to your unsettled state of mind, you may find yourself struggling with unfounded worries about your baby's health and well-being.

At this stage, your self-image depends a great deal on the attitude you bring to your pregnancy. Some women love being pregnant and regret that this special time is drawing to a close. As their bulk grows, these women delight in the extra attention and pampering that comes their way during pregnancy. Others feel unattractive and unwieldy and often over-react to the slightest hint of rejection.

This is a good time for you and your partner to concentrate on nurturing your relationship. Even if you don't feel sexy right now, make an effort to keep the romance going. Find time for kissing and cuddling, and for paying attention to the little things that make you both feel special. Take advantage of this time to plan for the months ahead and discuss ways to share the workload when the baby comes. This will help alleviate your anxiety and may make you feel less overwhelmed by the prospect of your impending motherhood.

Your Developing Baby

Let's take a look at what's happening with your baby in the third trimester.

The Seventh Month

If you enjoy the thought of singing or playing music for your unborn baby, this is the time to start. By the seventh month, your baby can hear sounds from outside the womb and is starting to open and close her eyes. She can even sense changes in light, as the world moves from day to night. The lanugo, or fine hair, is starting to disappear from your baby's face and the brain is developing rapidly. The nervous system is now capable of controlling many body functions, and the respiratory system has matured to the point where some function is possible. A baby born at this stage is not in as much danger as one born at six months, but the possibility of complications and death is still quite high. Your baby is now about 15 inches (38 centimetres) long and weighs between 2.5 and 3 pounds (1.1 and 1.4 kilograms).

The Eighth Month

During the last two months of pregnancy, your baby will add a great deal of body fat, gaining approximately 1 ounce (28 grams) per day. Her bones are getting stronger and the brain is still developing at a rapid pace. The brain is forming the different regions needed to control physical and mental activity, and the nervous system is almost fully functional. Your baby can now respond to light, sound, and pain. Even the tiny taste buds are ready to distinguish between sweet and sour.

Space is at a premium, as the fetus's arms and legs crowd all the available room in the uterus. Movement is becoming restricted, although the baby still kicks and stretches often and can frequently be felt rolling from side to side. Your baby has grown to 18 inches (45 centimetres) in length and may weigh as much as 5 pounds (2.3 kilograms) by the end of this month. A baby born at this stage is still considered preterm but has an excellent chance of survival.

The Ninth Month

At 38 weeks, your baby is considered full term. As you enter your ninth month, the baby is still laying down fat in preparation for birth, making the skin appear smooth and healthy. The arms and legs look round and full, and small breast buds appear on both sexes. As the hair on the head becomes thicker and coarser, the fine hair on the body rapidly disappears. Although most of the bones are quite strong by now, the bones of the baby's head remain soft and pliable to allow for easy passage through the birth canal. Antibodies are also flowing rapidly from your bloodstream through the placenta, giving your baby a final dose of immune protection against disease.

At this point, all the space in your uterus is completely filled, and the baby has little room to move. As the final weeks approach, the baby naturally moves into the birth position. For a normal birth, the baby will be lying head down in your pelvis, with her body curled into a tiny ball, legs tucked up to the chest. This is known as the fetal position.

The baby's lungs are fully mature, so there is little risk of complications if she is born a week or two early. Most babies are born between the 37th and the 42nd week. As the due date approaches, your baby should be about 20 inches (50 centimetres) long and will weigh between 6 and 8 pounds (2.7 and 3.6 kilograms).

Health Care in the Third Trimester

As you enter the third trimester, prenatal checkups follow the same routine as in earlier months. Your doctor will check your weight gain, the height of your uterus, and your blood pressure, as well as monitor the fetal heartbeat. If you have swelling, varicose veins, digestive problems, or other symptoms, be sure to raise them during these prenatal checkups.

If you haven't already discussed labour and delivery with your doctor, the third trimester is a good time to review your options. Find out what your doctor wants you to do when you think you are going into labour. Should you call your doctor or go directly to the hospital? Should you go as soon as you start to feel contractions, or should you wait until contractions reach a specific duration or frequency? Make a point of asking about your doctor's approach to pain management, too. You certainly don't want to be making critical decisions about epidurals and episiotomies when you're in the throes of active labour.

By the 32nd week of pregnancy, your doctor will start monitoring your pregnancy more closely. Prenatal checkups will be every two weeks, rather than once a month. By the 36th week, you can expect to see your doctor on a weekly basis. In addition to the normal routine, your doctor will add new features to your regular checkups. As you approach your due date, the doctor will start to monitor:

- The size of the fetus

- Whether the baby has dropped or engaged

- The baby's position: is she facing to the front or to the back of the birth canal?

- The baby's presentation: is she approaching the birth canal head first, buttocks first, or feet first?

- Whether your cervix has begun to efface (thin) and dilate (open)

- The frequency and duration of your Braxton-Hicks contractions

Prenatal Testing

Most of the prenatal screening and diagnostic testing is carried out during the first and second trimesters. However, pregnancies can run into trouble at any point and may require more in-depth investigation during the last few months. There are three tests you might be asked to consider in your third trimester.

Non-Stress Test

If the baby is not very active or you are past your due date, your doctor may recommend a non-stress test. This test measures the baby's heart rate over a period ranging from 20 minutes to one hour. You will be asked to wear an electronic heart monitor that straps around your belly. The monitor records the baby's heart patterns on a graph and displays them on a computer monitor. Your doctor will be watching the fetal heart patterns to see if they increase or accelerate when the baby moves.

A baby's heart normally beats between 120 and 160 times per minute. The non-stress test will show a positive result if the baby's heart rate can be seen to increase by at least 15 beats per minute, for a 15-second time period during the test. If the baby's heart rate does not accelerate or slows down considerably, it might mean that the baby is sleeping or that you are having a very mild contraction. However, your doctor may request a biophysical profile if the results of the non-stress test are not as reassuring as they should be.

Biophysical Profile (BPP)

A biophysical profile combines information from a non-stress test and an ultrasound to assess your baby's overall health. The ultrasound can last for up to half an hour and is used to monitor the baby's activities in your womb. The test gives a good picture of her physical condition by measuring:

- Breathing movements
- Body movements
- Muscle tone
- Heart patterns
- The amount of amniotic fluid surrounding the baby

The scores on the BPP are combined with the scores on the non-stress test. A high score means your baby is in good condition. A low score may suggest that further testing is necessary or may be an indication that the baby needs medical attention and should be delivered.

Group B Streptococci Test (GBS)

Sometime between the 35th and 37th week of pregnancy, you may be offered a Group B streptococci test. Group B streptococci (GBS) is a common bacteria that can be found in the vagina and rectum. While this bug is harmless to you, it can cause meningitis, pneumonia, or blood poisoning in your baby.

To test for the presence of GBS, your doctor will take a swab of your vagina and rectum. If you test positive for the bacteria, you will be given intravenous antibiotics during labour to prevent transferring the bacteria to your baby. It is ineffective to treat GBS in early pregnancy. Even if you do take antibiotics in the first or second trimester, the bacteria would probably return before the baby was born, so don't complicate your pregnancy by taking unnecessary medications to try to avoid this problem.

7

⟨⟨⟨⟩⟩⟩

Eating Your Way Through
Pregnancy: A Nutrition Plan

N ow for the how to, what to, when to eat guide for your pregnancy. Hopefully, you've had time before your pregnancy to read the opening chapters of this book. If you've done so, and followed my suggestions, then you're already on the right track. My goal was to get you eating healthy before you conceived, so you need to make only minor adjustments to your diet now.

If you didn't pick up this book until after you learned you were pregnant, there's no need to worry. Now is the most important time to improve your diet to meet the needs of your changing body and developing baby. Whether you're in the first, second, or third trimester, it's never too late to fine-tune your eating habits. And a good way to start is by reading the nutrition advice provided in Chapter 2.

You might be wondering why I have not given you a trimester-by-trimester guide to nutrition. With the exception of calories, protein, and recommended weight gain, little else changes throughout the course of pregnancy. As you'll read below, there are only a few small modifications you will need to make as you enter the second and third trimesters. The diet you follow today will pretty much be the same diet you follow in the final weeks of pregnancy (with an extra helping of calories and protein).

In the pages that follow, you will learn how much you need to eat, nutrient by nutrient. I start with the bigger issues: weight gain, calories, protein, and fat, then moving on to the key vitamins and minerals you need to pay attention to during your pregnancy. But there's more to a healthy pregnancy than just making sure your diet includes all the nutrients you need. Food safety is paramount for pregnant women. So I have included a section addressing concerns about food poisoning, drinking water, artificial sweeteners, and herbal remedies.

In this chapter I sometimes refer to information presented earlier in the book. You may find it helpful to review the charts listing the folate and iron content of selected foods, and sources of caffeine. Since nutrients aren't eaten in isolation but, rather, come from a variety of foods, I've translated my nutrition advice for pregnancy into a 14-Day Meal Plan, which can be found in Part Four. If you decide to follow this meal plan day by day, you can be sure you're getting everything you need, from calories and protein to folate and fibre.

Weight Gain During Pregnancy

How much weight you need to gain during your entire pregnancy will depend on how much you weighed before you became pregnant. You may need to turn back to Chapter 1 to calculate your pre-pregnancy body mass index (BMI). If you don't know how much you weighed before you became pregnant, determine your BMI based on your weight as early in your pregnancy as possible. The recommended weight gain guidelines below are associated with the lowest risk for pregnancy and delivery complications.

WEIGHT GAIN GUIDELINES FOR PREGNANCY

Pre-pregnancy BMI less than 20	28 to 40 pounds (12.5 to 18 kilograms)
Pre-pregnancy BMI between 20 and 27	25 to 35 pounds (11.5 to 16 kilograms)
Pre-pregnancy BMI higher than 27	15 to 25 pounds (7 to 11.5 kilograms)

Nutrition for a Healthy Pregnancy: National Guidelines for the Childbearing Years. Health Canada (Ottawa, 1999). Adapted and Reproduced with the permission of the Minister of Public Works and Government Services Canada, 2004.

Gaining too little or too much weight can be harmful to you and your baby. Women who gain the right amount of weight are less likely to have low-birth-weight babies (less than 5.5 pounds or 2500 grams). There are two types of low-birth-weight babies. Preterm, or premature babies, are born before the end of the 37th week of pregnancy. The earlier a baby is born, the less developed his organs will be, and the less he is likely to weigh. Small-for-date babies are born full term but are underweight. These babies are born small in part from a slowing or temporary halting of growth in the womb.

As newborns, low-birth-weight babies are more likely than normal-weight babies to have health problems, including breathing, digestive, and vision problems. Some of these medical problems are mild and resolve themselves with no or few lasting effects. Serious medical problems are more common in very low-birth-weight babies—babies born weighing less than 3 pounds 5 ounces (1500 grams). Complications such as mental retardation and vision or hearing loss can have lasting effects.

Women who are overweight and have a high BMI before pregnancy are more likely to develop gestational diabetes (see Chapter 9) and to give birth to high-birth-weight babies—babies born weighing more than 8.8 pounds (4000 grams). Studies suggest that heavy babies have a higher risk for adult weight problems. Giving birth to a large baby also increases the risk of complications at delivery.

If your pre-pregnancy BMI was too low or too high, it does not necessarily mean your baby will be born under- or overweight. What's important is that you closely monitor your weight gain throughout your pregnancy in order to put on the appropriate number of pounds to match your weight before conceiving. Please keep the following point top-of-mind: *weight reduction during pregnancy is not recommended*. Weight loss during pregnancy can harm your baby. The weight gain guidelines listed above are associated with the healthiest pregnancy outcomes for both you and your baby.

WHERE DOES ALL THE WEIGHT GO?*

Blood	4 pounds (1.8 kilograms)
Breasts	2 pounds (0.9 kilogram)
Womb	2 pounds (0.9 kilogram)
Baby	7.5 pounds (3.4 kilograms)
Placenta	1.5 pounds (0.7 kilogram)
Amniotic fluid	2 pounds (0.9 kilogram)
Body fat	7 pounds (3.2 kilograms)
Water retention	4 pounds (1.8 kilograms)

*Based on a weight gain of 30 pounds (13.6 kilograms)

A Weight Gain Guide for the First Trimester

Few of your total pregnancy pounds are gained during the first trimester. Even though your baby is developing rapidly, he is not growing very large. Most women gain between 2 and 8 pounds (1.0 and 3.5 kilograms) during this time. If you were overweight before pregnancy (a BMI higher than 27), aim for a weight gain at the lower end of the range. Conversely, if you started your pregnancy underweight (a BMI less than 20), try to gain closer to 8 pounds (3.5 kilograms).

As long as your weight gain is within the range, there's no need to worry if you don't hit the lower or upper end of the range. Keep in mind, though, that excess weight gained during the first trimester is not easily lost after the baby is born (an incentive to avoid "eating for two"). I usually advise my clients who were at healthy pre-pregnancy weights to strive for a weight gain of 3 to 5 pounds (1.5 to 2.5 kilograms). By weeks 10 to 12, you might start to feel your waistband become a little snug, but you really shouldn't need to move into maternity wear until you're into the second trimester.

A Weight Gain Guide for the Second and Third Trimesters

After the first trimester, weight gain is usually steady and incremental. And studies indicate that the weight gained during these six months is easily lost after birth. If you were at a healthy weight before you became pregnant, you should gain approximately 3/4 pound (0.4 kilogram) per week. If you were underweight, a weekly weight gain of 1 pound (0.5 kilogram) is appropriate. And if you were overweight prior to pregnancy, putting on 1/2 pound (0.2 kilogram) per week is better for you and your baby.

The average rate of weight gain is usually greater during the second trimester than it is during the third; many women find that their weight gain slows during the third trimester. Some women even lose a few pounds in the final few weeks. This is common. At no point in your pregnancy should you try to limit weight gain.

If you notice a rapid gain of more than 2 pounds (0.9 kilogram) in one week, report it to your doctor right away. It could signal edema—excess fluid retention—and the onset of pre-eclampsia, a potentially serious pregnancy disorder (see Chapter 9).

Calories: Trimesters 2 and 3, Add 300 Calories Per Day

I'm sure you've heard the phrase "I'm eating for two." And in one sense, it is perfectly true. After all, your developing baby depends solely on you for her nourishment. She gets all her calories and nutrients from your body. But eating for two does not mean you can eat all the ice cream you want. Pregnancy does not double your daily calorie requirements. My good friend Sandra once told me, if you think like this and eat for two, once the baby is born, you'll quickly realize how much your baby ate and how much you ate. Eating too much not only will add more fat to your body, it will also increase the chance you'll give birth to a heavy baby.

Calorie Needs for the First Trimester

Since your body's energy expenditure changes only slightly and weight gain is minor during the first trimester, your calorie needs don't change. If you followed the pre-pregnancy eating plan outlined in Chapter 2, you already know how many calories you are taking in each day. If you were in the process of losing weight before you became pregnant, you will now need to boost your intake from the 1600 calories suggested to 1900 calories per day. If you were happily maintaining your weight before pregnancy, stay at the same calorie level. (For most women, this is around 1900 calories per day.) And if you were underweight, trying to gain a little weight by following the 2200-calorie plan, stick with that.

Taking in enough calories during the first trimester is critical for the healthy development of your baby's organs and the placenta, the blood- and nutrient-rich sac that transfers all nutrients from you to your baby. If the placenta isn't properly developed, your baby will have a more difficult time getting nutrients from you later in the pregnancy.

FIRST TRIMESTER MEAL PLAN: 1900 CALORIES

Breakfast:

1 Protein Serving (optional)

Starchy Food Servings: 2

Fruit Serving: 1

Milk Serving: 1

Water: 2 cups (500 ml)

Morning Snack:

Fruit Servings: 1

Milk Servings: 1

Water: 1-2 cups (250-500 ml)

Lunch:

Protein Servings: 3

Starchy Food Servings: 2

Vegetable Servings: 1 or 2

Fat Servings: 2

Water: 2 cups (500 ml)

Afternoon Snack:

Fruit Servings: 1

Milk Servings: 1

Fat Serving: 1

Water: 2 cups (500 ml)

Dinner:

Protein Servings: 4

Starchy Food Servings: 2

Vegetables: 2 to 3

Fat Servings: 2

Water: 2 cups (500 ml)

Every woman's calorie requirements are different, both before and during pregnancy. How many calories you need to eat will depend on your metabolism and your activity level. You might find that you need to eat a little more than 1900 calories each day to achieve your recommended weight gain. Here's a guide to follow:

- Start at the 1900-calorie level. For those of you who were underweight, start at 2200 calories. On page 112, you'll see how much food this means you have to eat each day.

- If your weight gain is slower than 1 pound (0.5 kilogram) every two to four weeks, add one to three 100-calorie snacks to your diet.

- If your weight gain is faster than 1 pound (0.5 kilogram) every two to four weeks, reduce your intake by 100 calories. You may find you need to cut back by 200 calories.

What do 100 calories look like? They're roughly the equivalent of a slice of whole-grain bread, a large banana, or a glass of low-fat milk. Not a bowl of ice cream! Below you'll find a handy list of a variety of nutrient-rich, 100-calorie snack choices.

100-CALORIE SNACK IDEAS*

Dairy and Alternatives

Egg, omega-3, hardboiled, 1

Milk, skim or 1%, 1 cup (250 ml)

Yogurt, 1% milk fat, 1 cup (250 ml)

Soy milk, plain, enriched, 1 cup (250 ml)

Bread and Other Grain Foods

Bodybuilder Cookie, 1 (page 297)

Whole-grain bread, 1 slice

Fruit and Vegetables

Apple, medium, 1

Applesauce, 1 cup (250 ml)

Apricots, 3

Banana, medium, 1

Blueberries, 1 cup (250 ml)

Chunky Pear Applesauce, 1/2 cup (125 ml)
(page 295)

Dates, 5

Figs, dried, 6

Fruit juice, unsweetened, 3/4 to 1 cup
(175 to 250 ml)

Orange, large, 1

Pear, medium, 1

Plums, 3

Prunes, dried, 5

Raisins, 1/4 cup (50 ml)

Strawberries, 1 cup (250 ml)

Veggies, raw, with 2 tbsp (25 ml)
Roasted Red Pepper Dip (page 271)

Legumes

Black beans, cooked, 1/2 cup (125 ml)

Chickpeas, cooked, 1/3 cup (75 ml)

Kidney beans, cooked, 1/2 cup (125 ml)

Lentils, cooked, 1/2 cup (125 ml)

Nuts

Almonds, unsalted, whole, 14

Cashews, unsalted, whole, 11

Peanut butter, 1 tbsp (15 ml)

Peanuts, unsalted, whole, 17

Pecans, halves, 10

*Calorie values range from 90 to 115.

Getting in your daily calories can be challenging if you experience morning sickness. The nausea and vomiting that many women suffer in the first trimester can make food unappealing and put a damper on their appetites. You'll find my recommendations to help you deal with morning sickness in Chapter 9.

Calorie Needs for the Second and Third Trimesters

Once you enter the second trimester, you do need to eat more food. Extra calories are needed to promote the growth of your baby and the placenta, as well the expansion of your own body's tissues. Your uterus, breasts, blood volume, and fat stores are all burning up calories as they expand during pregnancy.

Throughout the second and third trimesters, you need to add 300 calories to your daily intake. In food terms, here's what 300 calories looks like.

300-CALORIE FOOD OPTIONS

Food	Calories	Food	Calories
1 cup (250 ml) skim or 1% milk	90–100	3/4 cup (175 ml) fruit-bottom 1% yogurt	150
1/2 cup (125 ml) cooked brown rice	115	2 ounces (60 g) cooked salmon	115
2 ounces (60 g) lean beef or poultry	100	1/2 cup (125 ml) cooked green vegetables	25
OR		OR	
1 cup (250 ml) plain 1% yogurt	100	1 cup (250 ml) calcium-enriched plain soy milk	75–100
5 asparagus spears	20	8 whole almonds and 6 dried apricot halves	100
3/4 cup (175 ml) cooked lentils	180	1 small veggie burger	100–120
OR			

Your additional calories should come from nutrient-dense foods, not sweets or junk food. The examples listed above will give you the extra calories you need, as well as protein, essential fatty acids, B vitamins, calcium, and zinc, all key pregnancy nutrients that you will read about later in this chapter. Don't waste your calories on processed, refined foods or junk foods that offer little nutrition beyond their calories.

To maximize your nutrient intake, I recommend that you add one milk serving and one or two protein servings to your daily diet (for a guide to serving sizes, see page 303). The remainder of your calories can come from an extra serving of fruit, vegetable, or whole grain. All you really need to do is increase your portion sizes slightly at one of your meals and add a small snack to your daily diet.

If you were following the 1900-calorie plan in the first trimester, it's now time to move to the 2200-calorie level. If you did well on 2200 calories, it's time to increase your food intake to get 2500 calories per day. You can choose to select these 300 calories yourself (wisely, of course), or you can follow the 2200-calorie guide below to ensure you're getting the energy and nutrients you need each day. The purpose of this meal plan is to show you how to spread your calories out over the course of the day. Eating three meals and three snacks will help prevent hunger by keeping your blood-sugar levels stable during the day. And it will ensure you get the important nutrients you need. If you need to boost your daily calorie intake to 2500, add these extra calories as bigger snacks, healthy desserts, or larger portions at meals.

If you don't want the hassle of coming up with your own meal ideas, I encourage you to follow the 14-Day Meal Plan for a Healthy Pregnancy. It's chock full of delicious recipes that take 30 minutes or less to prepare. Each day's worth of meals and snacks add up to meet the calorie recommendations below. And you will be sure that you're getting plenty of iron and folate each day. Follow it day by day, as presented, or use only the recipes that appeal to you.

SECOND AND THIRD TRIMESTER MEAL PLAN: 2200 CALORIES

Breakfast (500 calories):

Protein servings: 1 (optional)

Starch servings: 2

Fruit servings: 2 (choose one citrus fruit to boost iron absorption)

Milk servings: 1

Water: 3 cups (750 ml) throughout the morning

Morning Snack (250 calories):

Fruit servings: 1

Milk servings: 1

Almonds: 10 whole

OR

1/4 cup (50 ml) Spa Trail Mix (page 300) with 1 cup (250 ml) low-fat yogurt

Lunch (500 calories):

Protein servings: 3

Starch servings: 2

Vegetable servings: 1 to 2

Fat servings: 2

Water: 1 cup (250 ml)

Water: 3 cups (750 ml) throughout the afternoon

Afternoon Snack (250 calories):

Herbed White Bean Spread (page 271), Baked Whole Wheat Pita Chips (page 277), and raw veggies

OR

1 Granola Baked Apple (page 294)

Dinner (500 calories):

Protein servings: 4

Starch servings: 2

Vegetable servings: 2 to 3

Fat servings: 2

Water: 1 cup (250 ml)

Bedtime Snack (200 calories):

Grain servings: 1

Milk servings: 1

OR

one of the following snacks:

2 Farmland Flax Cookies (page 298)

1 Bodybuilder Cookie (page 297)

2 Apple Crisp Mini-Muffins (page 297) with 1 cup (250 ml) low-fat milk or calcium-enriched soy milk

Chocolate Banana Pudding (page 294)

Pure and Simple Vanilla Pudding (page 291)

Frozen Orange-Vanilla "Cream" (page 299)

What If You're Gaining Too Much or Too Little Weight?

If you find you're gaining weight too quickly, reduce your daily calorie intake by 100, just as I outlined in Chapter 2. Experiment until you find what works for you. I suggest you start by cutting back on grain portions; this includes bread, pasta, and rice. This way, you'll still get the protein and calcium you need each day. If you find you're gaining weight too slowly, add an extra 100 calories to your daily diet. Use the list above to help you do this.

As your pregnancy continues and your metabolism changes, you may need to continue fine-tuning your intake. As your baby and your stomach grow bigger, you may find your exercise level changes. If you power walk for 45 minutes most days during the first and second trimesters, your changing body will demand that you slow the pace during the third trimester. If, over the course of your pregnancy, you burn fewer and fewer calories through physical activity, you may need to reduce your food portions slightly to prevent gaining too much weight.

Protein: Trimesters 2 and 3, Add 25 Grams Per Day

Foods such as fish, poultry, lean meat, milk, and tofu supply essential amino acids, the building blocks that all cells and tissues need in order to grow. Proteins are constantly being broken down in our bodies. Most of the amino acids are reused, but we must continually replace some of those that are lost. This process is known as protein turnover. Our need to keep this process going begins at our own conception and lasts throughout life. Without dietary protein, growth and all bodily functions would not take place.

Protein-rich foods also supply you with vitamin B6 and zinc, two nutrients that help form your developing baby's tissues. And it's important to meet your daily protein requirements for the healthy development of the placenta; you may recall from Chapter 2 that a low protein intake can compromise the development and functioning of the placenta.

During the first trimester, your protein requirements remain unchanged from your pre-pregnancy diet. It is not until the second and third trimesters that you need more protein, an additional 25 grams each day. That's roughly the amount found in 3 ounces (90 grams) of cooked lean meat, poultry, or fish. Or, if you're a vegetarian, it means adding to your daily diet 1 cup (250 ml) of soy milk along with one veggie burger or with 3/4 cup (175 ml) of cooked lentils.

You know now that you must get an additional 300 calories each day during the second and third trimesters. The extra food you eat to achieve this should provide protein, too. Let's take another look at those 300-calorie food options, this time adding in the protein factor.

300-CALORIE AND 25-GRAM PROTEIN FOOD OPTIONS

Food	Calories	Protein (Grams)
1 cup (250 ml) skim milk	90	8
1/2 cup (125 ml) cooked brown rice	115	2.5
2 ounces (60 g) lean beef or poultry	100	14
Total:	*305*	*24.5*
1 cup (250 ml) plain 1% yogurt	100	9
5 asparagus spears	20	2
3/4 cup (175 ml) cooked lentils	180	15
Total:	*300*	*26*
3/4 cup (175 ml) fruit-bottom 1% yogurt	150	9
2 ounces (60 g) cooked salmon	115	14
1/2 cup (125 ml) cooked green vegetables	25	2
Total:	*290*	*25*
1 cup (250 ml) calcium-enriched plain soy milk	75–100	9
8 whole almonds and 6 dried apricot halves	100	3
1 veggie burger (soy protein–based)	100	12
Total:	*275–300*	*24*

As you can see from the list above, your best food choices for calories and protein are lean meat, poultry, fish, legumes, soy foods, dairy products, soy milk, and nuts. Fruit contains almost no protein. Grain foods such as rice, cereal, pasta, and bread offer a little—about 2 grams per serving.

Essential Fatty Acids: Daily

It is important to include sufficient amounts of two essential fatty acids (EFAs), linoleic acid and alpha-linolenic acid, in your daily diet. These fatty acids are considered essential because your body cannot manufacture them, so they must be obtained from the foods you eat. In this way, EFAs are similar to vitamins, which we cannot manufacture in our bodies but must get from external sources. The difference is that we need EFAs in much larger quantities than we do vitamins.

Alpha-linolenic acid belongs to the omega-3 family of fats. It is found in certain vegetable oils (hemp, flax, canola, and walnut), soybeans, tofu, and omega-3 eggs. Linoleic acid is a member of the omega-6 family. It's found in nuts and seeds and certain vegetable oils, including canola, safflower, soybean, and corn. Meat also contains some linoleic acid.

Think of linoleic acid and alpha-linolenic acid as the parents of the omega-6 and omega-3 families, respectively. Each "parent" can be used to create other members of its family. For instance, when you consume alpha-linolenic acid, it can be used to make EPA and DHA, two important members of the omega-3 fat family. Given linoleic acid, the body can make other members of the omega-6 family.

Your body uses these omega-3 and omega-6 fatty acids to build cells and eicosanoids, hormone-like substances that regulate our blood pressure, blood cholesterol, and immune function. But these fatty acids are also crucial for proper brain and nerve function. As such, they are essential for proper brain growth and development in growing babies and children. In fact, deficiencies have been linked to impaired learning abilities and poor memory in children. You may recall from Chapter 2 how the omega-3 fatty acid DHA, found in oily fish, is so important for your baby's brain development, especially during the third trimester.

In 2002, the Institute of Medicine at the National Academy of Science released new recommended intakes of fat, including the omega-3 and omega-6 fats. Here's how much omega-3 fat you need every day, and how to get it.

RECOMMENDED INTAKES OF OMEGA-3 AND OMEGA-6 FATS

Type of Fat	Non-Pregnant	Pregnant	Food Sources
Omega-3s	1.1 grams	1.4 grams	Oily fish, omega-3 eggs, canola oil, flax oil, walnut oil, flaxseed, soybeans, tofu, walnuts, wheat germ
Omega-6s	11–12 grams	13 grams	Nuts, seeds, borage oil, corn oil, safflower oil, sesame oil, soybean oil, sunflower oil, meat

National Academy of Sciences, Institute of Medicine, Food and Nutrition Board. *Dietary reference intakes for energy: carbohydrate, fiber, fat, fatty acids, cholesterol, protein, and amino acids (macronutrients).* Washington, DC: National Academy Press, 2002.

Normally, vegetable oils and meat supply enough essential fats to meet the body's needs. However, you may be at risk for not getting enough linoleic acid if you get most of your oil from baked or fried foods made with hydrogenated vegetable oils. Hydrogenated oils, found in commercial baked goods, snack foods, and fried fast food, lack essential fatty acids. And if your cupboards are full of fat-free salad dressings, you might not be getting enough. You need some fat for good health.

Wondering how much fish it takes to get your daily omega-3 fix? Remember, you need 1.4 grams each day during pregnancy. Let's take a look.

OMEGA-3 FAT CONTENT OF FISH AND SEAFOOD (GRAMS)

Per 3-ounce (90-g) serving, cooked

Cod, Atlantic	0.1
Crab, Alaska king	0.4
Pollock, Atlantic	0.4
Salmon, Atlantic, farmed	1.8
Salmon, chinook	1.5
Salmon, chum	0.7
Salmon, coho, wild	0.9
Salmon, pink, canned	1.0
Salmon, sockeye	1.0
Scallops	0.3
Shrimp	0.3
Tuna, white, canned in water	0.7

US Department of Agriculture, Agricultural Research Service, 2001. USDA Nutrient Database for Standard Reference, Release 16. Nutrient Laboratory Home Page, www.nal.usda.gov/fnic/foodcomp.

Follow the tips below to get your essential fats each day:

• Eat oily fish two to three times per week.

• Include 1 to 2 tablespoons (15 to 25 ml) of healthy oil in your daily diet.

• Snack on a handful of nuts and seeds.

• Reach for omega-3 enriched eggs. These eggs are laid by hens fed a diet containing 10 to 20 percent ground flaxseed. One large egg has 0.4 gram of omega-3 fat, 10 times more than a regular egg.

Folic Acid: 600 Micrograms Per Day

By now you know how important this B vitamin is for you both before and during pregnancy. Prior to becoming pregnant, you needed 400 micrograms of folic acid from a multivitamin each day to help prevent neural tube defects. Now that you are pregnant, you need more folic acid to support your expanding blood supply and the growth of your baby, as well as to reduce the risk of birth defects. Your need for folic acid remains high right up until the end of your pregnancy, when it helps prevent preterm birth. That's why a minimum of 600 micrograms of folic acid is recommended throughout your pregnancy.

You might recall that folic acid refers to the synthetic form of the B vitamin, a form that is absorbed well by the body. Multivitamin pills contain folic acid (usually 400 micrograms). Enriched white flour and pasta products also have folic acid added, enough to increase your daily intake of the nutrient by about 100 micrograms. A daily prenatal vitamin supplement typically provides 1 milligram of folic acid. Or you may be taking a separate folic acid supplement to be sure you're getting 600 micrograms of folic acid.

Folate in Foods

Just because you're getting all the folic acid you need in your supplement does not mean you can forget about getting good sources of folate in your diet. Quite the contrary. During pregnancy you need to get folic acid from your daily supplement as well as folate from a healthy diet. Folate-rich foods such as legumes and leafy greens also provide you with iron and calcium, notable nutrients for a healthy pregnancy.

When it comes to boosting your intake of folate during pregnancy, my recommendation remains the same as it was before you became pregnant: aim to include at least two folate-rich foods in your daily diet. Here's a list to remind you of the top folate foods (you'll find a more detailed list in Chapter 2). One serving, providing 55 micrograms or more, equals 1/2 cup (125 ml) cooked vegetable, 1 cup (250 ml) raw vegetable, 3/4 cup (175 ml) fruit juice, 1/2 cup (125 ml) cooked legumes, or 1/4 cup (50 ml) nuts or seeds.

Vegetable

Asparagus
Collard greens
Romaine lettuce
Spinach, cooked
Turnip greens

Fruit

Avocado, 1/2
Orange juice
Pineapple juice, canned

Legumes, Nuts, and Seeds

Black beans
Chickpeas
Kidney beans
Lentils
Navy beans
Peanuts
Pinto beans
Soybeans
Soy nuts
Sunflower seeds

Iron: 27 Milligrams Per Day

This noteworthy nutrient makes red blood cells, supplies oxygen to cells for energy and growth, and builds bones and teeth. This mineral is so crucial in pregnancy because your body must produce extra blood to support your growing baby. During pregnancy, iron requirements increase from 18 to 27 milligrams per day. If you're a vegetarian, your iron requirements are higher, since iron from plant foods is poorly absorbed by the body. Your iron daily requirements increase from 32 milligrams before pregnancy to 48 milligrams while pregnant.

If your iron stores were normal before you became pregnant, a healthy diet containing plenty of iron-rich foods is sufficient to meet your increased needs. However, because so many women have inadequate iron stores before pregnancy, a low-dose iron supplement of 30 milligrams is routinely recommended for the second and third trimesters.

Your iron requirements don't actually increase until the 12th week of pregnancy. Despite this, it is important to focus on boosting your iron intake throughout the first trimester. You need to build up your stores so you'll be ready for the months ahead. If you're taking a prenatal supplement (see below), you're getting between 30 and 60 milligrams of elemental iron, depending on the brand. If you can't tolerate a prenatal supplement during the first trimester, make sure you add iron-rich foods to your daily diet. Once your digestive system settles toward the end of the first trimester, add a prenatal supplement to your daily nutrition routine.

Iron deficiency, with or without anemia, is common during pregnancy (see Chapter 9), and it's important to prevent your stores from becoming too low. Iron deficiency anemia is linked to poor fetal weight gain, preterm delivery, and low birth weight.[1] Anemia can affect how you feel, too. You'll feel more fatigued and not be able to perform at your peak. Iron deficiency anemia also decreases your body's resistance to infection.

If your doctor detects an iron deficiency at any time during your pregnancy, he or she may prescribe larger doses of iron to improve your iron status. In Chapter 2, you'll find a list of iron-rich foods, advice on how to enhance your body's absorption of this mineral, and information on iron supplementation.

Vitamins and Minerals

Besides folate and iron, your body requires additional amounts of other vitamins and minerals to support a healthy pregnancy. Many of these nutrients work together to build a healthy baby. You've already heard that protein, with the help of vitamin B6 and zinc, is needed to make your baby's developing tissues. And while calcium is necessary to maintain your bone strength and build your baby's skeleton, it's vitamin D that helps your body use the mineral more efficiently.

Here are the key nutrient players during pregnancy, how much you need, and how to get them in your diet.[2] (Your prenatal vitamin supplement will also include some of these nutrients.) The RDAs below represent the recommended daily intake for healthy women, pregnant and non-pregnant, aged 19 to 50 years.

VITAMIN AND MINERAL RECOMMENDED DIETARY ALLOWANCES (RDAS) DURING PREGNANCY

Nutrient	Non-Pregnant	Pregnant	Daily Upper Limit[a]	Best Food Sources
Vitamin A	2330 IU	2566 IU	10,000 IU	Butter, cheese, egg yolk, milk; dark green and orange vegetables (which contain beta-carotene, converted to vitamin A in the body)
Vitamin B6	1.3 mg	1.9 mg	100 mg	Lean meat, poultry, fish, whole grains, avocado, banana, potato
Vitamin B12	2.4 mcg	2.6 mcg	None established	Meat, poultry, fish, dairy products, egg, enriched soy or rice beverage
Folate	500 mcg	600 mcg	1000 mcg (1 mg)[b]	Kidney beans, lentils, peanuts, artichoke, asparagus, avocado, spinach
Vitamin C	75 mg	85 mg	2000 mg	Cantaloupe, citrus fruit, kiwifruit, mango, strawberries, broccoli, Brussels sprouts, cauliflower, red pepper, tomato juice
Vitamin D	200 IU	200 IU	2000 IU	Milk, fortified soy and rice beverages, oily fish, whole eggs
Calcium	1000 mg	1000 mg	2500 mg	Cheese, milk, yogurt, calcium-enriched soy milk, calcium-enriched orange juice, tofu, almonds, bok choy, broccoli
Iron	18 mg	27 mg	45 mg[c]	Lean beef, baked beans, ready-to-eat breakfast cereals, Cream of Wheat, wheat germ, molasses, dried apricots, raisins, prune juice, spinach
Magnesium	320 mg	350–360 mg	350 mg[d]	Black beans, navy beans, lentils, wheat bran, wheat germ, nuts, seeds, tofu, dates, figs, leafy greens
Zinc	8 mg	11 mg	40 mg	Lean beef, poultry, pork, seafood, oysters, yogurt, wheat germ, baked beans, chickpeas, pumpkin seeds

a. The upper limit refers to the maximum daily intake of nutrient that is likely to pose no risk of adverse effects. Unless otherwise stated, the upper limit refers to total intake from food, water, and supplements.

b. The upper limit refers to folic acid from supplements and fortified foods.

c. Many prenatal supplements contain 60 milligrams of iron, more than the daily upper limit. For many pregnant women, this amount of iron does not cause stomach upset and is well tolerated. As such, it is safe and appropriate to take 60 milligrams of iron during pregnancy to treat or prevent an iron deficiency.

d. The upper limit refers to magnesium from supplements. Too much supplemental magnesium can cause diarrhea.

National Academy of Sciences, Institute of Medicine, Food and Nutrition Board, Committee on Nutritional Status During Pregnancy and Lactation, Subcommittee on Dietary Intake and Nutrient Supplements During Pregnancy, Subcommittee on Nutritional Status and Weight Gain During Pregnancy. *Nutrition during pregnancy*. (Part I—Weight gain. Part II—Nutrient supplements.) Washington, DC: National Academy Press, 1990.

Prenatal Supplements

Now that you're pregnant, you might be wondering whether to switch from a regular multivitamin and mineral supplement to a prenatal (pregnancy) formula. Perhaps you made the switch when you were trying to conceive. If you have not done so, I recommend that you start taking a prenatal vitamin supplement now.

This is especially important for pregnant women who are vegetarians. A diet that lacks animal food can be low in vitamin B12, vitamin D, calcium, iron, and zinc. A prenatal multivitamin can help vegetarian moms-to-be get a nutrient boost. However, when it comes to meeting calcium requirements, be sure to include three servings of calcium-fortified soy or rice beverage in your daily diet. (These beverages are also fortified with vitamins A, D, and B12, riboflavin, and zinc.) Not all soy and rice beverages are fortified, so be sure to check the label.

Most prenatal multivitamin and mineral supplements have 1000 micrograms (1 milligram) of folic acid, enough to cover your increased needs throughout your pregnancy. There's no need to take more folic acid, unless you have had a previous pregnancy affected by a neural tube defect. (In this case, your doctor may prescribe a higher dose of folic acid.) Taking more than 1 milligram of folic acid each day can hide an underlying vitamin B12 deficiency. Some evidence also suggests that high doses of folic acid can cause a B12 deficiency to progress, leading to nerve damage. As is the case with many things, more is not better. That's why the safe upper daily limit for synthetic folic acid is 1000 micrograms (1 milligram).

There are other important reasons to switch to a prenatal formula. First, you'll get more iron from these products than from regular multivitamins. As you've already read, iron requirements increase when you're pregnant, and getting extra iron in a supplement is an important strategy to prevent iron deficiency anemia. Second, prenatal supplements offer enough, but not too much, vitamin A, a key nutrient for cell growth, healthy skin, and mucous membranes, and for resistance to infections.

Here's a look at the popular prenatal formulas and how much of each key nutrient they contain.

NUTRIENTS FOUND IN POPULAR PRENATAL FORMULAS

Nutrient	Materna	Orifer-F	Rexall Prenatal	Jamieson Prenatal
Beta-carotene	1500 IU	None	1500 IU	1800 IU
Vitamin A	1500 IU	1600 IU	1500 IU	1000 IU
Vitamin B6	10 mg	9 mg	10 mg	10 mg
Vitamin B12	12 mcg	None	12 mcg	10 mcg
Folic Acid	1 mg	0.8 mg	1 mg	1 mg
Vitamin C	100 mg	50 mg	100 mg	150 mg

Nutrient	Materna	Orifer-F	Rexall Prenatal	Jamieson Prenatal
Vitamin D	250 IU	200 IU	250 IU	200 IU
Vitamin E	30 IU	None	30 IU	30 IU
Calcium	250 mg	125 mg	250 mg	200 mg
Iron	60 mg	60 mg	60 mg	30 mg
Zinc	25 mg	20 mg	25 mg	20 mg

Prenatal multivitamins come in regular tablets, chewable tablets, and capsules. They are usually taken once a day. Follow the directions on the prescription or package label carefully, and ask your doctor or pharmacist to explain any part you do not understand. Take prenatal multivitamins exactly as directed. If you forget to take your supplement one day, there's no need to worry. Just resume the next day. Do not take a double dose to make up for a missed one. Do not take more than one per day.

When you're trying to decide which prenatal vitamin is right for you, ask your dietitian, doctor, and pharmacist for their recommendations, and keep the following in mind:

- Prenatal vitamins do not make up for a poor diet. The goal of prenatal vitamins is to supplement your diet, not replace it. In fact, prenatal vitamins work better when you are eating a healthy diet that includes a variety of foods.

- No prenatal vitamin will contain all the calcium you need.

- Too much vitamin A can cause birth defects, so be sure you're using a prenatal vitamin supplement (or regular multivitamin) with no more than 5000 IU vitamin A listed as retinol or retinyl esters.

Many expectant mothers find that taking a prenatal multivitamin increases nausea in early pregnancy and sometimes beyond. It may help to change how and when you take the multivitamin. I always recommend that my clients take their prenatal supplement with a snack before bedtime. Based on my clinical experience, women who take it at this time have little or no stomach upset (they sleep through any queasiness).

If you tried this and still can't keep the prenatal multivitamin down, consider switching brands. Some of my clients have found that switching from Materna to Orifer-F solves the upset stomach problem. If swallowing a large pill is difficult, cut it in half or talk to your health care provider about a smaller tablet or capsule that can be opened and sprinkled on food.

If you've tried different brands, at different times of the day, and you still can't stomach a prenatal multivitamin, try to take a regular multivitamin and mineral supplement. As hard as they may try, few mothers-to-be get a nutritionally balanced diet every day. And during the first trimester, this may become even more challenging when morning sickness suppresses your appetite and fatigue makes you skip eating in exchange for a power nap. Make sure your all-purpose multivitamin gives you 0.4 to 1.0 milligram of folic acid and less than 5000 IU of vitamin A.

If morning sickness plagues you, buy a multivitamin in capsule form. Capsules are the most popular type of multivitamin at my clinic. The lack of taste, smell, and the smaller size make taking these multivitamins easy to swallow.

Toward the end of the first trimester, once your queasiness subsides, try switching to a prenatal formula once again. This is the time when your iron requirements really start to climb.

Avoid Large Doses of Vitamin A

In 1995, a large study was published in the *New England Journal of Medicine* that brought the old adage "Too much of a good thing can be harmful" into the headlines. Prior to the study, it had been known that high doses of vitamin A can cause birth defects. That's why medications containing vitamin A–like compounds are not prescribed for women who might become pregnant (e.g., Accutane for acne). Then along came an American study that suggested the dose at which you're at risk is lower than previously thought.

Researchers from the Boston University School of Medicine analyzed the dietary and supplement habits of almost 23,000 pregnant women. They found that compared with women who consumed less than 5000 IU of vitamin A each day, those getting more than 15,000 IU from food and supplements were three times more likely to deliver babies with birth defects including cleft palate and heart abnormalities. And women who took over 10,000 IU of vitamin A in the form of supplements more than quadrupled the risk of birth defects in their babies.[3]

To put this in perspective, some multivitamins contain 5000 to 10,000 IU of vitamin A. So taking one or two multivitamins each day could be dangerous. The only way you would be at risk for getting too much vitamin A from your diet is if you eat liver. Three ounces (90 grams) of cooked calf's liver packs 30,689 IU of vitamin A. While the study did not determine that liver causes birth defects, it is definitely a food worth avoiding before and during pregnancy.

Since these findings were reported, many vitamin companies have removed or reduced vitamin A in their products and added beta-carotene, which is safe. Beta-carotene is a natural plant chemical found in bright orange and green fruit and vegetables. Once consumed, some beta-carotene is converted to vitamin A in the body. High levels of beta-carotene in the diet, as well as supplements containing beta-carotene, do not pose a risk for birth defects. So if you love carrots, that's great.

Caffeine: None or Less than 150 Milligrams Per Day

The effects of caffeine on pregnancy remain unclear. Researchers have found that high levels of caffeine, equivalent to more than six small cups of coffee per day, are associated with miscarriage.[4] And according to Canadian researchers, even less might be harmful. An analysis of studies conducted from 1966 to 1996 concluded that consuming as little as 150 milligrams of caffeine each day (one to two small cups of coffee) slightly increases the risk of miscarriage and low-birth-weight babies.[5] However, the researchers did note that they were unable to determine whether this finding was related to the woman's age at pregnancy, cigarette smoking, or alcohol use. In yet another study, researchers followed 5144 pregnant women and found no link between drinking three small cups of coffee per day (300 milligrams of caffeine) and miscarriage during the first trimester.[6]

Despite these conflicting findings, I recommend you play it safe. If you enjoyed a large coffee each morning before you became pregnant, it's time to cut back now that you're expecting. Based on the evidence at hand, limit your caffeine intake to a daily maximum of 150 milligrams—about one 8-ounce (250-ml) cup of coffee.

Chapter 2 lists foods and beverages that contain caffeine. Don't forget to consider the size of cup you use when estimating your caffeine intake—that grande-size cup at Starbucks delivers 16 ounces (500 ml) of coffee.

Fluids

Now that you're pregnant, you need to drink an extra cup (250 ml) of fluid each day to help your body keep up with the increases in your blood volume. This fluid should come from non-caffeinated, non-alcoholic beverages such as filtered or bottled water, milk, enriched soy milk, unsweetened fruit and vegetable juices, and certain herbal teas (more on the use of herbs during pregnancy below). Try to drink at least 9 cups (2.2 litres) of fluid each day. When you exercise, keep a water bottle with you so that you can easily replace the fluid you lose through sweating.

Alcohol

I am sure this comes as no surprise: alcohol and pregnancy do not mix. No safe level of alcohol during pregnancy has been established. For this reason, it is prudent to avoid alcohol during your pregnancy. Many women say no to alcohol before they become pregnant, in the months they are trying to conceive.

It is well established that heavy and continuous drinking can cause birth defects by affecting the growth and proper formation of a baby's body and brain. The effect of alcohol-related damage depends on how much is consumed during pregnancy.

Once you drink alcohol, it crosses the placenta quickly and enters your developing baby's bloodstream, in the same concentration as in your bloodstream. But a developing baby has immature organs and cannot detoxify alcohol effectively. As a result, alcohol stays around longer in an unborn baby's body than it does in your body.

Since about half of all pregnancies are unplanned, and many women drink alcohol, you may have enjoyed a few glasses of wine before you knew you were pregnant. Be reassured that having an occasional drink or two, before you realize you are pregnant, poses a very low risk to your baby. What's most important is that you abstain from drinking alcohol as soon as you suspect you are pregnant. An occasional drink during pregnancy is not thought to harm a developing baby.

Watch out for alcohol in foods and medications: liquor-filled desserts and chocolates, rum and fruit cakes, apple cider, fruit punches, cheese fondues, and cough medicines may contain alcohol.

Food Safety During Pregnancy

Foods contaminated with salmonella and E. coli can cause nasty bouts of food poisoning. Although it is always important to prevent food-borne illness, when you are pregnant you must be vigilant with safe food-handling practices. During pregnancy, you are more vulnerable to certain types of food poisoning, which can have serious, even life-threatening, effects on your developing baby.

Listeria Food Poisoning

Listeriosis is caused by *Listeria monocytogenes*, a type of bacteria found everywhere—in soil, ground water, and on plants. The hormonal changes of pregnancy affect a woman's immune system, making her more susceptible to listeriosis. Pregnant women are 20 times more likely to get this type of food poisoning than other healthy adults. Even if a woman is not showing signs of the illness, listeriosis can be transmitted to the fetus through the placenta. Food-borne illness caused by listeria-contaminated food can result in preterm delivery, miscarriage, fetal death, and severe illness of a newborn.

The symptoms of listeriosis can take a few days or a few weeks to appear. They can be so mild that you might not suspect you have the infection. Signs include flu-like symptoms, fever, muscle ache, and sometimes diarrhea and stomach upset. If the infection spreads to the nervous system, symptoms include headache, stiff neck, and confusion. If you think you might be infected, consult your doctor, who can perform a blood test to determine whether you have listeriosis.

The risk of listeriosis is slight. However, to reduce your risk of getting this infection, it is generally recommended that pregnant women avoid:

- Soft cheeses: feta, brie, Camembert, blue-veined cheese such as Roquefort, and Mexican-style cheeses (e.g., queso blanco, queso fresco). Hard cheeses are safe to eat.

- Refrigerated pâté or meat spreads. Canned, or shelf-stable, products can be safely eaten.

- Refrigerated smoked seafood (e.g., salmon, trout, whitefish, cod, tuna, mackerel). Smoked seafood is safe to eat if it is part of a cooked dish, or if it is canned and shelf-stable.

- Hot dogs, packaged luncheon meats, and deli meats, unless reheated until steaming hot

- Foods made with unpasteurized milk

Toxoplasmosis

This infection is caused by a parasite called *Toxoplasma gondii*. It causes no symptoms or only mild flu-like symptoms. In fact, many people carry the parasite but show no signs because their immune systems keep the bug at bay. Because the hormonal changes of pregnancy affect the immune system, pregnant women are at greater risk for getting toxoplasmosis. If you contract this infection when pregnant, there's about a 40 percent chance that you will pass it on to your baby.

Toxoplasmosis can be contracted in the following ways:

- Accidental ingestion of contaminated cat feces (e.g., if you accidentally touch your hands to your mouth after gardening or cleaning a cat's litter box). Because cats are a host for this parasite, pregnant women should avoid contact with cat litter; use rubber gloves or have someone else do the chore.

- Ingestion of raw or partly cooked meat, especially pork, lamb, or venison

- Ingestion of other raw foods, including fruit and vegetables

- Contamination of knives, utensils, and cutting boards that have had contact with undercooked meat

Safe Food Practices

The following food safety tips will help you prevent listeriosis, toxoplasmosis, and other types of food poisoning:

- *Wash your hands* often.

- *Keep raw foods and ready-to-eat foods separate.* Use separate utensils for handling raw foods and cooked foods to prevent cross-contamination.

- *Cook all meat thoroughly.* Cook meat to an internal temperature of 160°F (71°C). Cook poultry to 170°F (77°C) and stuffed poultry to 180°F (82°C). Use a meat thermometer to ensure meat and poultry is cooked to a high enough temperature. The best meat thermometers give a temperature reading rather than just a doneness range. Take the temperature from the thickest part of meat, away from the bone, within 1 minute of removal from heat for thin meats and 5 to 10 minutes for roasts (leave the thermometer in the meat for at least 30 seconds).

- *Refrigerate foods promptly, and keep at below 40°F (4.5°C).* Bacteria flourish between temperatures of 45 and 140°F (7 and 60°C). Avoid keeping foods in this temperature zone, called the danger zone. Keep hot foods hot and cold foods cold.

Lead and Other Heavy Metals

You may recall that I advised you in Chapter 2 to filter tap water to remove potentially harmful chlorine by-products. But there's another reason to filter. Naturally occurring substances such as arsenic, cadmium, iron, manganese, and uranium can leach into water from rock formations. Heavy metals such as copper and lead can also make their way into tap water from pipes and holding tanks in the distribution system or from plumbing in your home. Significant levels of lead have been found in areas with soft or very acidic drinking water supplies and in older (pre-1950) homes with lead distribution lines and newer homes, which have lead or brass plumbing. Pipes in newer homes may leach lead from solder for the first several years until a protective oxide layer has formed on the pipes.

Although the risk of lead poisoning in Canada is extremely low, exposure to lead during pregnancy can increase the risk of miscarriage and stillbirth, decrease your baby's birth weight, and interfere with his brain and nerve development. The main source of lead is water fed through lead pipes or pipes with lead solder. To minimize your exposure to heavy metals in water, practise these strategies:

- Run tap water freely for about two minutes each morning. Lead and copper tend to accumulate in the water pipes overnight; running the water for a few minutes will help flush them out.

- Do not drink water from the hot water tap; it may contain more lead than water that passes through the pipes cold.

- Use a pitcher-type product to filter tap water used for drinking and cooking. The Brita Water Filtration Pitcher is certified to reduce lead, copper, and mercury in tap water.

- Consider switching to bottled spring water or purified water for drinking and cooking. Because bottled water is not distributed through pipes, it does not contain lead or copper.

Other sources of lead include beverages stored or served in lead crystal decanters or glasses, foods consumed from ceramic dishes with improperly applied leaded glaze, and imported foods packaged in cans with lead solder.

Artificial Sweeteners

With a few exceptions, artificial sweeteners are safe to consume in moderate amounts during pregnancy. Artificial sweeteners in diet sodas, yogurts, and other sweet foods include aspartame (NutraSweet), sucralose (Splenda), and acesulfame K (Sunett). These sweeteners have not been shown to cause birth defects and are safe to use during pregnancy.

If you add those little packages of fake sugar to tea or decaffeinated coffee, I advise you to stay clear of saccharin and cyclamate (Sucryl, Sweet N' Low, Sugar Twin, and Weight Watchers). Studies have linked these two artificial sweeteners to bladder cancer in animals. That's why manufacturers are not allowed to add these sweeteners to foods; instead they are sold only as tabletop sweeteners.

Of the two, saccharin is of greater concern. Once consumed, it crosses the placenta into the baby's bloodstream. According to research, a baby is not able to detoxify as quickly as its mother. If you consume large quantities of saccharin each day, the potential exists for it to accumulate in your baby's body, increasing the risk of bladder cancer.

Women with the genetic condition phenylketonuria (PKU) should avoid using all products sweetened with aspartame. This disease prevents women from breaking down phenylalanine, an amino acid found in the diet. Aspartame is made up of two amino acids, phenylalanine and aspartic acid. If a special diet that excludes aspartame is not adhered to, phenylalanine will accumulate in the body and seriously harm a developing baby.

The main concern for healthy pregnant women is that a steady diet of artificially sweetened products will be lacking nutrient-dense foods and beverages. If you use these products, do so in moderation.

Herbal Supplements and Herbal Teas

It's estimated that 35 percent of Canadians use herbal remedies. Although herbs are considered natural, not all herbs are safe to take during pregnancy. As a matter of fact, few herbs are considered safe for pregnant women. (Although no research has been done on whether herbs are safe to take while trying to get pregnant, they are probably safe.) Herbs may be milder than prescription medications, but many contain natural ingredients that can cause miscarriage or preterm birth, harm your developing baby, and even jeopardize your health. Few studies have tested the safety of herbal supplements in pregnancy. If you use herbal products, do so cautiously.

HERBAL SUPPLEMENTS TO AVOID DURING PREGNANCY

Alder buckhorn	Ephedra (Ma huang)	Pleurisy root
Aloe vera	Essential oils	Pokeroot
Angelica	Feverfew	Rhubarb (safe as a food)
Barberry	Ginger root* (safe in cooking)	Rue
Birthroot		Sage (safe in cooking)
Black cohosh	Ginseng	Sarsaparilla
Blessed thistle	Goldenseal	Scotch broom
Bloodroot	Gotu kola	Senna
Blue cohosh	Juniper berries	Shepherd's purse
Cascara sagrada	Kava kava	Southernwood
Coltsfoot	Licorice root	Squill
Comfrey	Mistletoe	St. John's wort
Cotton root	Mugwort	Tansy
Damania	Nutmeg (safe in cooking)	Wild yam
Devil's claw	Osha	Wormwood
Dong quai	Parsley (safe in cooking)	Uva ursi
Echinacea	Pennyroyal	Yarrow

*Ginger may be safe when taken appropriately, for a short period, to treat severe morning sickness. See Chapter 9 for more about ginger and morning sickness.

HERBAL SUPPLEMENTS CONSIDERED SAFE DURING PREGNANCY

Bilberry	Ginkgo biloba	Raspberry leaf
Cranberry	Green tea extract	Valerian root
Evening primrose oil		

American Botanical Council. *Herb Reference Guide*. 2003. www.herbalgram.com/default.asp?c=reference_guide.

Although these supplements are considered safe to use during pregnancy, keep in mind that little research has been conducted on pregnant women. Be sure to inform your doctor if you take an herbal product. Use the following guidelines to ensure you buy a high-quality product:

- Choose a brand manufactured by a company with a strong reputation for producing high-quality products. Ask your dietitian, naturopath, doctor, pharmacist, or health food retailer for a list.

- Consider buying an herbal product manufactured by a company that also produces pharmaceuticals; it will likely have high-quality control standards.

- Unless it is not possible, always buy a standardized extract that clearly states the percentage of active ingredient or marker on the label.

- Check the expiry date; make sure the product will not expire over the period you intend to use it.

- Check to see if the product has an unbroken safety seal.

SAFE HERBAL TEAS

Citrus peel	Linden flower*
Ginger	Orange peel
Lemon balm	Rosehip

*Not recommended if you have a pre-existing heart condition

Because herbal teas often possess drug-like properties, it's wise to brew them weakly and consume no more than two to three mugs per day during your pregnancy. What about chamomile tea? Take it from me, it's difficult to sort through the conflicting reports on the safety of this popular beverage. Some experts, including Health Canada, report that chamomile may have adverse effects on the uterus and, therefore, don't recommend its use during pregnancy. Other sources make no mention of chamomile or say it is okay to use during pregnancy. According to the literature I have read, chamomile appears safe to drink in moderate amounts during pregnancy.

If you have a plant or pollen allergy, be careful not to use teas that can contain herbs related to plants to which you have known allergies. For instance, if you're allergic to plants in the Asteracease-Compositae family (ragweed, daisy, marigold, and chrysanthemum), avoid chamomile and echinacea.

Your Pregnancy Nutrition: A Summary

1. During the first trimester, follow the 1900-calorie meal plan (see page 109). If you gain weight too quickly or too slowly, use the 100-calorie snack list to adjust your diet to achieve a weight gain of about 1 pound (0.5 kilogram) every two to four weeks. When you enter the second trimester, add 300 calories to your daily diet. For the remainder of your pregnancy, follow the 2200-calorie level (see page 112).

2. Add 25 grams of protein to your daily diet throughout the second and third trimesters. Plan your extra 300 calories to provide the extra protein you need. Choose lean meat, poultry, fish, legumes, soy foods, and dairy products. The list of protein-rich foods in Chapter 2 can help you achieve this.

3. To get essential fatty acids, use healthy vegetable oils in cooking, snack on nuts and seeds, and eat oily fish two to three times each week. Refer to Chapter 2 for advice on safe fish to eat.

4. Take a prenatal supplement each day to get 600–1000 micrograms of folic acid and 27 milligrams of iron. Make sure your vitamin supplement does not exceed 5000 IU of vitamin A per daily dose. If your stomach can't tolerate the iron in such a supplement in the first trimester, take a regular multivitamin and mineral. Switch to a prenatal formula when you enter the second trimester and your stomach has settled.

5. Continue to include folate-rich foods in your diet every day. Reach for spinach, asparagus, avocado, artichokes, lentils, and chickpeas, to name just a few excellent sources.

6. Add iron-rich foods to your daily diet. Lean beef, spinach, dried fruit, and legumes are good choices.

7. Eliminate or reduce your caffeine intake to no more than 150 milligrams per day (one 6-ounce or 175-ml cup of coffee).

8. Continue to avoid all alcoholic beverages and alcohol-containing foods and medications.

9. To prevent listeriosis and other food-borne illnesses, be vigilant about using safe food-handling practices.

10. Use herbal products very cautiously. Use only those supplements and teas considered safe. Don't drink more than three mugs of herbal tea per day.

11. Minimize your intake of trans fat and pesticide residues.

12. And finally, continue to follow my nutrition strategies outlined in Chapter 2 to help you meet your calcium, fibre, and fluid requirements.

8

⚬⚬⚬

Eating Your Way Through
a Multiple Pregnancy:
A Nutrition Plan

More and more women today are giving birth to twins, triplets, even quadruplets. These are considered multiple pregnancies. If recent statistics are any indication, there's a good chance you know someone who has had a multiple birth. According to Multiple Births Canada, since 1974, the birth of twins has increased by 35 percent, triplets by 300 percent, and quadruplets by more than 400 percent. Every year in Canada, more than 4000 sets of twins and 75 sets of triplets, quadruplets, and quintuplets combined are born.[1]

Why are multiple births on the rise? The fact that more women are delaying their pregnancies until after the age of 30 accounts in part for the increase. That's because women over 30 are more likely to conceive multiples. But for the most part, it's because of the increased use of fertility treatments such as fertility enhancing drugs and assisted reproductive techniques (e.g., in vitro fertilization).

If your pregnancy is showing much sooner than you expected, it's natural to wonder if you're carrying twins. Signs that you might be pregnant with multiples include:

- You have severe morning sickness.
- You put weight on more quickly than anticipated in the first trimester.

- Your uterus is growing more quickly than would be expected for a single pregnancy.

Some women are more likely to have a multiple pregnancy than others. Risk factors include the following:

- You have already given birth to twins.

- You have a family history of fraternal (non-identical) twins.

- You have been undergoing fertility treatment.

- Your body mass index (BMI) prior to pregnancy was higher than 27.

In the days of our grandparents, having twins was usually a surprise, learned only in the delivery room. But today, most couples learn the news long before giving birth. Your prenatal ultrasound, done early in the second trimester, can detect almost all multiple pregnancies. Your doctor may also suspect multiples from an abnormal result on your triple screen test done in the second trimester (see Chapter 5 for more about prenatal testing in the second trimester). And then there's always the good old extra heartbeat your doctor may hear during a routine prenatal checkup. Sometimes it's the mom-to-be who gets the first clue, when she feels more fetal movement than in her previous single pregnancy.

A multiple pregnancy automatically puts a woman in the high-risk category. But that does not necessarily mean there will be problems during pregnancy or delivery. Your doctor will watch for potential problems such as preterm labour, high blood pressure and pre-eclampsia, gestational diabetes, and one or more miscarriages. With proper medical and nutritional care, these conditions can be managed and usually don't pose a major risk to the babies or mother.

Multiples, whether they're twins, triplets, or more, are usually born preterm (before 37 weeks) and, as a result, are often low birth weight (less than 5.5 pounds, or 2500 grams) or very low birth weight (less than 3 pounds 5 ounces, or 1500 grams). It's estimated that half of twins are born early and half are low birth weight.[2] According to studies, the average birth weight of twins ranges from 5 to 5 pounds 10 ounces (2300 to 2600 grams) at 37 weeks. Triplets weigh on average 4 pounds, or 1800 grams, each at a delivery date of about 33 to 34 weeks.[3] The duration of a woman's pregnancy decreases with each additional baby she is carrying.

AVERAGE DURATION OF PREGNANCY

Single	40 weeks
Twins	37 weeks
Triplets	34 weeks
Quadruplets	32 weeks

Being born early accounts for many of the problems multiple babies may experience as newborns. And the more babies a woman carries at one time, the greater the risk for complications. In Chapter 7, I discuss the potential health complications faced by low-birth-weight babies. Fortunately, with today's technology, the outlook for such tiny babies has brightened considerably. You'll read later in this chapter that adequate weight gain, especially in the first half of a multiple pregnancy, benefits multiple babies throughout pregnancy.

While some of the risks of a multiple pregnancy may not be entirely preventable, proper prenatal care that includes regular doctor visits, good nutrition, proper hydration, and plenty of rest are essential for a healthy pregnancy. There is no sense in worrying about possible complications; this will only add unnecessary stress. Instead, focus on taking the best possible care of yourself.

Prenatal Care

If you are pregnant with multiples, you can expect to see your doctor more often than women carrying one baby. This allows for close monitoring of you and your babies. The doctor will check for potential complications and help ensure you carry your babies for as long as possible. You will visit your doctor twice monthly during the second trimester and weekly during the third.

As a mom-to-be of multiples, you'll have more prenatal tests than if you were carrying one baby. These are precautionary tests to detect and minimize potential problems. Your doctor will check you regularly for signs of pre-eclampsia, a serious medical condition characterized by high blood pressure (see Chapter 9). Since gestational diabetes and iron deficiency anemia are more common with multiple pregnancies, you can expect your blood-sugar and iron levels to be measured regularly.

Your doctor will also closely monitor your babies via ultrasounds and other tests. Prenatal ultrasounds are an exciting way for you to get to know your babies and watch them grow. Your doctor will be able to tell what kind of multiples you're having. Monozygotic twins (identical twins) develop from one fertilized egg, which splits either before or after it implants in the lining of the uterus. Identical twins may share a placenta or they may not. Dizygotic twins (fraternal twins) come from two fertilized eggs.

It's important for your doctor to determine early on what kind of multiples you are carrying, since identical twins with a shared placenta have an increased risk of developing twin-to-twin transfusion. This condition occurs because the babies share blood vessels, sometimes resulting in one twin getting too much blood flow and the other too little. This condition can also happen in monozygotic multiples in a higher-order multiple pregnancy (e.g., triplets, quadruplets).

The doctor will use ultrasounds to check your babies' internal organs, monitor placenta movement, and determine your babies' positions. If you're expecting twins, your babies' positions help determine whether a vaginal or Caesarean delivery is more likely. Roughly one-half of all women having twins can experience natural childbirth if both babies are in a normal, head-down position. However, all triplets and quadruplets are born by Caesarean.

Preterm Labour

One of the most common complications of a multiple pregnancy is preterm labour, labour that begins before 37 weeks. Starting around the 20th week, your doctor will examine you carefully for signs of preterm labour. He or she will do an internal exam to check your cervix to be sure it's not opening too soon. It's important to know the signs and symptoms of preterm labour so you can call your doctor immediately:

- Cramps or stomach pain that doesn't go away
- Bleeding or fluid leakage from the vagina
- Increased amount of vaginal discharge
- Fever, chills, bad headache, dizziness, vomiting
- A significant change in your babies' movements
- Strong contractions, pain, or pressure in your vagina or pelvis

Bedrest

If you've had signs of preterm labour, you may be put on bedrest. Staying in bed will help increase blood flow to the uterus and prevent contractions stimulated by activity. The length of time your doctor tells you to rest in bed will depend on how far along you are in your pregnancy, if there are changes in your cervix, your general health, and the health of your babies.

There's no question that bedrest can be boring. If you are stuck in bed, use the time to plan ahead. You won't be able to paint the nursery or shop for baby clothes, but you can use the phone and make lists to help you get organized for what lies ahead—being a mother to more than one baby.

Activity Restrictions

Even if you don't have any signs of preterm labour, your doctor may advise that you cut back on your activities between the 20th and 30th weeks of your pregnancy. If you're expecting triplets or quadruplets, you may be asked to cut back even sooner. Depending on how physically demanding your job is, you may be told to change the nature of the work you do, or start your maternity leave early.

If you have been active and want to continue to exercise during your pregnancy, ask your doctor what's safe for you to do and how to modify your program as your pregnancy progresses. Low-impact activities such as walking or swimming tend to be the safest. Some doctors advise discontinuing exercise at 24 weeks if you're expecting twins, and at 20 weeks for a triplet pregnancy. You'll find you can do less and less as your pregnancy progresses. The size of your expanding uterus may cause you to feel short of breath, not to mention have difficulty moving around. Women pregnant with multiples can expect to be more uncomfortable than women expecting one baby.

A Nutrition Plan for a Multiple Pregnancy

Getting proper nutrition is widely accepted as being a key component of care for women expecting multiples. Yet the topic of diet and multiple pregnancy is one that is under-studied. Because limited nutrition research exists, there are no clear-cut diet guidelines for women expecting twins, triplets, or quadruplets. The recommendations made today are adapted from studies on single and twin pregnancies, as well as being based on the clinical experience of doctors.

Consult a Registered Dietitian

The recommendations below are meant as a guide to you and your health care provider. I strongly recommend that you work one on one with a registered dietitian throughout your pregnancy. Two studies have revealed that twin pregnancies have a healthier outcome if the moms-to-be receive nutrition education and counselling from a dietitian. Researchers from the University of Michigan Medical School interviewed 928 mothers of twins and found that those who received their nutrition advice from a dietitian had the highest weight gains and the lowest proportion of low-birth-weight babies.[4]

Another study from the Montreal Diet Dispensary compared 354 twin pregnancies served by a dietitian with 686 twin pregnancies that were not. The researchers found that the women receiving diet counselling consumed more calories and protein each day, gained more weight, and were 30 percent less likely to deliver preterm. As well, these women delivered 25 percent fewer low-birth-weight babies and half as many very-low-birth-weight babies.[5]

A dietitian will help modify your nutrition plan in order for you to achieve adequate weight gain and the proper intake of all the nutrients you need for your pregnancy. And if you encounter any complications along the way, such as anemia or diabetes, a dietitian will be able to advise you about specific diet modifications. Ask your doctor for a referral to a dietitian who has experience working with pregnant women, preferably multiple pregnancies. The Dietitians of Canada can also help you find a dietitian in your community. See the Resources section (page 304) for more information about this national organization.

Weight Gain Goals

Of all the nutritional factors influencing a multiple pregnancy, weight gain has received the most study. And it's not only how much weight you gain but also when you gain it that makes a difference in a multiple pregnancy. Studies indicate that gaining adequate weight at critical periods during pregnancy can reduce the chance that multiples will be born weighing less than 5.5 pounds (2500 grams).

Early weight gain is important since multiple pregnancies are shorter. Research in twin pregnancies shows that it is especially important for underweight and normal-weight women to gain adequate weight before 20 weeks to reduce the risk of delivering low-birth-weight babies.[6] A higher rate of weight gain at the 20th week and on to delivery can improve the birth weight of twins born to normal-weight and overweight women.[7]

When it comes to triplet pregnancies, research indicates that gaining adequate weight before the 24th week of pregnancy is associated with the best fetal growth rate and birth weight.[8] These studies reveal that women expecting triplets have healthier pregnancy outcomes if they gain at least 1.5 pounds (0.7 kilogram) per week for the duration of their pregnancies.

How much weight you should gain throughout your pregnancy will depend on the number of babies you are expecting. Based on the evidence to date, here is a general guide used for weight gain goals during a multiple pregnancy:

WEIGHT GAIN GUIDELINES FOR MULTIPLE PREGNANCIES

	Twins	Triplets
Total gain	35 to 45 pounds (16 to 20 kilograms)	45 to 55 pounds (20 to 25 kilograms)
First trimester	4 to 6 pounds (2 to 3 kilograms) total	1.5 pounds (0.7 kilogram) per week
Second and third trimesters	1.5 pounds (0.7 kilogram) per week	1.5 pounds (0.7 kilogram) per week

Keep in mind that these targets serve as a guide; how much weight your doctor wants you to gain will also depend on your pre-pregnancy weight. If you were overweight before becoming pregnant (a BMI higher than 27), you should gain at the lower end;

underweight women (a BMI less than 20) should strive for the higher end of the weight gain range. Underweight women should also aim for a steady weekly weight gain of 1.75 pounds (0.8 kilogram) after the 20th week.

Calories and Food Intake

When it comes to diet, little research has been done to establish the exact nutrient needs of women expecting multiples. We do know that your calorie needs increase tremendously to support the growth of your babies and all the hard work your body is undertaking. You will need to eat at least an additional 500 calories per day, over and above your pre-pregnancy calorie intake. This means you'll need to consume a minimum of 2700 calories each day. Underweight women may need to consume more calories and overweight women less. However, 2700 calories is a good starting point. Here's what these calories look like in terms of food (for serving sizes, see , page 303):

FOOD SERVINGS FOR 2700 CALORIES

Milk	Protein	Fruit	Vegetables	Grains	Fats
5	10	6	4	8	6

This is actually not as much food as it might seem at first glance. Here's how you might incorporate this food into your day.

Breakfast:

1 cup (250 ml) 1% or skim milk

1 1/2 cups (375 ml) whole-grain breakfast cereal with 2 tablespoons (25 ml) raisins

1 slice whole-grain toast with 1 tablespoon (15 ml) peanut butter

3/4 cup (175 ml) unsweetened fruit juice

Morning Snack:

1 cup (250 ml) low-fat yogurt

1 banana

Lunch:

Sandwich on whole-grain bread with 4 ounces (115 g) turkey breast and sliced tomatoes

1 cup (250 ml) lentil soup

6 whole-grain crackers

1/2 cup (125 ml) baby carrots with hummus dip

1 cup (250 ml) 1% or skim milk

Afternoon Snack:

Smoothie made with milk, frozen berries, small banana, plus 2 teaspoons (10 ml) flax oil

Dinner:

5 ounces (140 g) grilled salmon

2/3 cup (150 ml) cooked couscous

5 spears asparagus

Green salad with 2 tablespoons (25 ml) oil and vinegar dressing

1 to 2 cups (250 to 500 ml) water

Bedtime Snack:

1 apple

1 ounce (30 g) cheddar cheese

1 cup (250 ml) low-fat yogurt or milk

According to some experts, certain women may need an additional 1000 calories each day. Many of the studies on diet in multiple pregnancies have come from the University of Michigan, where doctors and dietitians work with expectant mothers in the university's Multiples Clinic. Women attending this clinic tend to give birth to twins and triplets that weigh more than the national average birth weight. Here's how much the clinic advises its patients to eat each day (for serving sizes, see , page 303).

DAILY CALORIES AND NUMBER OF RECOMMENDED SERVINGS FOR MULTIPLE PREGNANCIES

	Calories	Milk	Meat	Eggs	Fruit	Vegetables	Grains	Fats
Twins	3500	8	10	2	7	4	10	6
Triplets	4000	10	10	2	8	5	12	7
Quadruplets	4500	12	12	2	8	6	12	8

Adapted from Luke, Barbara, and Tamara Eberlein. *When You're Expecting Twins, Triplets, or Quads.* New York: Harper Collins, 1999.

The amount of food it takes to get the calories you need may seem overwhelming. But here's the bottom line: you need to eat a lot of nutrient-dense foods each day. Work with your dietitian to map out an eating plan and schedule that allows you to maximize your nutrient intake. I realize that eating more food may be easier said than done. Some women find it helpful to add nutritional supplement drinks to their diet. Drinks such as Ensure and Boost offer protein, carbohydrate, fat, vitamins, and minerals, and anywhere from 250 to 300 calories per can. You'll find these products in the nutrition section of your local drugstore.

If you are extremely nauseated, it can be a real struggle to meet your nutritional needs. Do the best you can. You'll find helpful tips for managing morning sickness in Chapter 9.

The study from the Montreal Diet Dispensary that I mentioned earlier concluded that nutrition counselling improves the outcome of twin pregnancies. The diet advice given to these women included eating an extra 1000 calories and 50 grams of protein each day after the 20th week of pregnancy. The additional calories and protein were above non-pregnant needs. This would mean bumping your intake from 2700 to 3200 calories in the second half of your pregnancy.

You can see that there is no clear-cut answer to how many calories you need to be consuming. At the end of the day, your recommended calorie intake will be determined by your rate of weight gain. You and your dietitian will likely modify your intake periodically throughout your pregnancy in order to achieve your target weight gain rate.

Protein

Women definitely need more protein to support the growth of twins. In fact, compared with women carrying one baby, women expecting twins need twice as much extra protein during their second and third trimesters. That translates into an additional 50 grams of protein each day. In food terms, this is roughly a 6-ounce (180-gram) chicken breast. (Women expecting one baby need to boost their daily protein intake by 25 grams during the last two trimesters.) At this time, there are no specific recommendations for women pregnant with triplets or more.

Women expecting twins will need to ensure a daily protein intake of 100 grams during the second and third trimesters. The 2700-calorie food plan I outline above provides 110 grams of high-quality protein. (The food intake guidelines for twins from the University of Michigan's Multiples Clinic provide 150 grams of protein each day.)

Here are the best food choices for boosting your protein intake:

Cheese:	1 ounce (30 g) = 7 grams protein
Eggs:	1 large whole egg = 6 grams protein
Milk or yogurt:	1 cup (250 ml) = 8 grams protein
Lean meat, poultry, or fish:	1 ounce (30 g) = 7 grams protein
Lentils, cooked:	1/2 cup (125 ml) = 10 grams protein
Soy nuts:	1/4 cup (50 ml) = 14 grams protein
Tofu, extra-firm:	3 ounces (90 g) = 9 grams protein

Essential Fatty Acids

Research suggests that the need for essential fatty acids is increased during a multiple pregnancy, even more so than for a singleton pregnancy. Essential fats are important for the healthy development of your babies' brains and vision (I discuss essential fatty acids in detail in Chapter 7). It turns out that multiple babies have much lower levels of essential fats in their bloodstreams than do singleton babies.[9] Based on this, women pregnant with multiples should include sources of these fats in their daily diets.

Linoleic acid and alpha-linolenic acid are two fatty acids vital to good health; your body uses these fats to produce immune compounds, among other things. However, your body cannot manufacture either linoleic acid or alpha-linolenic acid, so they must be supplied from your diet (that's why they're called *essential* fatty acids). Both these fatty acids are found in omega-6 and omega-3 fats. One type of essential fat you've probably heard lots about is DHA, the omega-3 fatty acid found in fish and seafood. It seems to play the most important role in brain and vision development during the last trimester of pregnancy and the first two years of life.

FOODS TO BOOST YOUR INTAKE OF ESSENTIAL FATS

Omega-6 Fatty Acids

Arachidonic acid	Meats; can also be made from linoleic acid
Linoleic acid	Corn oil, cottonseed oil, safflower oil, sesame oil, sunflower oil, leafy vegetables, nuts, seeds

Omega-3 Fatty Acids

Alpha-linolenic acid	Canola oil, flax oil, hemp oil, walnut oil, walnuts, wheat germ, omega-3 eggs, soybeans, leafy green vegetables
DHA and EPA	Breast milk, oily fish; a little can also be made from alpha-linolenic acid

Fluids

Keep drinking your water! Carry a water bottle with you so you can sip on fluids throughout the day. Dehydration can increase the risk of preterm labour, so aim for 12 to 16 cups (3 to 4 litres) of fluid each day.

Minerals and Vitamins

Calcium and iron are two particularly significant minerals during pregnancy. A prenatal supplement also plays an important role in your pregnancy nutrition regime.

Calcium: 2000 Milligrams Per Day

Just like non-pregnant women, women pregnant with one baby need to get 1000 milligrams of calcium each day. Although no study has been done to pinpoint an exact amount, it is reasonable that women pregnant with multiples need more calcium. Calcium not only helps build strong bones in both a mother and her babies, it's also been shown to reduce the risk of developing pre-eclampsia, a potential complication of a multiple pregnancy.

There's one more reason why some women carrying multiples might need more calcium. Magnesium sulfate is a drug often used to quiet the uterus and reduce the risk of preterm labour. But this medication also causes large amounts of calcium to be lost in the urine. So if you're taking magnesium therapy, you need to pay special attention to your calcium intake.

Aim to get 2000 milligrams of calcium each day from your diet and supplements combined. You'll come close to your target if you consume five servings of milk, yogurt, or a calcium-enriched beverage each day (5 × 300 mg = 1500 mg calcium). And cheese counts, too. One and one-half ounces (45 grams) of hard cheese provides roughly 300 milligrams of calcium. The safe upper limit for calcium is 2500 milligrams per day.

You will still need to supplement. Most prenatal supplements provide 250 milligrams of calcium. Assuming you are getting your five daily milk servings, that puts your calcium intake at 1750 milligrams a day. To make up the difference, take a calcium citrate supplement with vitamin D added. These are sold in 300- or 600-milligram tablets (the higher dose tablets are handy if you find it difficult to get all your milk servings). Do not take more than 600 milligrams at one time. If you need to take more than one supplement, spread the dose out over the course of the day. If you are taking iron supplements to treat anemia, do not take calcium at the same time. Take them at least two hours apart.

Iron: 30 Milligrams Per Day

Iron deficiency anemia is more common in multiple pregnancies than in singleton pregnancies. In addition to a prenatal vitamin supplement that supplies 30 milligrams of iron, be sure to include iron-rich foods in your daily diet. Animal foods contain the most absorbable form of the mineral (heme iron), whereas plant foods contain iron that's less efficiently absorbed (non-heme iron). If you are not a vegetarian, make a real effort to include heme iron foods in your diet each day. If you are a vegetarian, add an iron absorption enhancer at each meal.

Heme Iron Foods	Non-Heme Iron Foods	Iron Absorption Enhancers	
Fish	Eggs	Bell peppers	Kiwifruit
Meat	Fruit	Broccoli	Mango
Poultry	Legumes	Brussels sprouts	Snow peas
	Nuts, seeds	Cantaloupe	Strawberries
	Vegetables	Citrus fruit	Tomato juice
	Whole grains		

You'll find a more detailed list of iron-rich foods in Chapter 2. If your doctor diagnoses iron deficiency anemia during your pregnancy, you will need to take an iron supplement to rebuild your body's iron stores. For more information about treating anemia, see Chapter 9.

Prenatal Supplements: Once Daily, After 12 Weeks of Pregnancy

Women carrying more than one baby should take a prenatal supplement that supplies:

- Calcium, 250 milligrams
- Copper, 2 milligrams
- Folic acid, 600 micrograms
- Iron, 30 milligrams
- Vitamin B6, 2 milligrams
- Vitamin C, 50 milligrams
- Vitamin D, 5 micrograms (200 IU)
- Zinc, 15 milligrams[10]

In Chapter 7, you'll find a list of prenatal supplement brands and what's in each. As you will see, Materna and Rexall Prenatal meet the criteria listed above.

Where to Go for Support

The prospect of giving birth to twins, triplets, or quadruplets can be overwhelming for many couples. Anxiety about the pregnancy and delivery, worry about finances, and distress over losing time with an older child are all common emotions in mothers expecting multiples.

It's important to know you're not alone. It can be extremely comforting to share your feelings and experiences with others who are also expecting multiples or who have already delivered a healthy set of babies. The national organization Multiple Births Canada provides useful information and can connect you with multiple birth families in your community. See the listing in the Resources section (page 304).

9

∞∞∞

Feeling Your Best:
Managing Pregnancy
Discomforts and Disorders

With each trimester come certain problems: some can make it difficult for you to eat healthy foods, others can make it challenging to get a good night's sleep, and still others can simply make you feel uncomfortable and unattractive. Morning sickness, fatigue, heartburn, hemorrhoids, leg cramps, swollen feet . . . the list goes on. You may not be able to avoid these problems altogether, but there's plenty you can do to ease the discomfort. Simple dietary changes and lifestyle modifications can go a long way toward lessening the severity of these common pregnancy problems.

While certain discomforts are unique to a particular trimester, others can occur in more than one. For instance, morning sickness is predominately a first trimester problem, whereas constipation and hemorrhoids can occur in the second or third trimesters, or both. Some women sail through pregnancy with few problems, others suffer a number of minor grievances. Some women will experience a pregnancy-related condition that is potentially serious, such as hypertension or gestational diabetes. Just as no two women are alike, no two pregnancies are alike.

On the following pages, common pregnancy-related discomforts and disorders are presented in alphabetical order for easy reference. For each pregnancy problem, I discuss its cause, symptoms, risk factors, and diet and lifestyle strategies to manage or alleviate its discomforts.

Constipation

If you're suffering from constipation, take comfort from the fact that you're not alone. At least 50 percent of all women have constipation problems during pregnancy.[1] There's no need to worry if you aren't having a bowel movement every day. Everyone's bowel habits are different. Some women have bowel movements as often as three times a day, others as infrequently as three times a week, but they are all still regular. But if you have fewer than three bowel movements a week and your stools are hard, small, and difficult to pass, you are likely constipated.

What Causes Constipation?

Under normal circumstances, your digestive system functions efficiently. During the digestive process, a series of wave-like muscle contractions move food through the intestine, where it is broken down into nutrients and absorbed. Another series of muscle contractions moves the remaining waste material along to the rectum. Eventually, these waste products are eliminated from the body as a bowel movement.

As your pregnancy progresses, your uterus expands rapidly. The extra weight of your growing baby puts unusual pressure on your rectum and lower intestine, interfering with the normal functioning of your digestive system. To make matters worse, your pregnancy hormones make digestion sluggish by slowing down those wave-like contractions that move food through your intestine. As a result, waste products linger in your bowel, where they lose moisture, becoming hard and dry. These two factors, coupled with a diet low in fibre, can leave you feeling uncomfortably constipated throughout most of your pregnancy. The high dose of iron in prenatal supplements can also cause or aggravate constipation.

Although constipation will often go away after pregnancy, it can be prevented, or at least minimized, by fairly simple strategies. However, if you don't treat it, too much straining or pushing to pass hard stools can result in hemorrhoids (discussed later in this chapter) or small tears around the anus.

Symptoms

Constipation has a number of symptoms:

- Less than three bowel movements a week or more than four days between movements
- Hard, dry stools that are difficult to pass
- A feeling that your rectum isn't fully emptied or that not all stools have been passed
- Slight bleeding from your rectum
- Gas pains, bloating, or abdominal cramps

Who's at Risk?

Pregnancy increases your risk of constipation. You are also more likely to become constipated if you spend a lot of time sitting or have a sedentary lifestyle. If your diet is low in high-fibre foods and you don't drink an adequate amount of water each day, constipation is almost inevitable. Pregnant women who take iron supplements are also at greater risk for constipation.

Strategies for Managing Constipation

Constipation can be prevented or minimized fairly easily.

Diet and Nutrition Tips

The following strategies are easy to implement in your daily diet:

- *Boost your intake of insoluble fibre.* Foods with a greater proportion of insoluble fibre, such as wheat bran, whole grains, nuts, seeds, and certain fruits and vegetables, are used to treat and prevent constipation. Once consumed, these fibres make their way to your intestinal tract, where they absorb water, help to form larger, softer stools, and speed evacuation. Sometimes psyllium, a soluble fibre that adds bulk to stools, is used to treat constipation. But I don't find it nearly as effective as the insoluble fibre found in wheat bran. And many of my clients complain that soluble fibre actually increases their symptoms of bloating.

  You may recall from Chapter 2 that you need 25 grams of fibre each day to prevent constipation. To treat constipation, add high-fibre foods such as bran cereal to your daily diet. Here's a look at the fibre content of selected high-fibre foods:

  - 1/2 cup (125 ml) 100 percent bran cereal provides 10 grams fibre.
  - 1/3 cup (75 ml) Kellogg's All-Bran Buds provides 13 grams fibre.
  - 2 tbsp (25 ml) natural wheat bran provide 3 grams fibre.
  - 2 tbsp (25 ml) ground flaxseed provide 4.5 grams (soluble) fibre.
  - 1/4 cup (50 ml) whole almonds provides 4.2 grams fibre.

  Increase your fibre intake gradually to prevent intestinal discomfort. To minimize possible side effects such as bloating and gas, spread your fibre intake over the course of the day, rather than getting it all at once. It is normal to experience some flatulence when starting a high-fibre diet. This usually resolves itself within a few weeks, once the bacteria residing in your large intestine adjust to a higher fibre intake.

- *Choose higher fibre fruits and vegetables.* The fruits and vegetables listed below are always good options.

FRUIT

High Fibre (5+ grams)

Apple, with skin, 1

Blackberries, 1/2 cup (125 ml)

Blueberries, 1 cup (250 ml)

Figs or dates, 10

Kiwifruit, 2

Mango, medium, 1

Pear, medium, 1

Prunes, dried, 5

Prunes, stewed, 1/2 cup (125 ml)

Raspberries, 1/2 cup (125 ml)

Medium Fibre (2–4 grams)

Orange, medium, 1

Raisins, 2 tbsp (25 ml)

Rhubarb, cooked, 1/2 cup (125 ml)

Strawberries, 1 cup (250 ml)

Tangerine, medium, 1

VEGETABLES

High Fibre (5+ grams)

Green peas, 1/2 cup (125 ml)

Snow peas, 10

Swiss chard, cooked, 1 cup (250 ml)

Medium Fibre (2–4 grams)

Bean sprouts, 1/2 cup (125 ml)

Beans, string, 1/2 cup (125 ml)

Broccoli, 1/2 cup (125 ml)

Brussels sprouts, 1/2 cup (125 ml)

Carrots, raw, 1/2 cup (125 ml)

Eggplant, 1/2 cup (125 ml)

Parsnips, 1/2 cup (125 ml)

© 2000, American Dietetic Association. *Manual of Clinical Dieticians,* 6th edition. Used with permission.

- *Drink water throughout the day.* Dietary fibre needs to absorb fluid in the intestinal tract in order to add bulk to stool. Drink 8 to 12 cups (2 to 3 litres) of fluid every day. Always include 1 cup (250 ml) of fluid with high-fibre meals and snacks. If you're also suffering from heartburn, sip water over the course of the day. Avoid drinking large quantities at meals. Some women find that warm or hot fluids are helpful in promoting a bowel movement.

- *Eat a fermented dairy product every day.* Fermented dairy products such as yogurt, kefir, and sweet acidophilus milk contain lactic acid bacteria (e.g., acidophilus, bifidobacteria) that may help prevent constipation. These friendly bacteria normally reside in your intestinal tract, where they perform a number of tasks that keep your bowel healthy. Scientists are learning that, to achieve the health benefits of these bacteria, it is important to consume them regularly. Eat 1 cup (250 ml) of fermented dairy product daily. All yogurts in Canada are made with lactic acid bacteria whether or not they are labelled as such.

- *Reach for prunes.* Prunes are high in fibre (1 gram fibre per prune); they also contain a natural laxative substance called dihydroxtphenyl isatin. Eat five dried or stewed prunes for a snack. Or if you'd rather, drink prune juice for a concentrated source of prune's natural laxative. For a morning bowel movement, drink prune juice at bedtime. If the evening is preferred, drink prune juice at breakfast.

- *Consider taking psyllium seed husks.* Psyllium is a bulk-forming laxative high in both insoluble and soluble fibres. The laxative properties of psyllium are due to the swelling of the husk when it comes in contact with water. Once consumed, it forms a gelatinous mass and keeps the feces hydrated and soft. The increased bulk stimulates a reflex contraction of the walls of the bowel. Take 5 to 10 grams of the husks with 2 cups (500 ml) water, one to three times per day. You'll also find psyllium in a product called Metamucil. However, in my clinical practice, only a small handful of clients respond to taking psyllium, most of whom are men. Many women report that psyllium causes them to feel bloated.

Lifestyle Tips

These tips will help prevent or relieve constipation:

- *Eat on a schedule.* Eating at regular intervals during the day helps promote bowel motility.

- *Listen to your body,* and always respond to the urge to have a bowel movement. If your busy schedule interferes with your ability to respond to your body's defecation signals, revise your schedule. Go to bed earlier in order to rise earlier, allowing time for breakfast and a bowel movement.

- *Don't worry excessively* about your bowel movements. Anxiety can aggravate constipation.

- *Exercise regularly* to promote bowel motility. Aim to walk briskly for 30 minutes at least four times per week, preferably every day.

If these simple strategies don't relieve the problem, your doctor may recommend laxatives to help make your stool softer and easier to pass. Don't use over-the-counter laxatives without consulting your doctor, and never use enemas when you're pregnant.

Edema (Swelling)

By the time you reach the third trimester, you may find that your feet are swollen, your ankles are puffy, and your rings won't fit on your suddenly pudgy fingers. These are the classic signs of pregnancy edema, or swelling. A certain amount of swelling is normal during pregnancy, especially in the later stages. You may notice swelling in your hands and face, too.

If your third trimester hits during warm, humid weather, you'll probably find that your edema worsens. But there's no need to worry: the puffiness of pregnancy is only temporary.

What Causes Edema?

During pregnancy, the body has a tendency to retain excess water. Changes in your blood chemistry also cause water to move from your cells into your tissue. This excess fluid accumulates in your legs and feet as a result of the pressure your growing uterus puts on the veins in your lower body. This pressure slows down circulation so that extra blood begins to pool in your veins. The pressure from the trapped blood forces fluid from your veins into the tissues of your feet and ankles. This causes the swelling and achiness associated with pregnancy edema.

Edema is common in pregnancy and usually has no effect on you or your baby. However, severe or rapid swelling can be a sign of high blood pressure or pre-eclampsia, two dangerous conditions. If you experience sudden, severe swelling, especially in your hands and feet, contact your doctor immediately. You'll find information on pregnancy-related high blood pressure and pre-eclampsia later in this chapter.

Symptoms

The signs of edema include:

- Swelling in the feet, ankles, hands, and sometimes the face
- Skin on the feet and ankles become slightly purple, due to the increased pressure
- Swelling that is usually less noticeable in the morning, becoming more pronounced as the day goes by
- Tired, aching legs and feet

Who's at Risk?

Edema is so common in pregnancy that it's safe to say that most pregnant women are at risk of developing the condition. But you're at greater risk if you:

- Gain excessive amounts of weight during pregnancy
- Are expecting twins (or more)
- Have a family history of high blood pressure (hypertension)

Strategies for Managing Edema

While you probably can't prevent edema altogether, you certainly can decrease the puffiness and discomfort by following simple guidelines.

Diet and Nutrition Tips

Simple changes to your diet will help relieve edema:

- *Drink plenty of water.* It may sound odd, but drinking adequate amounts of fluid actually helps you retain less water. Aim to drink 9 cups (2.2 litres) of fluid each day. Drink more when exercising and during warm, humid weather. This fluid should come from non-caffeinated, non-alcoholic sources. Carrying a water bottle with you during the day, whether you're at home, at the office, or running errands, will help you remember to drink water.

- *Don't cut back on salt.* If you're following a healthy diet (one not loaded with salty, processed foods), chances are that you're getting somewhere between 2000 and 3000 milligrams of sodium per day. That's about 1 teaspoon (5 ml) of salt, and it's the amount your body needs to maintain its fluid balance.

  It might sound logical to limit your intake of salt if you experience fluid retention and swelling. But cutting back too much can be harmful to you and your baby. Salt contains sodium, chloride, and potassium, the three minerals that help regulate fluid in your cells. As you know, during pregnancy your blood volume expands by about 50 percent, even more if you're expecting twins. As your blood volume expands, the amount of water held inside your cells also expands. The added fluid requires more, not less, sodium, potassium, and chloride.

  Research in animals has shown that when sodium is drastically restricted during pregnancy, normal blood expansion cannot occur. This limits the fetus's supply of nutrients, resulting in smaller babies.[2] The bottom line: women need more salt when pregnant. Maybe that's why pregnant women often crave pickles, chips, and other salty foods. You should be consuming at least 2000 milligrams of sodium per day. But there's no need to start calculating your sodium intake: this amount can be achieved by following a varied diet. There's no need to add more salt or drastically cut back on salt.

Lifestyle Tips

A number of small lifestyle changes will also help relieve edema:

- *Lie down, with your legs raised higher than your heart,* as often as possible.

- *Sleep, read, and watch television lying on your left side* to take pressure off the vena cava, a large vein on the right side of your body that receives blood from your lower limbs and carries it back to the heart. The pressure slows down circulation and causes blood to pool in your legs, forcing fluid from your veins into the tissues of your feet and ankles.

- *If you have to sit for a long time, place a small stool under both feet* so your knees are at a 90-degree angle to your hips. Try not to sit with your legs crossed, as this causes pressure in the veins in your legs, which can slow down circulation, in turn causing blood to pool in your legs and forcing fluid from your veins into the tissues of your legs and feet.

- *If you're driving for a long time, take regular breaks* to stretch and promote circulation.

- *Wear low-heeled shoes that fit properly.* Shoes that are too narrow or too tight will restrict your circulation.

- *Consider wearing waist-high maternity support stockings.* These are put on *before* you get out of bed in the morning so blood has no chance to pool around your ankles.

- *Don't wear clothing or jewellery that binds,* such as stockings with tight leg bands, rings, or watches.

- *Continue with your regular exercise program,* whether it's brisk walking, swimming, or dancing. Exercise improves circulation.

Fatigue

One of the complaints I hear most often about pregnancy is how tired it makes one feel, especially during the first and third trimesters of pregnancy. Even if you've always been a night owl, pregnancy can make you think of tucking in many hours before your usual bedtime. Forget about those late-night parties and long days at the office: your body is working extra hard to accommodate the changes taking place within you and your baby.

The irony of pregnancy is that just when you need sleep the most, it can seem impossible to get a good night's rest. I've heard from many of my clients that the farther along they are in their pregnancy, the more elusive sleep becomes. Even if you can fall asleep, staying asleep can be a real challenge, particularly in the last trimester. Getting adequate rest is an important part of a healthy pregnancy. It may not be in your nature, but, if you aren't getting enough sleep at night, give yourself permission to nap or lie down during the day.

What Causes Fatigue?

Many factors contribute to the fatigue of pregnancy. Fluctuating hormone levels change your metabolism, lower your blood pressure, and disrupt your blood-sugar level. One of those pregnancy hormones, progesterone, has a sedative effect. As well, there are many physical and mental demands on your body that can tire you out at every stage of pregnancy. All your systems are operating in overdrive, which can quickly use up your energy stores and leave you running on fumes, instead of a full tank. Morning sickness and mood swings can also drain you of much-needed energy.

And let's not forget the sleep disruptions. The need to urinate more frequently, heartburn, and leg cramps can compete with your nightly slumber. Some women also find that the anticipation of birth and the worry about labour keeps them from letting their minds relax easily into sleep. And I've had several clients report that once sleep sets in, they are woken by exceptionally vivid dreams. It's no wonder that fatigue is one of the most common complaints of early and late pregnancy.

The normal fatigue of pregnancy is nothing to worry about. It certainly won't harm your baby. The worst that will happen is that you may not have the energy to socialize or concentrate at work. And your schedule may be altered by midday naps. Sometimes fatigue can interfere with your emotions, causing mood swings or crying jags. This, too, is normal and shouldn't be cause for concern. Just get the rest you need.

Fatigue is so common in pregnancy that it's easy to ignore. Naturally, some fatigue is normal, but excessive tiredness and lack of energy may be an indicator of anemia. You can read more about iron deficiency anemia later in this chapter. If you think you're more tired than you should be, tell your doctor.

Symptoms

Symptoms of normal pregnancy-related fatigue include:

- A strong urge to sleep, often in the middle of the day or early evening

- An obvious lack of energy

- Inability to concentrate, decreased mental alertness

- Mood swings; increased tendency to cry

Who's at Risk?

Fatigue is a ubiquitous problem in pregnancy. It's more pronounced in the first and third trimesters. In the second trimester, you'll probably sleep more soundly and have more energy.

Strategies for Managing Fatigue

If you're tired, try to sleep. Go to bed early; your body will thank you. Plan your day around a nap, if possible. If you're at work, go out to your car for a catnap at lunchtime, or find a comfy chair in the staff room and put your feet up for a while. Even a 15-minute break can boost your energy level for the rest of the day.

Diet and Nutrition Tips

Try implementing these suggestions to help you get a better night's sleep and boost your energy level:

- *Avoid caffeine in the evening.* This includes tea, iced tea, chocolate, diet cola, or that one small cup of coffee you still may be drinking.

- *Don't eat a* large *meal right before bedtime.* This will also help prevent heartburn.

- *Focus on your iron intake.* Take your prenatal vitamin each day to ensure you are getting the iron your body needs. Your increased iron requirement becomes more pronounced during the second and third trimesters. If you feel exceptionally tired, short of breath during daily activities (climbing stairs, brisk walking), and have difficulty concentrating, ask your doctor for a blood test to measure your iron stores. The best test for iron deficiency is serum ferritin; it gives an indication of your body's iron stores. Ask your doctor to run this test in addition to the usual hemoglobin test, which measures the level of iron in your red blood cells.

- *Eat every three hours* to prevent your blood-sugar level from plummeting. That means you need to plan for three meals and three snacks each day. If you're the type of person who gets so involved in what you are doing that you forget to eat, set a timer on your computer or watch. It will remind you that you need to stop for calories and nutrients.

- *Include protein foods in your meals.* Protein helps slow down digestion, causing a sustained release of energy. Add a few ounces of lean meat, poultry, or omega-3–rich fish to your meals. Enjoy an omega-3 egg, low-fat yogurt, or 1 percent cottage cheese at breakfast. If you're a vegetarian, make a point of adding a serving of beans, lentils, or soy foods to each meal.

- *Boost your intake of chromium-rich foods,* such as unpeeled (washed) apples, green peas, chicken breast, refried beans, mushrooms, oysters, wheat germ, and brewer's yeast. Chromium works with insulin in the body to help stabilize blood-sugar levels. Some prenatal supplements provide 25 micrograms of chromium; you need 30 micrograms when pregnant. Reach for foods that will make up the difference.

Lifestyle Tips

These simple lifestyle changes will also help alleviate pregnancy-related fatigue:

- *Avoid drinking fluids after dinner.* This will reduce the number of trips you make to the bathroom in the middle of the night. But make sure you're still drinking 9 cups (2.2 litres) of fluid every day to keep your body hydrated.

- *Rest on your left side when you lie down.* You will be more comfortable, as the pressure will be taken off the vena cava, a vein on the right side of your body that receives blood from your lower limbs and carries it back to the heart. Pressure slows down circulation and causes blood to pool in your legs, forcing fluid from your veins into the tissues of your feet and ankles.

- *Elevate your feet periodically during the day* to reduce fluid retention and aching in your legs at night.

- *Exercise at a mild to moderate pace* for 20 to 30 minutes in duration, no matter how tired you might feel. Getting a little exercise every day can boost your feeling of energy and stabilize blood-sugar levels. Plan to work out at a time during the day when you feel the most energetic. For many women, this means taking a brisk walk on their lunch hour.

Food Cravings and Aversions

There is plenty of truth to the notion that women crave certain foods during pregnancy, though it may not be for a bowl of ice cream topped with dill pickles. A food craving is an intense desire for a particular food. It is not an increased appetite (which you will definitely encounter during your pregnancy) but, rather, a need for a specific food, right then. While most women crave sweets, others seek out salty snacks. And others long for the sour taste of green apples, oranges, and—yes—pickles.

Food cravings occur most often in the first trimester. According to an Internet-based survey, about 85 percent of women report craving at least one type of food during their pregnancy.[3] Usually, the food being craved has one of three ingredients: fat, sugar, or salt. The foods most commonly craved by pregnant women include desserts, ice cream, candy, chocolate, fruit, and fish. When it comes to food aversions, or turn-offs, women often report a new-found dislike for meat, chicken, coffee, and sauces flavoured with oregano.[4]

What Causes Food Cravings and Aversions?

It's hard to say what causes food cravings and aversions in pregnancy. There are a few theories, but not one that experts agree on. It's possible that the powerful hormonal changes associated with pregnancy can trigger desires for certain foods. After all, hormones can affect your sense of taste and smell. But if all women go through the hormonal changes of pregnancy, why don't all develop the same cravings and aversions? It may be that hormones only intensify cravings that women experience when they are not pregnant.

Another interesting theory links morning sickness to food aversions. Research suggests that a woman's strong dislike for the taste or smell of a food occurs early in pregnancy, often in the first week that nausea hits.[5] This does not seem to be the case for food cravings, though. And according to some scientists in Seattle, cravings for sweet foods were more common in the second trimester, not the first.[6]

One of the most commonly held beliefs about food cravings is that they are a way of telling you your body lacks certain nutrients. If you crave meat, you're lacking iron. If you crave chocolate, your body lacks magnesium. This theory, however, has not been substantiated. And if it were true, why is it that we seldom crave foods that are good for us?

Your food cravings may be in part a response to a low blood-sugar level and hunger. If it's 4 P.M. and you're craving a chocolate bar, your body is probably telling you that it needs fuel, not necessarily magnesium.

Sometimes food cravings aren't really food cravings. That is, they don't have a physiological basis. Instead, they may be a psychological reaction to a negative mood or stress. A better term for this is "comfort eating"—something I'm sure we've all done. In this case, craving a food becomes a way to deal with negative moods, such as stress, upset, or boredom. Studies show that, ironically, many cravers feel guilty after they give in to their cravings. Foods cravings may also be a response to your environment: you always feel like snacking when watching television, or you crave pizza when you walk by a pizza stand.

Symptoms

Food cravings vary among women, and may be different in one woman's first and subsequent pregnancies.

- An intense desire for a certain food immediately (food craving)
- Nausea at the sight or smell of a certain food (food aversion)

Who's at Risk?

If you're pregnant, you're more likely to experience food cravings or food aversions or both. But research suggests that you might be even more susceptible if you suffered with morning sickness in your first trimester or if you experienced food cravings or food aversions before you became pregnant.

Strategies for Managing Food Cravings and Aversions

It is important to know if your craving is a physical need for food or a psychological need for food. That way, you may be able to prevent strong cravings from occurring in the first place.

Diet and Nutrition Tips

Here are strategies that may help you pass up the chocolate bar or bag of potato chips you're craving, and keep food aversions to a minimum:

- *Eat breakfast every day* to fuel your body and help prevent hunger and cravings later in the day. Skipping breakfast often sets the stage for overeating at meals and indulging in too many snacks.

- *Eat every three to four hours* to prevent your blood sugar from dropping too low. Make sure you get your between-meal snacks. Choose snacks with protein and carbohydrate; these will give you longer lasting energy. Reach for a low-fat decaffeinated latte, yogurt and fruit, fruit and nuts, whole-grain crackers and low-fat cheese, or an energy bar.

- *Choose a healthy substitute.* If you crave ice cream, have a small bowl of fruit sorbet or low-fat frozen yogurt instead. Or keep a box of fat-free Creamsicles or Fudgsicles in the freezer. If you want chips and salsa, buy baked tortilla chips, rather than the regular deep-fried ones. Replace that chocolate bar with a glass of low-fat chocolate milk. If you're craving cake or cookies, try one of my healthy recipes, such as Farmland Flax Cookies (page 298) or Bodybuilder Cookies (page 297).

- *Sample high-fat foods.* If that craving for junk food is too overwhelming to ignore, allow yourself to have a small serving. Avoid the urge to buy the economy-sized packages.

- *Plate your snacks.* Food cravings play a role in excess weight gain during pregnancy. So if your cravings are too strong to resist, pay attention to how much you are eating. Never, ever, snack out of the bag. When you continually reach your hand into that bag of cookies, you can't get a sense of how much you're eating, and you end up eating far more that you should. Whether your snack is crackers and low-fat cheese, popcorn, or apples slices, measure out the portion and put it on a small plate.

- *Buy good-quality chocolate* in small serving sizes if you think you're becoming a chocoholic. Dark chocolate has antioxidants that may help prevent heart disease. The healthiest chocolate contains 70 percent cocoa solids. High-quality chocolate bars state the percentage of cocoa solids on the label.

- *To avoid triggering an aversion, eat your food cold rather than warm;* warm food usually has a stronger smell, which may cause you to feel nauseated. Instead of grilled chicken and steamed vegetables, try a chicken breast sandwich with spinach leaves and tomato.

- *Drink pure vegetable juice* if the sight of vegetables turns your stomach. You'll get the same nutrients, but in a form that's more palatable. Also eat more fruit, since many contain the same vitamins and minerals found in vegetables.

- *Take a prenatal vitamin supplement* if food aversions are limiting your intake of important nutrients. But keep in mind that a supplement is not a substitute for wholesome foods. When your aversions to healthy foods subside, be sure to reintroduce them in your diet.

Lifestyle Tips

Along with the diet and nutrition tips above, these lifestyle tips can help you manage food cravings:

- *Brush your teeth and gargle with an antiseptic mouthwash* if your cravings have nothing to do with hunger. This works for many of my clients who crave foods and snack endlessly after dinner. Not only does doing so signal the end of eating, but nothing will taste good after you've gargled with a strong mouthwash.

- *Distract yourself* if it is potato chips or other junk food you are continually craving. Take yourself out of the situation for 45 minutes. If you still crave that unhealthy food, allow yourself a small serving.

- *Talk it out.* If your mood swings cause you to turn to food, seek out emotional support from those around you. Let your family and friends know how you're feeling. So often the simple act of expressing pent-up emotions can make you feel much better. And it will help those around you to understand you better.

- *Avoid situations that trigger cravings,* if possible. Instead of passing by the bakery on the way to work every morning, choose a different route. If watching television prompts constant nighttime munching, cancel the cable (seriously). Reading a book works, too.

- *Avoid foods and smells that trigger nausea.* Ask your partner or a friend to cook the meals if preparing foods sets off unpleasant feelings.

Gestational Diabetes

Gestational diabetes is a type of diabetes that develops only in pregnant women. In fact, almost 1 in every 20 pregnant women will develop diabetes for the first time during pregnancy.[7] Diabetes is a medical disorder that disrupts your body's ability to regulate blood sugar by impairing its ability to produce or use insulin, the hormone that converts blood glucose into food or energy. Unlike other types of diabetes, gestational diabetes is not permanent. In 97 percent of women, the condition disappears within a few days of delivery.

Although it's a temporary condition, it is not a disorder to be taken lightly. It can jeopardize both your health and your baby's health. If your doctor tells you that you have gestational diabetes, I strongly advise you to visit a registered dietitian (see Resources, page 304) for nutrition advice and a meal plan.

What Causes Gestational Diabetes?

Like all forms of diabetes, gestational diabetes interferes with your body's ability to process food effectively. Every time you eat or drink, food is passed through your digestive system, where it is broken down into simple sugars called glucose. Glucose is the body's main source of fuel and is used to power most of your bodily functions. Without an adequate supply of glucose, your body simply won't have the energy to operate efficiently.

Once the food has been broken down, glucose is transferred from your small intestine to your bloodstream, where it is carried to your cells to fuel energy and growth. To help your body use the glucose that's in your bloodstream, your pancreas produces insulin. Without insulin, glucose can't pass through your cells' membranes. If your body can't manufacture an adequate supply of insulin, glucose stays trapped in your bloodstream, depriving your cells of the energy source they need for healthy activity. If your body does not produce enough insulin to maintain normal blood-sugar levels, you have diabetes.

During pregnancy, the hormones produced by the placenta can change the way insulin works by blocking the interaction between insulin and glucose. As the placenta grows, it produces higher and higher levels of hormones, making it increasingly difficult for your body to use insulin. This is a problem known as insulin resistance.

Your pancreas compensates for insulin resistance by increasing its insulin production. During the second and third trimesters of pregnancy, hormonal disruptions, coupled with the growing demands of the fetus, can trigger your pancreas to produce up to three times as much insulin as normal.[8] These hormonal changes are a natural part of every pregnancy and usually don't cause any health problems for you or your baby. Gestational diabetes develops only if you have difficulty producing or using all the insulin you need during pregnancy, causing your blood glucose to rise to unacceptably high levels.

How Gestational Diabetes Affects You and Your Baby

Gestational diabetes is usually detected late in your pregnancy, often between the 24th and 28th week of pregnancy. If your diabetes is left untreated, you are at risk of developing:

- Pre-eclampsia or pregnancy-induced high blood pressure
- An increased number of urinary tract infections
- An oversized baby, which may require delivery by Caesarean section

By the time gestational diabetes is detected, your fetus is fully formed but still actively growing. This makes your baby vulnerable to the risks associated with untreated diabetes. As extra glucose builds up in your bloodstream, it crosses the placenta easily, which means that your baby develops high glucose levels, too. This stimulates the baby's pancreas to bring glucose levels back to normal by manufacturing more insulin. Because your baby is getting more energy than it needs to grow, it stores the extra energy as fat. Babies born to mothers with gestational diabetes are unusually large and fat at birth, a condition commonly known as macrosomia. Gestational diabetes exposes your baby to other risks as well, including:

- Shoulder damage (birth trauma), caused by the baby's large size at delivery

- Low blood sugar at birth, caused by the elevated insulin levels

- Prolonged jaundice as a newborn

- Low blood calcium

- Respiratory distress syndrome

Once you've had gestational diabetes, there's a good chance you'll develop it again in future pregnancies. And many women who have gestational diabetes go on to develop type 2 diabetes in their later years. Children born to women with gestational diabetes are also more prone to developing type 2 diabetes, and becoming obese, as they get older.

Symptoms

Gestational diabetes causes few symptoms and may go undetected without proper screening during prenatal exams. If you experience any of the following symptoms, check with your doctor, as they may indicate an increase in blood sugar:

- Increased thirst

- Frequent urination

- Unusual weight loss

- Excessive hunger

- Extreme fatigue or lack of energy

- Blurred vision

- Recurring infections, especially of the skin, gums, and bladder

Who's at Risk?

You are at risk of developing gestational diabetes if:

- You have a close relative with diabetes.

- You are obese (your pre-pregnancy body mass index [BMI] was higher than 29).

- You become pregnant after the age of 25.

- You developed gestational diabetes in an earlier pregnancy.

- You had a baby with a birth defect in an earlier pregnancy.

- You had a baby weighing more than 9 pounds (4 kilograms) in an earlier pregnancy.

- You had a stillbirth or miscarriage in an earlier pregnancy.

- You are of Hispanic, Aboriginal, or African-American descent.

Diagnosis

The Society of Obstetricians and Gynaecologists of Canada recommends testing all pregnant women for gestational diabetes between the 24th and 28th week of pregnancy.[9] Your doctor will screen you for gestational diabetes by administering an oral glucose tolerance test, a simple and relatively painless procedure. First, you will be asked to drink a full glass of a sugar drink. After approximately one hour, a sample of your blood will be tested to determine the sugar (glucose) levels. If your blood-sugar levels are higher than normal, chances are good that you have gestational diabetes. You may be asked to take a second oral glucose test to confirm the diagnosis.

Treatment

Treatment of diabetes involves diet management and exercise. You may also need to monitor your blood glucose level at home.

Registered Dietitians

The cornerstone of diabetes management is diet therapy and, as such, I strongly recommend you consult with a nutrition expert. A registered dietitian is a key member of the diabetes health care team and will help you develop a healthy meal plan tailored to your food preferences, activity level, lifestyle, and insulin requirements (as medication). Research shows that following the advice of a dietitian trained in diabetes management results in significant improvements in blood-sugar control.[10] See the Resources section (page 304) for details on how to find a dietitian in your community.

Meal Planning

Eating consistent amounts of food at regular intervals is important to promote proper weight gain and consistent blood-sugar levels during pregnancy. Your dietitian may develop a meal plan that distributes carbohydrate evenly among your meals and snacks, to prevent large rises in blood sugar. He or she will also explain which food groups and specific foods impact blood sugar the most.

If you do not use insulin, eat smaller meals more often during the day. If you take insulin, you need to carefully control the amount of carbohydrate (from starch, fruit, milk, and sugar) you consume at each meal. How much carbohydrate you eat, and how often, will be determined by your activity level and insulin requirements. Eating a bedtime snack is important to reduce the risk of having a low blood-sugar reaction overnight.

Low Glycemic Index Carbohydrates

Carbohydrate-containing foods provide glucose to your bloodstream. That means starchy foods (rice, bread, pasta, legumes, and potatoes), fruit, sweet vegetables (winter squash, sweet potatoes, carrots, green peas), dairy products, and sweets all impact your blood-sugar level. Both the type and amount of carbohydrate you eat will affect your blood-sugar level.

The term "glycemic index" is used to express the ability of a carbohydrate-containing food to raise blood sugar. Over the years, we have learned that some foods cause your blood sugar to rise quickly (high glycemic index) and others more slowly (low glycemic index). Studies have found that incorporating foods with a low glycemic index value into the diabetes diet improves blood-sugar control by resulting in a gradual rise in blood sugar.[11] Lentils, kidney beans, barley, whole-grain pumpernickel bread, oatmeal, 100 percent bran cereal, whole wheat pasta, yogurt, and soy milk are low glycemic index foods that can help optimize blood-glucose control. Ask your dietitian for a list of low glycemic foods.

Exercise

Moderate exercise becomes even more important when you have gestational diabetes. By following a program of regular physical activity, you can help lower your blood-glucose levels naturally. Exercise reduces the amount of insulin you need to keep blood-glucose levels normal. Even something as simple as taking a short walk after each meal will make a difference. Before you add any strenuous activities to your schedule, speak to your doctor or dietitian; he or she will know how much activity is right for you.

Home Monitoring

You may need to check your blood glucose often during the day to make sure it is at a normal level. (Your doctor will tell you how often to check.) Glucose meters measure the level of sugar in your bloodstream by analyzing a small drop of blood from your fingertip.

These are acceptable blood-sugar levels:

- Fasting (before breakfast) < 5.3 mmol/L

- One hour after a meal < 7.8 mmol/L

- Two hours after a meal < 6.7 mmol/L

If diet and exercise fail to keep your blood glucose within these ranges, especially in the fasting state, your doctor may prescribe insulin shots. However, most women with gestational diabetes are able to manage their condition with diet and exercise and do not require insulin. And most go on to deliver healthy babies.

You should test your urine once or twice a week for the presence of ketones, compounds caused by the breakdown of fat stores. Test first thing in the morning. If ketones in your urine are too high or are present on a regular basis, you may not be eating enough. Your diet many need to be altered, more food may need to be added, or your nighttime snack may need to be changed.

Heartburn (Gastric Acid Reflux)

Heartburn is not pleasant—just ask any pregnant woman who's had it. Heartburn is exactly what the name suggests: a burning sensation behind the breastbone. It tends to start in the pit of the stomach, quickly rising to the throat. Sometimes it can feel as though the food is coming back into your mouth.

Unfortunately, heartburn is a complication that affects as many as 80 percent of all pregnancies.[12] Just like many of pregnancy's discomforts, it's one of those annoying facts of life that you will inevitably encounter on the road to motherhood, usually in the second or third trimester.

What Causes Heartburn?

A small band of muscle surrounds the bottom of your esophagus, the long tube that carries food from your mouth to your stomach. This band, the lower esophageal sphincter, acts like a valve during normal digestion, opening to allow food to pass into the stomach and closing to prevent food and stomach acid from flowing back into the esophagus.

During pregnancy, the hormones that relax the pelvic muscles also relax the esophageal sphincter. Because the muscles no longer close tightly, stomach acid leaks into the esophagus, inflaming the tissues and causing a surprising amount of pain, as well as belching. Heartburn often hits, or is worse, after eating, when going to bed, or stooping over. (When you lie down, gravity helps stomach acid flow backwards out of your stomach.) Sometimes the pain can spread into the upper chest, back, and neck.

Heartburn is irritating and can even be quite painful. But it doesn't pose any problems for you or your baby. Since it goes away as soon as you deliver your baby, heartburn rarely continues long enough to cause any permanent damage to the esophagus.

Heartburn is most common during the last months of pregnancy, when the baby is compressing your stomach and forcing it out of place. Certain foods are more likely to cause acid reflux than others, so you can minimize your symptoms by making simple changes to your diet.

Symptoms

The following are common symptoms of heartburn:

- A burning sensation in your chest after eating a meal, the discomfort worsening when you lie down or bend over

- Pain in your chest that may extend into your neck and arms (sometimes mistaken for a heart attack)

- A sour taste in your mouth or a sensation of food backing up into your throat
- Belching
- Bloating
- Stomach pain

Who's at Risk?

Most pregnant women suffer from heartburn during their third trimester. Women who eat a high-fat diet may be more at risk of developing heartburn than others.

Strategies for Managing Heartburn

Small changes in your diet and your lifestyle can make a big difference when it comes to controlling the discomfort of heartburn. Certain foods can help reduce heartburn by preventing reflux and irritation of your sensitive, inflamed esophagus.

Diet and Nutrition Tips

Avoiding certain types of food can go a long way toward reducing heartburn:

- *Avoid fatty foods.* High-fat foods remain in the stomach longer than low-fat foods and increase the time the esophagus is exposed to the acidic stomach contents. Cream, ice cream, milkshakes, fatty desserts and pastries, gravies, butter, margarine, vegetable oil, fried meats, sausage, cream soups, French fries, and potato chips are often poorly tolerated.

- *Avoid chocolate and coffee.* Chocolate contains the compound methylxanthine, which relaxes the esophageal sphincter and increases the likelihood of reflux. Coffee also relaxes the esophageal sphincter and stimulates acid secretion by the stomach, which can worsen symptoms. If you are drinking that one small cup of coffee each day and are suffering heartburn, it's time to go cold turkey.

- *Avoid spearmint, peppermint, spicy foods, tomatoes, citrus fruit, onions, garlic, and carbonated beverages.* All these can irritate the esophagus.

- *Eat smaller meals more often during the day.* Instead of eating three large meals, eat five or six mini-meals. Too much food (and fluid) in your stomach at one time can add pressure on your esophageal sphincter, increasing the likelihood of heartburn.

- *Drink your fluids between meals,* rather than with meals. And drink slowly. Too much fluid at once can overfill your stomach.

- *Chew gum or suck on a hard candy.* This stimulates saliva, which helps control the release of stomach acid.

Lifestyle Tips

Minor changes in your lifestyle will also help reduce heartburn:

- *Wear loose fitting clothing.* Clothing that's tight around the waist puts extra pressure on your abdomen.

- *Don't smoke.* (Chances are you don't smoke anyway, especially now that you're pregnant.) Smoking increases stomach acid secretion.

- *Avoid exercising immediately after eating.*

- *Avoid lying flat* for one to two hours after eating.

- *Avoid bending or stooping* after eating.

- *Sleep with your head elevated* by raising the head of your bed by 6 inches (15 centimetres). This will help keep stomach acid where it belongs—in your stomach. Put blocks under the legs of your bed or pile pillows under your head to keep your upper body higher than your stomach when you lie down.

- *Try to avoid stress,* which slows down digestion and encourages esophageal reflux; try relaxation techniques to help reduce heartburn.

If these simple strategies don't work, consider taking an antacid to keep your heartburn under control. Not all antacids are safe during pregnancy, so be sure to discuss the options with your doctor before trying any over-the-counter solution.

Hemorrhoids

Hemorrhoids are common during pregnancy, showing up in the second or third trimester. Many women experience them for the first time when they're pregnant.

Hemorrhoids are swollen veins that develop in your anus and lower rectum, similar to varicose veins in your legs. *Internal hemorrhoids* develop in the upper area of the anal canal. They can't be seen and usually cause little discomfort. However, too much straining can push an internal hemorrhoid out through the anal opening, causing it to become irritated and painful. *External hemorrhoids* are swollen, skin-covered blood vessels that form outside the anus. They are itchy and painful and may be felt as a swollen mass near your rectum. They may even cause rectal bleeding.

What Causes Hemorrhoids?

Hemorrhoids tend to develop when the blood vessels in the anal area stretch and swell under pressure. And what causes that extra pressure during pregnancy? You guessed it:

that heavy baby in your uterus. The weight of your baby puts pressure on the pelvic veins that carry blood back to your heart. This slows down the return of blood to your heart, adding extra pressure to your veins below your uterus. As a result, your veins become swollen and dilated. At the same time, the hormone progesterone has a relaxing effect on your vein walls, allowing them to swell. If you stand or sit for long periods, gravity will only make the situation worse.

Constipation can also lead to hemorrhoids, especially if you push and strain during a hard bowel movement. And, of course, nothing causes you to push and strain more than delivering a baby. All that effort puts enormous pressure on the delicate tissues of blood vessels, so hemorrhoids are almost inevitable after birth. I tell my patients that hemorrhoids are an occupational hazard of motherhood!

Symptoms

Symptoms of hemorrhoids include:

- Itching and burning in the anal area
- Pain or discomfort around the anus and rectum
- Slight bleeding from the rectum; rectal bleeding can be a sign of other, more serious medical conditions, so report any bleeding to your doctor, even if you suspect it is a sign of hemorrhoids only.

Who's at Risk?

The very nature of pregnancy puts you at high risk of hemorrhoids. If you have poor bowel habits, become constipated, or stand or sit for long periods, the chances are good that you'll have hemorrhoids before your pregnancy is over. If you have a history of hemorrhoids, you have a higher risk of getting them when you are pregnant.

Strategies for Managing Hemorrhoids

Just because hemorrhoids are common during pregnancy, don't despair. There are several things you can do to either prevent getting them or reduce their symptoms.

Diet and Nutrition Tips

Diet can have a big impact on the management of hemorrhoids. You'll find the following suggestions helpful:

- *Follow a high-fibre diet to prevent constipation.* If your hemorrhoids are the result of straining to have a bowel movement, read the section on constipation in this chapter for tips on how to treat that condition. Make sure your daily diet includes an excellent source of insoluble fibre and plenty of fluids.

- *Add citrus bioflavonoids to your diet.* These natural compounds are found in the inner peel of citrus fruit. When consumed, they help strengthen blood capillaries. Research suggests that a special formulation of two bioflavonoids, diosmin and hesperidin, is effective in reducing the duration and severity of hemorrhoid episodes.[13] Another citrus bioflavonoid, called rutins, may also be useful.

    Although bioflavonoid supplements are sold in health food stores, their safety has not been evaluated in pregnant women. For this reason, it's wise to avoid using amounts greater than those found in foods. Eat one whole orange or grapefruit each day. Grate citrus peel and add to a morning smoothie, muffin and loaf recipes, pancake and cookie batters, and puddings.

Lifestyle Tips

Hemorrhoids can be relieved by implementing a few minor lifestyle changes:

- *Avoid standing or sitting for long periods.* If you sit at a desk all day long, get up and walk around for a few minutes every hour.

- *Elevate your legs periodically* during the day.

- *Sleep on your left side* to help increase the flow of blood back to your heart. Sleeping on your side will also take pressure off the rectal veins.

- *Take a warm sitz bath* for 15 minutes, two or three times a day. Soaking in warm water can really help ease the discomfort of hemorrhoids. A sitz bath (also called a hip bath) is a type of bath in which only the hips and buttocks are soaked in water. Its name comes from the German verb "sitzen," meaning to sit. It is usually taken in a small plastic tub that sits on top of the toilet (available at drugstores), but it can also be taken in a regular bathtub. The bath should be filled with 3 to 4 inches (8 to 10 centimetres) of warm water. Do not add bubble bath or oil.

- *Apply cold compresses* to the anal area to ease pain and swelling.

- *Apply witch hazel or other soothing lotions* to help relieve the itching.

- *Practise Kegel exercises every day.* Tense the muscles around your vagina and anus and hold for 10 seconds before relaxing. Repeat 25 times. This will increase circulation in the rectal area and strengthen the muscles around the anus. (See Chapter 10 for more details on Kegel exercises.)

Hypertension (High Blood Pressure)

It's estimated that between 5 and 10 percent of all pregnancies are complicated by pregnancy-induced hypertension (PIH).[14] Hypertension, or high blood pressure, develops most often during first-time pregnancies. Even mild hypertension can cause serious complications in your pregnancy, putting you and your baby at serious risk, so I can't emphasize enough how important it is to have your blood pressure monitored at each prenatal checkup.

If you don't get prompt medical treatment or manage it properly, hypertension can progress rapidly and may lead to life-threatening conditions such as eclampsia or HELLP syndrome. Hypertensive disorders are responsible for approximately one-third of all maternal deaths in Canada and are a leading cause of fetal mortality.[15] Unfortunately, despite extensive research and medical advancements, this statistic has improved little since the early 1970s.

What Causes Hypertension?

Every time your heart beats, it forces blood through your arteries. Blood pressure is calculated by measuring the amount of force, or pressure, your blood exerts against the walls of your arteries as it circulates through the body. With each heartbeat, the pressure in your arteries rises. This is known as *systolic pressure,* the pressure when your heart muscle is contracting. In between beats, your heart relaxes and the pressure in your arteries falls—this is *diastolic pressure*. Your blood pressure is a measurement of both the systolic pressure and the diastolic pressure in your arteries. For example, a normal resting blood pressure is 120/80. The top number is the systolic reading and the bottom number is the diastolic reading.

When your blood pressure levels are high, it means your heart is working hard to pump blood through your system. If your diastolic blood pressure during pregnancy is consistently 90 mg Hg or higher, you have hypertension. Some women have hypertension before they become pregnant, a condition known as chronic hypertension. However, most women with pregnancy-induced hypertension (PIH) have no history of blood pressure problems. PIH usually develops sometime after the 20th week of pregnancy, and most symptoms go away within six weeks after delivery.

The main hypertensive disorders that occur in pregnancy are pre-eclampsia, eclampsia, and HELLP syndrome.

Pre-Eclampsia

Pre-eclampsia, sometimes referred to as toxemia, develops during the last three months of pregnancy. The main indications of pre-eclampsia are high blood pressure and one or more of the following symptoms: protein in the urine, headache, blurred vision, and intense stomach pain. Other symptoms include swelling or fluid retention (edema). However, it is possible to develop pre-eclampsia and have no obvious symptoms at all. Often pre-eclampsia is detected only through a routine prenatal examination.

Eclampsia

Pre-eclampsia can quickly progress to eclampsia, a dangerous medical condition that causes convulsions and coma. Eclampsia occurs in approximately 1 in 1500 pregnancies and usually develops when pre-eclampsia is either undetected or untreated.[16] It can permanently damage vital organs and may be fatal to you or your baby.

HELLP Syndrome

Approximately 10 percent of all women with severe pre-eclampsia go on to develop HELLP syndrome.[17] HELLP is an acronym for hemolysis, elevated liver function, and low platelet count. Like eclampsia, HELLP syndrome can quickly progress to a life-threatening condition if you don't receive proper treatment for your high blood pressure. This disorder causes abnormalities in your liver and blood and can seriously damage vital organs. If you develop HELLP, you will probably be advised to deliver your baby early, to prevent serious complications in your pregnancy.

How Hypertension Affects You and Your Baby

All types of hypertension restrict the flow of blood through your arteries. Naturally, that means less blood reaches the placenta and uterus, which may restrict your baby's growth and development. If you have hypertension, your baby may be underweight and small at birth.

Hypertension also reduces the blood flow to your kidneys. When your kidneys aren't functioning properly, toxic waste material remains in your system, causing swelling and a buildup of body fluids. (That's why pre-eclampsia is often referred to as toxemia.)

PIH can also put you at risk for placental abruption, a condition that causes the placenta to separate prematurely from the uterine wall. Severe abruption causes heavy bleeding and shock and is dangerous to both you and your baby.

If hypertension progresses, you may experience seizures or convulsions. You could also go into a coma, have a stroke, or permanently damage vital organs, such as your brain, liver, and kidneys. In the most serious cases, hypertension can be fatal to you and your baby.

Symptoms

Hypertension often causes no noticeable symptoms, so you may not discover that your blood pressure is high until you go to your doctor for a checkup. However, symptoms that have been associated with PIH include:

- Excessive swelling of the hands and feet

- Sudden weight gain of more than 1 pound (0.5 kilogram) per day

- Severe headaches

- Drowsiness or dizziness

- Blurred vision, double vision, or flashing lights before your eyes

- Excessive nausea or vomiting

- Severe abdomen pain

- Rapid heartbeat

- Smaller amounts of urine or no urine

- Change in your mental status (e.g., decreased alertness)

Who's at Risk?

Doctors don't really know what causes PIH. But they do know that you are more likely to develop it if:

- You are pregnant with your first child.

- You have a family history of hypertension or pre-eclampsia.

- You have a personal history of chronic blood pressure, kidney disease, diabetes, or lupus.

- You are expecting twins (or more).

- You are younger than 20 years old or older than 35.

- You were overweight before you became pregnant.

According to the Heart, Lung and Blood Institute in the United States, the incidence of pre-eclampsia has increased by nearly one-third over the last 10 years.[18] This may be because more women over 35 are giving birth and multiple pregnancies are becoming more common, two risk factors for pre-eclampsia.

If you develop pre-eclampsia, the chances are good that you'll develop it again in future pregnancies. The risk is even greater for women who developed pre-eclampsia before their 30th week of pregnancy or developed it in a pregnancy other than their first.

Diagnosis

There is currently no test for PIH. The most effective way to diagnose the problem is to have your doctor monitor your blood pressure at each prenatal visit. A urine test can detect protein in your urine, an indicator of pre-eclampsia. If your doctor suspects hypertension, he or she may request additional blood tests to confirm the diagnosis.

Treatment

The only cure for PIH is delivering your baby. But, if your baby is too young to be born safely when your hypertension is diagnosed, your doctor will try to manage your condition with a comprehensive treatment plan. If your blood pressure is 140 to 150 mg Hg (systolic) or 90 to 99 mg Hg (diastolic), it is possible to control blood pressure without medication. If your condition is more severe, your doctor may recommend blood pressure medication.[19]

Calcium Supplements

Observational studies have revealed that women who have higher calcium intakes have a lower risk of developing high blood pressure during their pregnancies. This finding triggered researchers to investigate the effects of calcium supplements on blood pressure in pregnant women. A number of studies have found that taking calcium pills after the 20th week of pregnancy significantly reduces the risk of pre-eclampsia.

When scientists evaluated a number of studies together, they found that calcium supplementation lowered the risk of hypertension by 54 percent.[20] Canadian researchers analyzed the results of 14 studies involving more than 2500 pregnant women and concluded that taking 1500 to 2000 milligrams of calcium lowers blood pressure and reduces the risk of pre-eclampsia by 62 percent.[21]

Based on the evidence, the Canadian Hypertension Society recommends a calcium intake of 2000 milligrams per day to help lower blood pressure in women with pregnancy-induced hypertension.[22] If you have a history of kidney disease or kidney stones, speak to your doctor before taking this much calcium.

To meet your needs for calcium, you should already be consuming 1000 milligrams of calcium each day from your diet (this requires 3 cups or 750 ml of milk, yogurt, or calcium-enriched beverage). And you'll also get about 250 milligrams of calcium from your prenatal supplement. To boost your intake to 2000 milligrams, take a 500-milligram calcium supplement twice daily. But do not take this at the same time as your prenatal vitamin, since calcium inhibits your ability to absorb iron.

Vitamins C and E

These two antioxidants might be helpful in managing blood pressure throughout the second half of pregnancy. Compared with pregnant women with normal blood pressure, it appears that women with pre-eclampsia produce more free radicals, harmful oxygen compounds that roam the body and damage cells. Free radicals are a normal by-product of metabolism, and our bodies have a built-in system of antioxidant enzymes to deal with them. Certain disease states, cigarette smoking, exposure to pollution, even heavy exercise, can increase free radical production. It's thought that free radicals impair the ability of blood vessels to relax and dilate and that this can lead to PIH.

After years of research, we have learned that your body needs a daily supply of dietary antioxidants to help extinguish harmful free radicals. That's where vitamins C and E enter the picture. As antioxidants, these natural substances act as scavengers, mopping up free radicals before they do harm. And it seems that getting more vitamin C and E in your diet can protect you from pre-eclampsia.

Researchers at Harvard University observed that, compared with women who consumed the most vitamin C, those whose diets provided less than 85 milligrams doubled their risk of pre-eclampsia. What's more, those women who got less than 35 milligrams per day had an almost fourfold higher risk for the condition.[23] British researchers studied women at risk for pre-eclampsia and found that taking vitamin C (1000 mg) and E (400 IU) supplements from weeks 16 through 22 of their pregnancies lowered the risk of pre-eclampsia by 75 percent.[24]

During pregnancy you need 85 milligrams of vitamin C each day. Vitamin C–rich foods include citrus fruit and juices, cantaloupe, kiwifruit, mango, strawberries, broccoli, Brussels sprouts, cauliflower, red pepper, and tomato juice. To supplement, take 500 milligrams of Ester C once or twice daily (studies in the lab have found that this form of vitamin C is more available to the body). The daily upper limit is 2000 milligrams.

Your vitamin E requirements don't change when you are pregnant. You should be getting 22 IU each day. Wheat germ, nuts, seeds, vegetable oils, whole grains, and kale are good sources of vitamin E. To supplement, take 400 or 800 IU of *natural* source vitamin E. The daily upper limit is 1500 IU.

Bedrest

If you have hypertension, your doctor will probably prescribe regular bedrest during the remaining months of your pregnancy. Just imagine—someone finally giving you permission to stay in bed all day. It's not as fun as it sounds. You'll probably get bored and want to move around, especially because PIH doesn't make you feel sick enough to stay in bed. But no matter how restless you feel, heed your doctor's advice and stay put.

Your high blood pressure is already restricting the flow of blood to vital organs and, when you stand up, the pressure of your heavy uterus significantly reduces blood flow to your legs. By resting in bed, you take the pressure off the leg veins and increase blood flow to the uterus and kidneys. Your baby needs a good blood supply to the placenta to grow healthy and strong—and you need good blood flow to keep your body functioning normally. Your doctor will probably recommend that you lie on your left side as much as possible to further improve the flow of blood through your arteries.

Exercise

There are conflicting reports about the effect of aerobic physical activity on hypertension in pregnancy. Some researchers suggest that women who exercised regularly before pregnancy were less likely to develop pre-eclampsia, and that exercising during pregnancy may help protect obese women from the condition. But others report that exercise does not alter the risk of getting pre-eclampsia.

While the jury is still out on the value of exercise in PIH, a regular program of gentle exercise is recommended during pregnancy. Before adding any exercise to your routine, check with your doctor to ensure you don't do anything that will worsen your high blood pressure.

Iron Deficiency Anemia

There's no question that iron deficiency anemia is the most common nutrient deficiency during pregnancy. Your increased blood volume, combined with the extra iron required by your developing baby and the placenta, can really take a toll on your iron stores. With all this activity going on, it doesn't take long before the demand for iron outstrips your normal supply.

What Causes Iron Deficiency Anemia?

If your diet and prenatal supplement do not provide enough iron to meet your increased needs, your iron stores will dwindle and anemia may eventually occur. If your diet lacked iron before you conceived, there's a good chance you began your pregnancy with low levels of iron. This naturally increases your risk for iron deficiency, with or without anemia, as your pregnancy progresses.

Your body needs iron to make hemoglobin, the main component of red blood cells that carry oxygen to all your cells and tissues. When you don't have enough red blood cells to transport oxygen to your tissues, your vital organs become starved of the energy they need to perform efficiently. For you, this translates into a lack of energy, loss of appetite, and an inability to work effectively. I've had women tell me that they don't have the energy to get out of bed in the morning or that simple chores, such as washing dishes, can drain them to the point of exhaustion. Severe anemia can also stress your heart and lower your resistance to infection. Even more worrisome, anemia can increase your risk of complications if you lose a lot of blood or require surgery during delivery.

Based on the premise that many women have low iron stores before they become pregnant, Health Canada recommends that women take a low-dose iron supplement of 30 milligrams during their second and third trimesters, in addition to eating a diet rich in iron. You'll get this amount of supplemental iron in a prenatal vitamin supplement.

If your stomach and bowel can't tolerate a prenatal supplement, there's good news. A recent Australian study suggests that even a smaller dose of iron can prevent iron deficiency anemia in pregnancy, without the side effects associated with iron pills. A total of 430 women were given either 20 milligrams of iron (as ferrous sulfate) or a dummy pill from the 20th week of their pregnancies to delivery. At delivery, women in the iron-supplemented group had a 70 percent lower risk of iron deficiency anemia.[25] Such lower dose iron supplements can be obtained over the counter in pharmacies and health food stores.

How Iron Deficiency Anemia Affects You and Your Baby

Your baby's needs for iron will be fulfilled long before yours. Normally, your anemia must be fairly advanced before your baby is seriously affected. However, there is evidence to suggest that even mild anemia can increase your risk of preterm delivery and low birth weight.[26] There's also a slight risk that your baby could be born with anemia or iron deficiency, which could cause developmental problems if not treated quickly.

Symptoms

Symptoms of iron deficiency anemia include:

- Extreme fatigue
- Pale skin and brittle, pale nails
- Light-headedness, dizziness, or fainting
- Headaches
- Shortness of breath
- Heart palpitations
- Cold hands and feet
- Poor appetite
- Susceptibility to infection

Who's at Risk?

You are at risk for developing iron deficiency anemia if you:

- Eat a diet low in iron
- Don't take a prenatal supplement containing iron
- Are plagued with frequent vomiting during your pregnancy

- Have had two or more pregnancies close together

- Are carrying more than one baby

- Had a heavy menstrual flow before conception

- Donate blood more than three times a year

- Are a teenager

Diagnosis

Routine blood tests included as part of your prenatal checkups will indicate whether your iron stores and hemoglobin are low. Fatigue is a natural part of pregnancy, so it's easy to overlook or ignore symptoms of anemia.

Treatment

Once you become iron deficient enough to be anemic, diet alone won't resolve the problem. Usually, your doctor will recommend that you take daily iron supplements throughout your pregnancy to build up your iron reserves. Depending on the extent of your iron deficiency, you will need to take a daily dose of 60 to 120 milligrams.

If you are advised to take an iron pill, take it on an empty stomach to enhance absorption. Most of my clients find that taking their iron supplement before bedtime reduces stomach upset (you sleep through any stomach upset that may occur).

Iron supplements can have a few unpleasant side effects. Iron is well known to cause constipation (refer to the section on constipation in this chapter for effective ways to stay regular). Don't be alarmed if you notice that your stools turn black while you're taking iron; this is quite normal and no reason for concern. If you have a pre-existing gastrointestinal disorder, such as ulcerative colitis, iron can cause complications that you should discuss with your doctor.

I routinely recommend the brand Palafer. I rarely hear a client complain about uncomfortable side effects with Palafer iron. You'll have to ask your pharmacist for this product, since it's kept behind the counter (as are all high-dose iron supplements).

Just because you are taking an iron supplement does not mean you can stop adding iron-rich foods to your diet; it is still important to include good sources of iron in your meals. You'll find a list of iron-rich foods in Chapter 2.

Over the next few months, your doctor will perform more blood tests to ensure that your iron supply has increased to a healthy level. When it comes to iron supplements, more is not better. Too much iron can cause indigestion and constipation. And excessive doses of iron can be toxic, causing damage to your liver and intestines. An iron overload can even result in death. If you have young children at home, keep iron tablets locked away.

Leg Cramps

It's estimated that almost 30 percent of pregnant women suffer from leg cramps.[27] These painful cramps become more frequent in the third trimester, plaguing you most often at night, when you're trying to get much-needed rest. Many of my clients complain that leg cramps wake them from a deep sleep. If leg cramps interrupt your rest, make sure you take time to nap or rest during the day.

What Causes Leg Cramps?

Although there are many theories about what causes leg cramps during pregnancy, so far, no single underlying cause has been found. It's most likely that this painful condition is the result of a combination of factors. Pressure of the baby's head on the nerves in the pelvis may cause the muscle fibres of your leg to fire spontaneously. Pressure from your growing baby also may reduce circulation to the legs, causing blood to pool in your veins and trigger painful spasms. As well, the changes in your weight and centre of gravity in later pregnancy may overtax your leg muscles, producing cramps and muscle pain.

Swelling, increased blood volume, and other physical demands of pregnancy may alter the levels of calcium and magnesium in your system, which is thought to be associated with muscle cramps. And too much phosphorus in your diet (often as a result of eating a lot of processed-meat snack foods or drinking a lot of soda pop), may lead to cramping.

For the most part, leg cramps are more of a nuisance than a health hazard. They may catch you unaware during the day, causing sharp pains that go away fairly quickly. While most leg cramps are harmless, some types of leg pain can signal a serious inflammation of the deep veins of your leg. This condition can be life-threatening, so make a point of reporting all leg pain to your doctor. The easy way to distinguish between ordinary, pregnancy-related leg cramps and dangerous leg pain is to squeeze your calf muscles when you aren't experiencing a cramp. You should feel no pain in your muscles between cramping episodes. If you do feel pain when you squeeze, if the muscle pain is constant, or if you notice any swelling or tenderness in your legs, see your doctor immediately.

Symptoms

Leg cramps can be quite painful and can be worsened by circulation problems in your legs that may occur as your uterus expands, affecting the pressure on blood vessels in the legs. If your muscle pain is constant, rather than just occasional, speak to your doctor. Signs of leg cramps are:

- Sharp, stabbing pains in your calves or feet, especially at night
- Charley horse feeling in the calves

- Cramping in the soles of the feet

- Cramps typically lasting from a few seconds to a few minutes

Who's at Risk?

Since we don't know what causes leg pain, it's hard to identify who is at risk. Too much phosphorous or too little magnesium in your diet may put you at increased risk.

Strategies for Managing Leg Cramps

Based on what little knowledge we have about the cause of leg cramps, the following strategies may decrease their frequency and intensity.

Diet and Nutrition Tips

Increasing certain nutrients in your diet may be effective in battling leg cramps:

- *Boost your magnesium intake.* Evidence suggests that magnesium might be useful for treating leg cramps. Swedish researchers gave 73 pregnant women suffering from leg cramps either a magnesium supplement or a placebo pill for three weeks. They found that, compared with the women not taking magnesium, the supplemented group experienced a significant reduction in leg cramps.[28] A recent British study also suggests that a 300-milligram magnesium citrate supplement can ease nighttime leg cramps (this study was not conducted in pregnant women, however).[29]

    It does make sense that magnesium might help. After all, this mineral is needed for muscle contraction and the transmission of nerve impulses. And it's a nutrient that is missing from many women's diets. Best foods for magnesium include legumes, lentils, nuts, leafy greens, figs, dates, wheat bran, and wheat germ. During pregnancy you need 350 milligrams (19- to 30-year-olds) or 360 milligrams (31- to 50-year-olds) each day. Most prenatal supplements provide 50 to 100 milligrams of the mineral.

    To supplement, try 100 to 150 milligrams of magnesium citrate once or twice daily. Do not exceed a daily total of 350 milligrams of supplemental magnesium; more than this can cause diarrhea. (I have had a few clients who experienced magnesium's laxative effect with less than 350 milligrams.) Be sure to include the magnesium that's in your prenatal supplement in your intake calculation.

- *Consider calcium supplements.* Many people think that leg cramps are caused by a lack of calcium and that calcium supplements will therefore relieve them. So far, there is no strong evidence that dietary calcium is related to muscle cramps. A scientific review of five trials involving 352 pregnant women concluded that the evidence that calcium reduces leg cramps is weak and any improvement was caused by a placebo-effect.[30] But, if you are not meeting your daily calcium requirements (1000 milligrams), reach for a calcium-rich food or supplement to bolster your intake. If your leg cramps disappear, that's great. Just because most women don't respond doesn't mean you won't.

- *Drink plenty of water*—8 to 12 cups (2 to 3 litres) per day to maintain adequate fluid levels.

Lifestyle Tips

In terms of lifestyle, there's not a lot you can do to prevent leg cramps. But there are several ways to alleviate them when they do occur:

- *Flex and point your feet several times* before going to bed at night. This simple exercise limbers the muscles and may prevent cramps.

- *Perform nightly stretching exercises* to prevent leg cramps. Stand about 30 inches (12 centimetres) from a wall and, keeping your heels flat on the floor, lean forward and slowly move your hands up the wall to achieve a comfortable stretch.

- *Keep the bedcovers loose* while in bed to prevent the weight of the covers from causing your toes and feet to point, which causes the calf muscles to contract and cramp.

- *If a cramp strikes, try to stretch it out;* start by straightening your leg, flexing your foot upward toward your knee, or grab your toes and pull them toward your knee.

- *Massage the cramped muscle* with long, steady strokes in the direction of your toes.

- *Put a hot water bottle or heating pad on the painful area* or take a hot bath.

- *Walk the cramp off* by pacing for a few minutes.

- *Include swimming and water exercises in your weekly workout routine;* these will help keep your muscles stretched.

Mood Swings and Emotional Disorders

Pregnant women can be unpredictable emotionally. Lovely stories about pregnant women glowing with happiness and serenity abound. Sure, you'll have many moments of joy as your baby grows and you anticipate the wonderful events of motherhood. However, if truth be told, pregnant women are more likely to be cranky, irritable, tearful, and just a teensy bit irrational as their hormonal overload plays havoc with their emotions.

The worst thing about mood swings is their unpredictability. Little things that normally wouldn't bother you can cause great distress. And something that was not a problem yesterday can be a big problem today. Unfortunately, you may not even realize how quickly your mood changes or how irrational you may seem to those around you. While pregnancy is a happy time in your life, don't be surprised if you don't always feel as happy as you think you should.

Although mood swings are common in pregnancy and are usually nothing more than a minor annoyance, as many as 10 percent of pregnant women become clinically depressed.[31] It's easy to miss a diagnosis of depression because many of the symptoms mimic those of pregnancy. Depression can interfere with your ability to work or carry out your daily activities. And it will certainly diminish the joyful aspects of your pregnancy. If you are having emotional difficulties during your pregnancy, don't keep it to yourself. You need to get prompt medical attention so that the symptoms don't become worse or linger after the birth of your baby.

What Causes Mood Swings and Emotional Disorders?

Mood swings can be caused by many factors. The hormonal changes of pregnancy can have a powerful effect on your emotions. Lack of sleep and changes in your eating habits can also contribute to mood swings. And the new life growing inside you can bring many joys and worries. The social, economic, physical, and emotional changes associated with pregnancy and parenthood may profoundly alter the way you view yourself and the world around you. Coming to terms with these monumental changes can trigger volatile mood shifts and may, in some cases, undermine your emotional well-being.

Fears and anxieties are normal in pregnancy, so you shouldn't feel guilty or blame yourself if you're feeling emotionally vulnerable. Make sure you keep the lines of communication open with those close to you and with your doctor. Talking things over with people who care about you can help you handle the emotional stresses and strains more confidently.

Sometimes, mood swings can progress to more severe emotional disorders, such as depression, generalized anxiety, and obsessive-compulsive disorders. These are serious problems that, if left untreated, may interfere with your ability to care for yourself and your unborn baby.

How Emotional Disorders Affect You and Your Baby

Emotional disorders can depress your appetite and prevent you from nourishing your body properly. You may lose sleep and find yourself unable to concentrate on work or daily activities. Some women become overly anxious and obsessive about the health of their unborn babies, while others go to the opposite extreme and lose interest in their pregnancy altogether. These types of disorders can seriously disrupt the emotional connection, or bonding, that naturally develops as your baby grows in your womb. Researchers believe that emotional disorders, both during and after pregnancy, may have lasting effects on the developing fetal brain, which extend into childhood.[32]

Symptoms

Mood swings can make you feel happy one minute and sad the next. But they generally don't interfere with your ability to work or carry out your daily responsibilities. If mood swings progress to a more serious emotional disorder, you may experience:

- Crying spells for no apparent reason

- Disturbed sleep and fatigue

- Changes in appetite

- Feelings of worthlessness

- Feelings of guilt or anger

- Excessive worries about your health or the health of your baby

- Nervousness or anxiety

- Depressed moods or chronic sadness

- Poor concentration, memory loss, and confusion

- Thoughts of death or suicide

As you can see, certain symptoms of depression are similar to the normal mood changes of pregnancy. That's why it is difficult for your doctor to diagnose an emotional disorder without your help. If you feel some combination of these symptoms every day for over two weeks, talk to your doctor. You could be experiencing a major depression and should get prompt medical attention to minimize the effects of your emotional state on your baby.

Who's at Risk?

Mood swings affect most women at some point in their pregnancy. However, you may be more at risk of developing a serious emotional disorder if you:

- Have a previous history of major depression

- Have a family history of major depression

- Are having troubles in your marriage

- Have recently suffered through a very stressful event in your life

Pregnant women are most vulnerable to emotional disorders in their third trimester. According to reports prepared by the British Columbia Reproductive Mental Health Program, women who are depressed in their third trimester are highly likely to continue their depression during the postpartum period.[33]

Treatment

Mood swings are a normal part of pregnancy and don't usually require any medical treatment. However, if you are feeling sad or depressed to the point where your moods are affecting your quality of life, there are treatments that may help you. Many women suffer needlessly because they are too afraid or embarrassed to admit that they are having emotional difficulties. Don't let those concerns stand in your way; ask for the help you need. Your doctor can put you in touch with people and programs that will help you manage your emotional challenges, both during pregnancy and after your baby is born.

Treatment may be as simple as learning new coping strategies or better ways to draw on your support network of family and friends. Individual therapy or couple counselling can help address problems in your marriage or personal relationships. If you are suffering from a serious emotional disorder, your doctor may also prescribe medications to help improve your mood and give you a more positive outlook on life. There has been a great deal of research in this area and there are antidepressants that are considered safe to take during pregnancy and breastfeeding.

Morning Sickness

Morning sickness refers to the episodes of nausea (and sometimes vomiting) that plague pregnant women, primarily during the first trimester. For some women, morning sickness is the first indication of their newly pregnant state. And for some, symptoms are worse in the morning and improve over the course of the day. But the term "morning sickness" is a misnomer, because it can strike at any time of the day. And sometimes the nausea can last all day long.

If you've managed to get through the first trimester of pregnancy without a single episode of morning sickness, consider yourself one of the lucky ones. It's estimated that about 200,000 Canadian women are affected by morning sickness each year.[34] To put that number into perspective, about 50 percent of all pregnant women suffer from nausea and vomiting—that's a lot of queasy women! Believe it or not, many doctors think morning sickness is a good sign because it means the afterbirth (the placenta and fetal membranes) is developing well.

What Causes Morning Sickness?

Researchers haven't discovered the exact cause of morning sickness, but it likely has to do with the hormonal changes that take place during pregnancy. Nausea tends to peak around the same time your hormones do. One theory suggests that it has to do with a rapid increase in the level of hCG (human chorionic gonadotropin), which overstimulates the part of the brain that controls nausea and vomiting. Increasing estrogen levels may also trigger nausea by causing an enhanced sense of smell and sensitivity to odours. It's also possible that morning sickness is linked to emotional stress and a high-fat diet.

As long as you can keep some food down and drink plenty of fluids, morning sickness shouldn't harm your baby. But morning sickness can become more of a problem if you can't keep any foods or fluids down and begin to lose a lot of weight. Fortunately, only 1 percent of Canadian women suffer symptoms severe enough to endanger their health and that of their babies.[35]

Symptoms

Most women with morning sickness complain of episodes of nausea and vomiting, sometimes accompanied by headaches and dizziness. Symptoms of severe morning sickness include:

- Persistent vomiting after eating or drinking anything, even water

- Weight loss

- Dehydration

- Concentrated, dark-coloured urine

Symptoms usually start around the 6th week of pregnancy and clear up by week 12. By the second trimester, morning sickness is usually gone. There isn't a set time for morning sickness to stop, since each woman is different and each pregnancy is different. An unfortunate 20 percent of all pregnant women continue to suffer from morning sickness for much longer than three months, and some women have to put up with it for the entire nine months of their pregnancy.[36]

If your symptoms seem severe, or you can't keep anything (including fluids) down for 24 hours, see your doctor. If your doctor is not available, make a trip to the emergency room. You may have a condition called hyperemesis gravidarum (HG), a severe form of morning sickness. Women with HG experience unrelenting, excessive nausea or vomiting that prevents proper nourishment. If severe or left untreated, the condition can cause weight loss, dehydration, nutrient deficiencies, metabolic imbalances, and difficulty with daily activities.

If your doctor determines you have HG, preventing and correcting dehydration and nutritional deficiencies are top priorities to promote a healthy outcome for mother and baby. Milder forms of HG are not associated with any harm to the mother or the baby. Women with more severe symptoms that lead to complications, severe weight loss, or prolonged nausea and vomiting are at the greatest risk of adverse outcomes for both mother and baby. The sooner a woman is diagnosed and treated with HG, the more likely she will be able to avoid severe symptoms.

Who's at Risk?

The majority of pregnant women are at risk of developing morning sickness. But experts believe that the following women may be more susceptible:

- Women pregnant with twins or higher multiples

- Women who have suffered nausea while taking birth control pills

- Women who have suffered motion sickness

- Women who have a mother or sister who experienced morning sickness

- Women with a history of migraine headache

Strategies for Managing Morning Sickness

Ask any pregnant woman and she's bound to have a few tips for dealing with morning sickness. Some of my pregnant clients never go anywhere without crackers or rice cakes—the only foods that seem to keep the nausea under control. Below are plenty of tried-and-true strategies to help ease a queasy stomach. Certain strategies may be more successful for you than others.

Diet and Nutrition Tips

Try these diet strategies to help prevent nausea:

- *Eat plain, bland carbohydrates before rising* each morning, to avoid hunger. Keep soda crackers or rice cakes by the bed and nibble on a few about 20 to 30 minutes before getting up. Eat a snack before bedtime.

- *Avoid foods and smells that trigger your nausea.* Have someone else cook meals for you when you feel lousy. You may find you tolerate cold foods, such as a sandwich, better than hot meals. If you don't know what makes you feel sick, evaluate your surroundings. It could be the smell of coffee brewing, the sight of raw food, perfume, patterned carpets, camera angles on television programs, and so on—it might not always be the obvious.

- *Eat several small meals during the day* (every two hours is a good target) so that you are never too full or too hungry. This will help to keep your blood-sugar levels more stable, which may prevent episodes of morning sickness. Don't lie down after you eat. Drink a small amount of unsweetened fruit juice (apple, grape, cranberry) every one to two hours.

- *Choose low-fat protein foods* (lean meat, canned light tuna, chicken breast, eggs, legumes) and easily digestible carbohydrates (fruit, rice, pasta, potatoes, toast, dry cereals).

- *Avoid fried foods and other high-fat foods.* Fatty foods take longer to digest (even longer when you are pregnant), so they will remain in your stomach longer and increase the likelihood of queasiness. Spicy and acidic foods may irritate your stomach and should also be avoided.

- *Drink water or other fluids between meals,* rather than with meals. This will prevent you from feeling too full. Be sure to get your fluids, though. Sip beverages slowly through-out the day. If your morning sickness includes vomiting, sip on drinks such as Gatorade or Powerade. These beverages provide a little bit of carbohydrate along with sodium, potassium, and chloride, electrolytes you lose when you're sick to your stomach.

- *Reach for foods and beverages that calm* an upset stomach—gelatin desserts, Popsicles, chicken broth, herbal teas, sports drinks, and ginger ale (let the ginger ale sit on the counter for 30 minutes to allow some of the gas to escape).

- *Take your prenatal vitamin with food or at bedtime.* Iron in prenatal supplements may irritate the stomach. If changing the time you take your supplement doesn't help, try another brand (see Chapter 7 for information on prenatal supplements). If you have to stop taking your prenatal supplement altogether, don't worry. Your morning sickness will likely subside by the end of the first trimester, just when your iron requirements begin to rise. You should then have no difficulty finding a brand you can tolerate.

- *Consider taking extra vitamin B6.* Studies suggest that vitamin B6 supplements ease pregnancy-related nausea and vomiting, especially severe forms of morning sickness.[37] One study done in the early 1990s found that low-dose B6 supplements improved nausea but not vomiting in early pregnancy.[38] The dose of vitamin B6 used in the studies was 10 to 25 milligrams, three times per day (25 milligrams every eight hours). Look for a low-dose B6 supplement (10 or 25 milligrams) or, alternatively, a low-dose B complex supplement that provides all the B vitamins. Choose a product that supplies 25 milligrams of B6. Do not exceed a daily dose of 100 milligrams.

- *Cook with ginger.* Ginger has been scientifically shown to reduce morning sickness. It's believed that the active ingredients in ginger root, gingerols and shogaols, speed the movement of food through the intestinal tract. Gingerol compounds may also improve appetite and digestion by their ability to reduce stomach acid secretions and increase the release of important digestive aids. Buy fresh ginger root and add to stir-fries and marinades. If you use a juicer, throw in a thick slice of ginger root along with the fruit or vegetables.

- *Use ginger supplements cautiously.* A few studies have found ginger supplements to reduce feelings of nausea in pregnant women.[39] Although the use of ginger during pregnancy is controversial, there is no conclusive evidence that ginger is harmful during pregnancy. You can buy ginger extract supplements in health food stores or pharmacies. The dose used in clinical studies is 250 milligrams, four times per day. If you do take ginger supplements, use them for a short period only and do not exceed 1 gram (1000 milligrams) per day. The effects of long-term high doses of ginger on the growing fetus are not known. (Adding fresh ginger root to meals is safe throughout pregnancy.)

Lifestyle Tips

Implementing a few changes in your daily routine will help reduce morning sickness:

- *Get a good night's sleep and take naps as needed,* since nausea gets worse if you're tired.
- *Keep room temperatures cool* and avoid hot places. If your body is overheated, you'll feel nauseated more easily. Avoid overdressing.
- *Try acupressure wristbands;* some women find they help keep nausea at bay. The bands apply pressure to specific points on the wrist and are often used to ease seasickness. You can find them at drugstores, health food stores, and travel stores.
- *Consider anti-nausea medications,* if nothing else seems to ease your nausea. Ask your doctor which are considered safe during pregnancy. If your case is severe, you may be prescribed doxylamine succinate/pyridoxine HCI (Diclectin), a drug specially for treating nausea and vomiting in pregnancy. According to the Society of Obstetricians and Gynaecologists of Canada, "it is the most studied medicine of its kind in the world" and is considered both safe and effective for managing morning sickness.

Varicose Veins

Varicose veins plague many women, pregnant or not. They develop most often in the legs, appearing on the inside of the leg, the back of the calf, or down around the ankles. During pregnancy you might also develop varicose veins in your vulva or vagina. Varicose veins that appear in your anal area are known as hemorrhoids (managing hemorrhoids is discussed earlier in this chapter).

What Causes Varicose Veins?

Varicose veins are partially inherited as a weakness in the valves of your veins, which pregnancy then overwhelms. They are caused by the increased weight of the baby on your leg and pelvic veins and the relaxing effect of progesterone on the vein walls. The combination of this added pressure and increased elasticity causes the veins to bulge and swell. The increased flow of blood that happens during pregnancy aggravates the problem since the veins must accommodate even more blood volume than usual.

As the veins stretch, they also grow longer. To fit into the same space, the veins begin to twist and bend under the skin, giving them the characteristic snake-like appearance that most women find unattractive.

Unlike hemorrhoids, varicose veins are usually permanent. They don't cause serious medical problems but they can make your legs ache and swell, especially if you stand or sit for long periods. In most cases, they tend to be more of a cosmetic concern than a medical one. Sometimes varicose veins can be signs of circulatory problems. Be sure to let your doctor know if you start noticing varicose veins developing on your legs.

Symptoms

You may not have any symptoms at all with varicose veins. However, common complaints include:

- Enlarged veins that can be seen under your skin
- Swollen feet and ankles
- A dull pressure or aching heaviness in your legs
- Muscle cramps
- Itchy skin near the affected veins

Who's at Risk?

Being pregnant naturally increases your risk for varicose veins. The risk is greater if you have a family history of the condition. You may be even more susceptible if you:

- Were overweight before becoming pregnant
- Gain more than the recommended amount of weight during pregnancy
- Are carrying more than one baby

Strategies for Managing Varicose Veins

A number of lifestyle modifications can help ease the discomfort of varicose veins and prevent the condition from becoming worse. When it comes to nutrition strategies, however, there are few.

Diet and Nutrition Tips

Ensuring your meals contain plenty of fibre may be the best way to reduce your risk of varicose veins through diet:

- *Eat high-fibre foods* such as whole grains, bran cereal, and fresh fruit and vegetables to promote regular bowel function. Research suggests that constipation can contribute to varicose veins. Straining to evacuate small, firm stools puts pressure in the abdominal muscles, which can be transmitted to the veins in the leg. To avoid constipation, make sure your daily diet provides 25 grams of fibre. You'll find lists of fibre-rich foods in Chapter 2 and in the section in this chapter on managing constipation.

- *Drink plenty of fluids* to help your body absorb the fibre from your diet.

- *Avoid excessive weight gain* during your pregnancy.

Lifestyle Tips

These tips will help prevent or alleviate varicose veins:

- *Follow a program of gentle exercise* to improve muscle tone and circulation; walking is a good place to start.

- *Avoid high-heeled shoes and don't wear tight clothes* around your waist, groin, and thighs. Clothing that constricts your upper leg can decrease blood flow and cause varicose veins to worsen or become painful.

- *Lie down and elevate your legs* above the level of your heart. Do this three or four times a day for 15-minute periods.

- *Avoid long periods of sitting or standing.* If your job requires this, change your position frequently.

- *Avoid sitting with your legs crossed.*

- *Purchase a pair of compression or elastic support stockings* if your legs ache, to keep your veins from stretching.

10

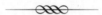

Exercising During Pregnancy: Dos and Don'ts

In the old days, pregnant women were told to put their feet up and take it easy. How times have changed. Today women are encouraged to be physically active during their pregnancies. Many women decide that pregnancy is the perfect time to start exercising. And if you exercised regularly before you became pregnant, it's only natural for you to want to continue doing so now. After all, improving your muscle strength and endurance can help you cope with the physical demands of pregnancy, not to mention labour.

Moderate exercise is safe and beneficial if you have an uncomplicated pregnancy and no serious medical problems. Exercising safely during your pregnancy will not harm you or your baby. If you're new to exercise, you can definitely start becoming active (but not until the second trimester). If you're a workout veteran, go ahead and continue exercising now that you're pregnant. But depending on how hard you exercised before pregnancy, you may need to make a few modifications so you don't overdo it or harm your baby.

No matter how fit you are right now, check in with your doctor first. Whether you were a regular gym-goer or a couch potato prior to pregnancy, talk to your doctor or midwife before you start or continue an exercise program. It's important to make sure you don't have any health conditions that could limit your activity. Keep checking in with your health care providers throughout your pregnancy to get advice on modifying your routine.

Reasons to Exercise During Pregnancy

No doubt you've already heard countless reasons why exercise is good for you. It makes you feel more energetic, it adds strength to your bones, it helps ward off heart disease and certain cancers, and so on. And when it comes to pregnancy, fitness has many additional benefits. Here are a few good reasons to lace up your walking shoes:

- Regular aerobic exercise during pregnancy will help you feel better about your body at a time when it is changing. Researchers have learned that pregnant women who exercise have better body images.[1]

- Regular exercise will boost your sense of well-being and self-esteem. Studies suggest that women who exercise during their pregnancies are less likely to feel depressed and anxious.[2]

- Being in shape can help your body cope with many of the discomforts of pregnancy: backache, muscle cramps, fatigue, and swelling. It can also help you sleep better.

- Being active can help prevent pregnancy-related constipation, hemorrhoids, and varicose veins.

- Regular exercise before and during the first trimester may lower the risk of pregnancy-induced high blood pressure.[3] A recent study out of Seattle reveals that women who engaged in light to moderate activity had a 24 percent lower risk of pre-eclampsia compared with inactive women. Brisk walking cut the risk by one-third.[4]

- Exercising during pregnancy may reduce the risk of neural tube defects in babies of women who did not take a multivitamin before becoming pregnant.[5]

- Being physically fit can speed up your recovery after labour. Exercise that promotes muscle tone, strength, and endurance will make it easier to get your body back in shape. And let's face it: it's a lot easier, both physically and mentally, to get back to exercising after your baby is born if you were doing it before.

When Not to Exercise

As you can see, exercise is an important part of a healthy pregnancy. But in some cases, exercise is forbidden during pregnancy to protect the health of the mother, the baby, and sometimes both. Your doctor will advise against any exercise for the duration of your pregnancy if you have any of these conditions:

- Preterm labour

- Preterm rupture of membranes (the membranes that hold the amniotic fluid rupture before labour)

- Persistent bleeding during the second or third trimester

- Pregnancy-induced high blood pressure or pre-eclampsia

- Evidence of intrauterine growth restriction (the baby's growth is less than excepted for that stage of pregnancy)

- High-order pregnancy (triplets)

- Uncontrolled type 2 diabetes, high blood pressure, asthma, or thyroid disease

- Heart disease

Certain other health problems require your doctor to carefully weigh the risks and benefits of exercise before giving you the green light. If you have one or more of the following conditions, talk to your doctor before starting any type of fitness program:

- Miscarriage or preterm labour in a previous pregnancy

- High blood pressure

- Asthma

- Anemia or iron deficiency

- Eating disorders

- Twin pregnancy after the 28th week

A Safe Exercise Program for Pregnancy

If you didn't exercise on a regular basis before becoming pregnant, it's best to wait until the second trimester to start a fitness regime. If you were physically active before pregnancy, it's fine to start right away. Just don't increase the intensity of your exercise program during the first trimester. This will prevent overheating your baby at a critical time in her development. And avoid strenuous exercise during the third trimester, when the demands of your growing baby are the greatest.

Experts agree that regular exercise is better than sporadic exercise. Short, frequent sessions are healthier than occasional bursts of activity. Once your doctor gives you the go-ahead to exercise, stay committed. Exercise three to five times per week, but don't overexert yourself. Your exercise program should consist of four components: a warm-up, aerobic exercise, strength exercise, and a cool-down.

I also strongly recommend that you consult with a personal trainer before starting a fitness regime. You don't have to belong to a gym to reap the benefits of a personal trainer; many will come right to your home. To consult a trainer in your area, contact the Canadian Personal Trainers Network (see Resources, page 304). Ask for a personal trainer who specializes in prenatal exercise. Tell them your goals, where you live, and whether you prefer a male or female trainer, and they'll set you up with a referral.

Warm-up

Before you jump right into your workout, it's important to begin with a 5- to 10-minute warm-up. This gets your heart, lungs, muscles, and joints ready for exercise so you'll be less likely to get injured. Start by walking, cycling, stepping, or swimming at a low intensity to get your blood flowing and your heart beating a little faster. During the last few minutes of the warm-up, gently stretch the leg muscles that you will be working the most during your aerobic workout. If you work out at a gym, ask a personal trainer to show you how to stretch your quadriceps, hamstrings, hip flexors, and calves. Be sure to inform your personal trainer that you are pregnant.

Aerobic Exercise: Three to Five Times Per Week

Often referred to as cardio exercises, aerobic activities get your heart, lungs, and circulatory system in shape. To improve your health and level of fitness, cardio exercise should involve large muscle groups (e.g., the legs) and should be maintained continuously. When you continuously exercise the big muscles in your legs, they require more oxygen than usual. This challenges your cardiovascular system to deliver more oxygen to your working muscles. Not only do your legs get a workout, your heart and lungs get fit, too.

The most comfortable aerobic exercises for pregnancy are those that don't require your body to bear extra weight. Swimming and stationary bicycling are great and can be continued throughout your pregnancy. Low-impact activities such as walking or aquafit are also well tolerated. Activities involving physical contact or the risk of falling should be engaged in with caution. And any exercises that put you at risk for a lack of oxygen should be avoided.

AEROBIC EXERCISES RECOMMENDED DURING PREGNANCY

Aerobic classes (low-impact)	Stepping
Brisk walking	Swimming
Cross-country skiing	Tennis (if you played before pregnancy)
Jogging (only if you did it before pregnancy)	Water aerobics
Stationary bicycling	

AEROBIC EXERCISES TO AVOID DURING PREGNANCY

Downhill skiing	Horseback riding
Climbing	Scuba diving
Contact sports (basketball, hockey, soccer)	Waterskiing
Hiking at high altitude	

If you're new to exercise, exercise three days per week, gradually working up to four or five times each week in your second trimester. Begin aerobic exercise for 15 minutes. Gradually increase the duration of your workout to 30 minutes. You should not exercise longer than 30 minutes in your target heart rate zone (see below) at any time during your pregnancy.

The aerobic portion of your workout must also include a three-minute cool-down to lower your heart rate and get the blood flowing from your working muscles to the rest of your body. To accomplish this, decrease the intensity level or slow the pace of your exercise.

Strength Exercise: Two to Three Times Per Week

Muscular strength, tone, and endurance are important to your overall health and physical fitness. And now that you're pregnant, strength exercises will help prepare your body for the physical changes you are about to experience. And they'll help get you ready for the work that's required to give birth to your baby. You can get your muscles in shape by using your body weight for resistance (push-ups, abdominals, squats, lunges) or working out with dumbbells, Dyna-Bands, and weight machines at the gym.

There are many different strength exercises that you can do in the comfort of your home—no weights or special equipment are required. All you will need is a floor mat to lie on, a chair to sit on, and a wall to support you. These exercises will condition your body for pregnancy:

- To improve posture and prevent back pain: standing pelvic tilt, upright rowing, upper back and neck stretch, abdominal exercises

- To support your breasts: push-ups, wall push-ups

- To prevent swollen ankles and varicose veins: ankle circles, toe raises, calf stretch

- To maintain bladder control and prevent hemorrhoids: pelvic floor exercises

- To prepare you for childbirth: pliés, quadriceps stretch, hamstring strengthening, hamstring stretch, inner and outer thigh conditioning

Kegel Exercises

Pelvic floor exercises are also known as Kegel exercises, after Dr. Kegel, who created the exercise. Your pelvic muscles are attached to your pelvic bone and act like a hammock, supporting the urethra, bladder, uterus, and rectum. During pregnancy, these muscles become weakened by the weight of your baby and your enlarged uterus. It's important to exercise these muscles, before and after childbirth, to help prevent urinary incontinence and hemorrhoids. What's more, strengthening your pelvic floor muscles will help in vaginal delivery and recovery afterwards.

Just how do you go about working these muscles? First, you need to find the right muscles. Here are three ways to do so:

1. Try to stop the flow of urine when you are sitting on the toilet. If you can do it, you are using the right muscles.

2. Imagine that you are trying to stop passing gas. Squeeze the muscles you would use. If you sense a pulling feeling, those are the right muscles.

3. Lie down and put your finger inside your vagina. Squeeze as if you were trying to stop urine from coming out. If you feel tightness on your finger, you are squeezing a pelvic muscle.

Now that you've found the right muscles, contract them and hold the contraction for up to 10 seconds. Don't hold your breath. Then relax for a count of three. Do this 20 to 30 times a day. But be careful not to tighten your stomach, legs, or other muscles. The beauty of Kegel exercises is that they can be done anywhere, anytime—while you're stretching, reading a book, cooking dinner, or talking on the phone.

Guidelines for Safe Strength Training

Follow these guidelines to ensure you are strength training in a safe manner:

- Warm up with five minutes of light aerobic activity and stretching to get your circulation going and joints moving.

- Exercise in a slow, controlled manner to the point where your muscle is working, but not to excessive fatigue. Avoid abrupt changes in direction and bouncing movements. During pregnancy, your body releases a hormone called relaxin that loosens your joints in preparation for childbirth. Quick, rapid movement can make your joints prone to injury.

- If you use weights, make sure the amount you lift is light.

- Breathe regularly when doing an exercise. Holding your breath can cause changes in your blood pressure and blood flow, which can in turn cause dizziness and fainting. Exhale on exertion and inhale on relaxation.

- Rest for at least one day between strength-training sessions to allow your muscles to recover.

- After the first trimester, avoid exercises that require you to lie on your back, as the weight of the baby may interfere with blood flow to your uterus. Modify these exercises so they are performed on your side, standing, or sitting.

- If you do any exercises on the floor, get up slowly and carefully. Because your centre of gravity changes during pregnancy, getting up too quickly can make you dizzy and increase your risk of falling.

- Do not perform any abdominal exercises if a diastasis recti (separation of the abdominal muscles) develops. To check for a diastasis recti, lie on your back and lift your head off the floor. Feel your abdominal muscles around your belly button area with your fingers. You should feel a hard abdominal wall. If instead you feel soft tissue in between your stomach muscles, you have a diastasis recti. Sometimes you can also see a bulge in the centre of your abdomen.

- Ask a certified personal trainer to show you proper exercise technique to protect your back and joints. A personal trainer also will instruct you on specific exercises and the appropriate amount of weight to use. I strongly recommend that you hire a personal trainer for at least a few sessions.

Cool-down

At the end of your workout, you need to cool down for 10 to 15 minutes to help get your body back to its resting state. Low-intensity calisthenics and gentle stretching will help prevent muscle soreness and increase flexibility. Try to include a few relaxation exercises, such as deep breathing or visualization, in your cool-down.

How Hard Should You Work Out?

Many women find they need to decrease their level of exercise during pregnancy. It's important to not overdo it when you're exercising. Now is not the time to go for the burn, or exercise to the point of exhaustion. Getting too hot from exercise, especially in the first trimester, may harm your baby. So play it safe and don't overexert yourself.

There are a few ways to tell if you're exercising at a safe intensity level. The first one is easy; it's called the talk test. As the name suggests, you are not overdoing it if you can comfortably carry on a conversation while you exercise. If you become winded at all while talking, you need to slow down the pace.

You can also judge your exercise intensity by how fast your heart is beating. According to the Canadian Society for Exercise Physiology, the following heart rate zones are the most appropriate for pregnant women:

TARGET HEART RATE ZONES

Age	Heart Rate Range (beats per minute)	Heart Rate Range (beats per 10 seconds)
Under 20	140 to 155	23 to 26
20 to 29	135 to 150	22 to 25
30 to 39	130 to 145	21 to 24
40 and over	125 to 140	20 to 23

Canadian Society for Exercise Physiology. *Active Living During Pregnancy: Physical Activity Guidelines for Mother and Baby.* Ottawa, 1999.

Remember that pregnancy is physically demanding. Your heart works harder to pump more blood to your tissues and those of your baby. As a result, your heart rate changes during pregnancy. It increases abruptly early in pregnancy and continues to increase moderately in the third trimester. Exercising within your target range ensures that your heart is supplying your body and your baby with oxygen-rich blood. If you are just starting an exercise program, stick to the lower end of your target heart rate range.

You might be wondering how to determine your heart rate during exercise. If you want to spend about $200, you can buy a high-tech heart rate monitor, which consists of a chest band that transmits your heart rate to a wristwatch. But it's a lot cheaper to count the number of times your heart beats in 15 seconds. Just hold two fingers (your pointer and middle finger) to the inside of your wrist or on your neck. Once you find your pulse, look at the second hand of your watch and count the number of beats in 10 seconds, starting at zero. (If you can't find your pulse, ask a fitness professional at the gym for help.) If you multiply that number by six, you'll get the beats per minute.

Another method to determine whether you are overdoing it is called the rating of perceived exertion. This test makes you think about how you feel during exercise—how hard you are breathing, how your muscles feel, and how you perceive your overall exertion. In the 1950s, Dr. Gunnar Borg, an emeritus professor at Stockholm University, developed a scale to quantify the exertion and pain (or lack of it) felt during exercise. Researchers, doctors, exercise physiologists, and sports professionals worldwide now use this rating scale.

BORG'S RATING OF PERCEIVED EXERTION

Exertion	Rating	Exertion	Rating
No exertion	0	Hard	4
Extremely light	0.5	Very hard	5, 6
Very light	1	Extremely hard	7, 8, 9
Light	2	Maximal exertion	10
Somewhat hard	3		

During pregnancy, aim for a rating range of 2 to 3. Experts from Queen's University in Kingston, Ontario, recently reviewed all published studies on pregnancy and exercise dating back to 1966. Their conclusions support the use of Borg's scale, together with your target heart rate zone, as the best way to estimate exercise intensity during pregnancy.[6]

When to Stop Exercising

Listen to your body during each workout. What's comfortable for one woman may not be comfortable for you. The following symptoms are warning signs to stop exercising and call your doctor or midwife immediately:

- Any pain, especially in the pelvic region
- Rapid heartbeat even after resting from exercise
- Severe headache that won't go away
- Dizziness
- Blurry vision
- Shortness of breath beyond what's usual for you during light to moderate exercise
- Excessive fatigue
- Feeling faint
- Vaginal bleeding
- Difficulty walking
- Contractions
- Unusual absence of your baby's movements

Avoid Overheating and Dehydration

Skip your workout, or exercise indoors, when the temperature is hot or the air is humid. Such weather makes you more prone to overheating, and though there's no evidence, this could harm your baby. If your hands are clammy or you experience hot and cold flashes, your body temperature is too high. Stop exercising right away.

To help stay cool, wear loose-fitting, breathable clothing. Layer your workout clothes so they are easy to shed when you work up a sweat. I also recommend you invest in a supportive maternity bra and running shoes that fit properly. If your shoe size changes as a result of swelling, invest in a new pair of shoes.

Be sure to drink plenty of water before, during, and after your workout. Drink water even if you don't feel thirsty. Dehydration can raise your body temperature to a dangerous level, and it may also cause contractions. Use a water bottle at the gym and carry one with you when you're out for a walk. Here's how much water you need to drink:

Fluid requirements for Exercise

Two hours before exercise:

- Drink 2 cups (500 ml) of fluid.

During exercise:

- Start drinking cool fluids early at a rate of 1/2 to 1 cup (125 to 250 ml) every 15 to 20 minutes.
- For exercise sessions lasting less than one hour, plain water is the best fluid for hydration.

After exercise:

- Drink 2 cups (500 ml) of fluid for every pound (0.5 kilogram) you lose during exercise. Weight loss after and exercise session should not exceed 2.2 pounds (1 kilogram).
- A sports drink containing sodium may improve recovery, but it's not necessary as long as sodium is in the foods you eat.[7]

You're now set to enjoy an active pregnancy. Don't forget to consult your health care provider. And keep in mind that exercise increases your calorie needs, so make sure you get those extra 300 calories each day.

Part Three

———⸺⸺———

After Your Pregnancy

11

⊛⊛⊛

Breastfeeding and a Nutrition Plan for Mom (and Baby, Too): 4 to 6 Months

If you're like most women, you probably decided how you were going to feed your baby during the first trimester of your pregnancy, or even before you became pregnant. If you have chosen to breastfeed your newborn, that's great. Breastfeeding offers many benefits to you and your baby. The Canadian Paediatric Society, the Dietitians of Canada, and Health Canada all recommend exclusive breastfeeding for at least the first four months of your baby's life. (The Society of Obstetricians and Gynaecologists of Canada and the World Health Organization recommend exclusive breastfeeding for a minimum of six months.) And experts recommend that women continue breastfeeding (along with complementary foods) for two years or longer.

Today, almost 75 percent of Canadian women report breastfeeding their babies (regardless of the duration). This statistic is certainly up from many of our mothers' generation—the early 1960s—when only 38 percent said they breastfed their infants.[1] When I was born, it wasn't a given that women would breastfeed. My mother's doctor didn't recommend one way or another how she should feed me. Despite this, my mother's decision not to breastfeed her children had mostly to do with the societal norms of the day. Back then, it was taboo to breastfeed in public or even in a group of friends (unless they all agreed it was okay to do so).

It was summertime, and my mom wanted to spend her days with me at the parks and beaches without worrying about where to feed me. So she followed the only piece of feeding advice her pediatrician offered: she fed me canned milk, as opposed to powdered formulas. So I was raised on a homemade formula of evaporated milk—definitely not something recommended today. The formula was provided on a piece of paper, passed from doctor to nurse to new mother.

How times have changed after almost 40 years of research, knowledge, and increased interest in health. Although breastfeeding has always been a healthy and natural way to feed a baby, attitudes have changed. If you decide that breastfeeding is right for you, you'll find it extremely easy to get the support you need every step of the way. How long you breast-feed your baby is a decision only you can make. While many mothers nurse for one year or longer, others stop after six months. Your lifestyle, work commitments, and other factors may enter into the decision. There is no right time to stop breastfeeding. Even if you breast-feed for a short time, your baby will benefit.

Breastfeeding Benefits Your Baby

Breastfeeding provides many benefits to your baby, including protection from infection and prevention of allergies, asthma, and sudden infant death syndrome. Breast milk has also been shown to play a role in the intellectual development of your baby.

Protection from Infection

Many studies have revealed that babies fed only breast milk for the first four to six months are less likely to get respiratory tract infections, ear infections, urinary tract infections, stomach infections, and diarrhea. Some studies even suggest that breastfeeding can protect infants from infections for years after nursing.[2]

Prevention of Allergies and Asthma

Hay fever, asthma, eczema, and food allergies are often referred to as atopic diseases or atopy. Atopic diseases have one thing in common: they're allergic disorders caused by the body eliciting an immune response. This immune reaction triggers the release of massive quantities of chemicals that cause symptoms in the skin, the cardiovascular system, the gastrointestinal tract, or respiratory system.

Plenty of evidence shows that exclusive breastfeeding for the first four months can lower your baby's risk of developing an atopic disorder, especially if you or the baby's father is affected by one.[3] Infants with a parent or sibling with an allergic disorder are at greater risk of developing atopy during infancy or childhood. A review in the *Journal of Pediatrics* of 12 studies found that exclusive breastfeeding reduced the risk of asthma by 30 percent in children without a family history of atopy, and by 48 percent in children with a family history.[4]

Prevention of Sudden Infant Death Syndrome (SIDS)

Sudden infant death syndrome (SIDS) is the sudden and unexpected death of an apparently healthy baby. Typically, a peacefully sleeping baby simply never wakes up, for reasons that remain elusive. SIDS affects 1 of every 750 babies born in Canada. It usually occurs between two and four months of age; it rarely occurs before two weeks or after six months.

It is heartening to know that over the past 15 years, the incidence of SIDS has fallen in Canada, mainly because researchers have identified strategies to help reduce an infant's risk. While one of the most important preventive measures a parent can take is to place the baby on her back to sleep, breastfeeding may also offer protection. A handful of studies have linked breastfeeding to a lower risk of SIDS. American researchers analyzed 23 studies on the risk of SIDS in bottle-fed infants compared with breastfed infants and found that bottle-feeding was associated with double the risk. Nineteen of the 23 studies favoured breastfeeding as a protective measure against SIDS.[5] It's not entirely clear why breastfeeding may cut the risk of SIDS; however, some researchers believe that the immune-enhancing properties of breast milk play a role.

Other studies suggest that compared with formula-fed infants, breastfed babies have lower blood pressure during childhood and adolescence, are less likely to be obese, and have a lower risk of leukemia.[6]

Promotion of Intelligence

Several studies have reported that nutrients in breast milk have a positive effect on intellectual development in childhood. Compared with babies who are not breastfed, those who are breastfed for at least four months score higher on verbal IQ and performance tests. And it seems that the longer a woman breastfeeds her child, the greater the effect. Researchers at the University of Chicago recently reviewed 40 studies on the subject and concluded that breastfeeding does indeed promote intelligence. Many studies measure infant IQ scores at 12 or 18 months of age. Other studies suggest that the positive effects of breastfeeding on intelligence persist into childhood and possibly even adulthood. Danish researchers studied 3250 young adults and found that the longer they were breastfed as babies, the greater they scored on IQ tests at 18 years of age.[7]

Breastfeeding Benefits You

Along with the advantages provided to your baby, breastfeeding provides the nursing mother with several benefits, including possible protection from certain types of cancer.

Bonding with Your Baby

Breastfeeding helps build a special bond between you and your baby. When you nurse, that skin-to-skin contact, cuddling, and holding can help your newborn feel more secure and comforted. Breastfeeding moms may also have increased self-confidence and feelings of closeness with their babies. However, there is no question that the act of feeding your baby—whether breast milk or formula—elicits warm, protective, and powerful emotions in mothers.

Convenience

Breastfeeding saves time and money. There is no buying, measuring, or mixing of formula. And there are no bottles to sterilize and warm. It takes just a moment to provide breast milk to your hungry baby. Breastfeeding is also environmentally friendly.

Getting Back into Shape

Immediately after birth, your baby's sucking causes your body to release oxytocin, a hormone that causes your uterus to contract. This helps shrink your uterus more quickly to its original size and lessens any bleeding a woman may have after giving birth. (Oxytocin also helps initiate the letdown of your milk by causing the tiny muscles around your milk glands to contract and squeeze.)

Breastfeeding burns up calories (as many as 500 per day), so it can make it easier to lose those pregnancy pounds. Nursing for at least five to six months mobilizes fat from your lower body, which can promote weight loss. After the first month, most breastfeeding women gradually lose 1 to 2 pounds (0.5 to 0.9 kilogram) per month, but some lose as many as 4 pounds (1.8 kilograms) each month. But not all women lose weight, and some may even gain a little during breastfeeding.

But be forewarned: breastfeeding alone won't necessarily help you get your pre-pregnancy figure back. Other factors seem to have a greater effect on your total weight loss: your age, your pre-pregnancy weight, and how you gained weight when you were pregnant. And let's not forget that exercise and healthy eating count, too.

Many of my clients report that breastfeeding makes them feel hungry all the time. It is sometimes difficult to lose that last 10 pounds when your appetite kicks into high gear.

Breastfeeding is not the time to diet. Eating too few calories will slow down your milk production and cause you to lose protein, not fat. But don't worry—you will lose the extra weight; you just need to be patient. In Chapter 14, I'll give you plenty of tips for getting your figure back.

Protection from Cancer

It turns out that breastfeeding for the first six months may protect your future health, too. Exclusive breastfeeding (no supplementing with formula) delays the return of ovulation and the menstrual cycle. This prolonged suppression of the menstrual cycle seems to be linked to a lower risk of breast, ovarian, and possibly uterine cancers.

There is evidence that breastfeeding reduces the risk of premenopausal breast cancer, so women with a family history of the disease may especially benefit from nursing. The *Lancet* medical journal recently reported an analysis of 47 studies in 30 countries that included more than 50,000 women with breast cancer and 96,973 women without the disease. The researchers concluded that the longer women breastfeed, the greater the protection from breast cancer. The researchers went on to say that the lack of or short duration of breastfeeding in developed countries is a major contributor to the high incidence of breast cancer in these countries.[8]

What Makes Breast Milk So Special?

The advantages that breastfeeding offers your baby suggest that breast milk contains beneficial substances not found in formula. Breast milk is a complete form of nutrition for infants. Your own milk has just the right amount of fat, sugar, water, and protein, in the right proportions, needed for your baby's growth and development. As your baby grows, the composition of your breast milk changes to meet your baby's changing nutritional needs. And many babies have an easier time digesting breast milk than they do formula.

Breast milk offers your baby a lot more than just important nutrients to grow on. It also provides special antibodies called immunoglobins, which help protect your baby from bacteria and viruses that cause infections. In the early days of breastfeeding, your baby feeds on a creamy high-protein, low-fat milk called colostrum. It is this first milk that's particularly rich with immunoglobins, which bolster your baby's immunity. These special compounds stimulate the growth of friendly bacteria in your infant's intestinal tract to help prevent penetration by potential allergy-causing substances (allergens).

Breast milk also contains two special fatty acids, DHA (docosahexaenoic acid) and AA (arachidonic acid). I discuss in Chapter 7 how these fatty acids, especially DHA, contribute to your baby's brain development in the third trimester. Well, your baby's brain continues to develop during the first few months of infancy. It's thought that DHA and AA in breast milk benefit the mental development and visual acuity of children. While it's true that these fatty acids occur naturally in breast milk, your diet plays an important role in the composition of fat in your milk. In the nutrition advice below, I offer suggestions on how to boost its DHA content.

Tips for Breastfeeding Your Baby

Breastfeeding often takes practice—it doesn't come naturally to all women. It calls for patience, experimenting, and, frequently, asking for help from experienced moms. Some women adjust to breastfeeding easily while others find it difficult to learn. The truth is, breastfeeding can be difficult, frustrating, and heart-wrenching. If you're feeling discouraged, it may help to know you're not alone. Here's my friend Ilda's story.

Breastfeeding was tough with both my children. A fact which came as a shock; I was blown away to discover that breastfeeding hurt. I called a lactation consultant and she gave me a list of things I was potentially doing wrong. My problem, she said, was most probably due to a bad latch. Desperate to learn what a good latch was, I hauled my newborn out to a breastfeeding class. Once there, the nurse helped me achieve a good latch, but much to my dismay, it still hurt. My heart sank. If I was doing it right— why did it hurt so much?

"It still hurts to feed him," I said.

"It shouldn't," the nurse nonchalantly replied and quickly moved on to the next hapless breastfeeder.

I cried all the way home. I was already a failure as a mother. I looked nothing like the serene and smiling mothers pictured with their suckling babes in the parenting books and magazines.

After the breastfeeding class, I went home and railed to my husband. I told him to run to the store as fast as his legs could carry him and get some formula. I was giving up. While he was gone, I called my one and only mommy friend and told her my deep, dark secret.

"I can't breastfeed."

"What do you mean, you can't?"

"It hurts like hell. I'm doing something wrong."

"It's supposed to hurt until your nipples toughen up. It usually gets better after about a week. Just hold on for a few more days. I promise it will get better."

That was all I needed to hear. Why had no one told me that? Epiphany! There was a light at the end of the tunnel. My breastfeeding future was secure.

Breastfeeding will hurt—at first. It takes about a week, but it definitely gets better. I've breastfed both of my children; all I needed was a little hope.

If you feel like giving up, get encouragement and advice from a friend or relative who's experienced breastfeeding. If you don't have friends who nurse their babies, contact your local public health unit; nurses are available to answer questions and give you plenty of advice. They can also direct you to other breastfeeding resources in your community. Talk to your doctor or midwife about any health concerns that may get in the way of successfully breastfeeding.

You might also consult a lactation consultant, who will come to your home (for a fee) to observe you and offer helpful tips. Lactation consultants are certified by the International Board of Lactation Consultant Examiners under the direction of the US National Commission for Certifying Agencies. You can visit its website to find a lactation consultant in your province. Or you might want to visit a La Leche League meeting in your area (see Resources, page 304).

While this chapter is by no means a comprehensive guide to breastfeeding, below are a few tips you might find helpful. Just remember to take it one day at a time.

- *Start within the first few hours of birth.* Your baby is most awake and ready to learn how to breastfeed in the first two hours after birth. Even if your milk hasn't come in yet, put your baby to your breast and let her nuzzle. Your baby has already developed a sucking instinct, so these practice sessions will help both of you begin to learn the mechanics of breastfeeding. Ask a nurse to help get you started.

- *To begin feeding, stroke your baby's lower lip with your nipple.* This triggers the rooting reflex that causes your baby to open her mouth wide.

- *Find a comfortable position* that won't make your back and arms sore. Many women find the cradle position works well, but you may find that another position is best for you. I highly recommend investing in a breastfeeding pillow (or ask for one as a shower gift). This pillow props your baby up to a comfortable position so you can concentrate on the latching-on.

- *Find a quiet, comfortable spot.* The more relaxed you are, the easier it will be to breastfeed. Your milk will flow more freely and easily. Avoid noisy distractions while you and your baby learn to breastfeed.

- *Use both breasts.* Feed with the first breast until it feels soft, then, if your baby is still hungry, offer the second breast. Alternate the side with which you start feeding.

- *Breastfeed often.* In the first month, your baby will breastfeed 8 to 12 times per day, usually every one and a half to three hours. The more often you breastfeed, the more milk you will produce. Breastfeed on demand, whenever your baby shows signs of hunger, such as sucking and licking mouth movements, putting her hands on her mouth, increased body movements, and making small sounds. If you can, try to breastfeed before your baby is too upset and crying loudly. Calming a crying baby will only further delay feeding. Feeding on demand may make your life a little chaotic but, after about a month or two, your baby will establish a feeding pattern.

- *Avoid rushing through feeding.* Don't watch the clock to see how long your baby is nursing. Let her set the pace. Your baby may pause during feeding to look at you or her surroundings. These short breaks don't mean there's a problem with feeding. Breastfeeding is a time to slow down and enjoy the closeness with your baby. When your baby is full, she will let you know. She will simply stop sucking, fall asleep, or let go of your nipple. However, if your baby needs burping, she might turn away from your breast. Try burping her, then wait a few minutes before returning to feeding. If there's no interest, your baby has had enough.

- *Take care of your breasts.* Let your nipples air dry after feeding. During the first few weeks, your nipples may be sore—perhaps very sore. Many women find that applying lanolin ointment to their nipples between feedings helps ease the discomfort. Other women find that using lanolin morning and night helps prevent cracking and bleeding. To deal with the dryness and cracking, one of my clients says she expresses just enough milk after feeding to spread on her nipples. Don't use soap on your nipples, as this causes them to become dry and cracked. A warm shower can go a long way to reducing the discomfort of breast engorgement (hard, lumpy, painful breasts caused by swollen milk glands).

- *Don't give your baby soothers or bottles* until four to six weeks after birth. Giving a soother or bottle before she learns how to breastfeed can cause her to have problems latching on to your breast.

- *Feed your baby only breast milk* for the first four to six months. Breast milk is all your baby needs at this time to grow strong and healthy. Providing extra foods, resulting in your baby not taking as much milk from your breast, will slow down your milk production.

Signs Your Baby Is Breastfeeding Well

If it's your first time breastfeeding, it's not uncommon to wonder if your baby is getting enough milk. Below are a few ways to help you feel confident that she is feeding well.

Can You Hear Deep, Slow Sucking Sounds?

At the start of a feed, your baby will suck quickly. Then, when your milk starts to flow, the sucks will become slower and deeper. During each suck, your baby should pause from sucking while her mouth is open at its widest. This tells you that your baby is drinking your breast milk. You should also be able to hear your baby swallowing. Your newborn should feed at least eight times in 24 hours, and each feeding should consist of at least 10 to 20 minutes of deep, slow sucking.

How Many Wet Diapers and Stools?

Here's a general guide to help you tell if your baby is getting enough milk:

1 day old	At least 1 wet diaper and 1 to 2 sticky dark green or black stools
2 days old	At least 2 wet diapers and 1 to 2 sticky dark green or black stools
3 days old	At least 3 heavy wet diapers and 2 to 3 brown, green, or yellow stools
4 days old	At least 4 heavy wet diapers and 2 to 3 brown, green, or yellow stools
5 days old	At least 5 heavy wet diapers and 2 to 3 stools, more yellow
6 days old	At least 6 heavy wet diapers and 2 to 3 large yellow stools (soft or seedy)

Toronto Public Health. *Breastfeeding Your Baby.* Toronto, 2000.

You might be wondering how heavy a wet diaper should feel. It should feel the same as if you poured at least 2 tablespoons (25 ml) of water on a dry diaper. A heavy wet diaper feels like a dry diaper with 4 or 5 tablespoons (60 to 75 ml) of water. Your baby's urine should be clear to pale and have almost no smell.

After one month, some breastfed babies have many stools each day, while others have one large stool every one to seven days. This is completely normal as long as the stool is soft and your baby is healthy.

How Much Weight Is Your Baby Gaining?

It's normal for breastfed babies to lose 5 to 7 percent of their weight in the first few days after birth. That's because they're born with a store of fat and water that they use up in the first few days of life. By the fifth day, they will start to gradually regain this weight, and by two weeks, most babies are back up to their birth weights. Your baby is feeding well if he gains at least 4 to 8 ounces (113 to 227 grams) per week during the first three months, and at least 3 to 5 ounces (85 to 142 grams) per week from four to six months.

Other signs that breastfeeding is going well include:

- Your breasts are being emptied and feel softer after nursing.

- Your baby has good colour and his skin bounces back after it's pinched (if your baby is dehydrated, his skin will stay puckered briefly after pinching).

- Your baby's mouth is wet and pink.

- Your baby looks relaxed and sleepy after breastfeeding.

Vitamin D Supplements for Breastfed Babies

Vitamin D helps maintain your bone density and helps your baby build strong bones and teeth. Without enough vitamin D, children develop bowed legs when they begin to walk because their weak bones cannot withstand their body weight.

We get vitamin D from two sources: foods and exposure to sunlight. When the sun's ultraviolet light hits the skin, a vitamin D precursor is formed. This compound makes its way to the kidneys, where it's transformed into active vitamin D. But the long Canadian winter means that your skin produces little or no vitamin D from October through March. Even in the summer, you may be making less vitamin D than you think. If you wear sunscreen, its sun protection factor (SPF) blocks the production of vitamin D by as much as 95 percent.

When it comes to foods, best sources for vitamin D are fluid milk (yogurt and cheese don't have any vitamin D), fortified soy and rice beverages, fatty fish, egg yolks, and margarine. Women who don't drink much milk or enriched soy beverage and have little exposure to sunlight are at increased risk for vitamin D deficiency. A baby born to a vitamin D–deficient mother will have limited stores of vitamin D and will be at higher risk for deficiency. Even if you are getting enough vitamin D from foods and sunshine, breast milk is not a reliable source of this important nutrient. And it's likely that your baby is not making much vitamin D from sunlight through protective clothing and sunscreen.

For these reasons, breastfed babies require a vitamin D supplement until their diets provide a source of vitamin D. Give your baby 400 IU (10 micrograms) of vitamin D each day. If you live in a northern community that receives little sunshine during the year, he needs 800 IU (20 micrograms) per day. You can purchase vitamin D supplements as liquid drops from a local pharmacy.

A Nutrition Plan for Breastfeeding Moms

When you are breastfeeding, you are still eating for two, just as you were while pregnant. In fact, during pregnancy your body stored extra nutrients and fat to prepare you for nursing. But you still need to take in more food and nutrients than usual to provide energy for milk production. And you still need to be concerned about how the foods you eat, or beverages you drink, will affect your baby. Here's what you need to know for the first four to six months of exclusive breastfeeding.

Calories

During breastfeeding, you need to consume more calories than at any other time in your life. The first four to six months are the most calorie demanding, since breast milk is your baby's only food during this time. When you gradually introduce solid foods into his diet at four to six months, your milk production will slow down, so your body won't be burning as many calories. This is the time when many breastfeeding moms get frustrated about their weight; if you don't reduce your food intake or add exercise, you will be more likely to gain weight.

For the first four to six months, you need an additional 500 calories per day for milk production. Some of these calories come from the breakdown of your body's fat stores (roughly 170 calories), but the rest must come from your diet. You'll need to eat an extra 330 calories above your pre-pregnancy calorie needs while you exclusively breastfeed.

For most women who maintained a healthy weight before pregnancy, this means following my 2200-calorie meal plan just as you did during the second and third trimesters of your pregnancy. (Refer to the meal plan in Chapter 7.)

You will need to eat more calories if you were underweight before you became pregnant, or if you didn't gain enough weight during your pregnancy. If you fall into one of these categories, increase your daily calorie intake to at least 2500. If you are breastfeeding twins or triplets, your calorie needs will be different. Some experts suggest that mothers of multiples require fewer calories to breastfeed than do mothers of single babies. Ask your dietitian for advice on what's best for you and your babies.

If you were overweight prior to pregnancy, you can follow the 1900-calorie meal plan, though not until six weeks after delivery. Stick to your pregnancy diet for the first six weeks until breastfeeding is well established. After this, you can reduce your calorie intake, but do not let your energy intake fall below 1800 calories per day. Eating less can make you feel tired and dizzy, impair your milk supply, and reduce the amount of immune-enhancing antibodies present in your breast milk.

After four to six months of breastfeeding, you will start introducing your baby to solid foods (you'll find a how-to guide for introducing solids in Chapter 13). During this time, breast milk production slows down and the calorie requirement to maintain your milk supply is slightly less than it was when you were exclusively breastfeeding. You need an additional 400 calories per day, rather than 500. Natural postpartum weight loss usually stabilizes in women after the first six months, which means your body's fat stores don't contribute to your daily calorie requirements. Bottom line: those extra 400 calories must come from your diet.

DAILY CALORIE REQUIREMENTS FOR BREASTFEEDING

The first 4 to 6 months (add 330 calories to pre-pregnancy diet)	Calories
Healthy pre-pregnancy weight	2200
Underweight prior to pregnancy	2500
Inadequate weight gain during pregnancy	2500
Overweight prior to pregnancy	1900

After 4 to 6 months (add 400 calories to your pre-pregnancy diet)	Calories
Healthy pre-pregnancy weight	2300
Underweight prior to pregnancy	2600
Inadequate weight gain during pregnancy	2600
Overweight prior to pregnancy	2000

The information in the table above is a general guide for moms breastfeeding one baby.[9] These calorie levels are good starting points for most women. If you find you are hungry all the time or you are losing more than 1 pound (0.5 kilogram) per week, you're not eating enough. Increase your food intake by 100-calorie increments until you feel comfortable. One serving of fruit, milk, or grains provides roughly 100 calories. Your activity level will also determine your calorie needs. Once you get back to a regular exercise program, you will need to eat more food.

Protein

Protein is the building block for muscles, organs, hormones, enzymes, and immune compounds. Dietary protein from foods such as lean meat, fish, poultry, beans, soy foods, and dairy products is important for you and your breastfeeding baby. You might be surprised to learn that the protein content of your breast milk is relatively constant. In other words, the amount of protein in your diet does not influence the amount of protein your baby gets from your breast milk.

But you do need more protein when you are breastfeeding. Just as in the last two trimesters of pregnancy, you need an additional 25 grams of protein per day. This extra protein is needed to help maintain muscle mass while your body burns extra calories to produce milk. If your diet lacks protein, or you aren't eating enough calories, your body will break down your tissues to maintain a steady supply of protein in breast milk.

As I mentioned in Chapter 7, 25 grams of protein can be found in 3 ounces (90 grams) of cooked lean meat, poultry, or fish (choose low-mercury), or, for vegetarians, from 1 cup (250 ml) of soy milk along with one veggie burger or 3/4 cup (175 ml) of cooked lentils. If you're getting it all from dairy, 25 grams of protein is found in 3 cups (750 ml) of yogurt or milk.

But you needn't worry about adding this food to your meal plan. The 1900- and 2200-calorie meal plans, as well as my 14-Day Meal Plan, all provide you with enough protein for breastfeeding. I've made sure to provide you with adequate calories from protein-rich foods.

Essential Fats

The composition of fats in your breast milk is controlled mainly by your diet during pregnancy and while breastfeeding. That means that the types of fat you eat are the same types of fat your baby gets. In Chapter 7, I encouraged you to boost your intake of foods rich in omega-3 fats to aid in the development of your baby's brain and eyes. (For a quick refresher course on essential fats, turn to that chapter.) These fats play an important role in brain development during infancy. As you can see below, now that you're breastfeeding, you need to include more healthy fat in your diet.[10]

FAT REQUIREMENTS DURING BREASTFEEDING

Type of Fat	Pregnant	Breastfeeding	Food Sources
Omega-3s	1.4 grams	1.3 grams	Oily fish, omega-3 eggs, canola oil, flax oil, walnut oil, flaxseed, soybeans, tofu, walnuts, wheat germ
Omega-6s	13 grams	13 grams	Nuts, seeds, borage oil, corn oil, safflower oil, sesame oil, soybean oil, sunflower oil, meat

To help you meet your requirements for essential fats, follow the same advice I gave you for during your pregnancy:

- Eat oily fish three times per week—salmon, trout, and sardines are good choices.
- Include 1 to 2 tablespoons (15 to 25 ml) of healthy vegetable oil in your daily diet.
- Snack on a handful of nuts and seeds.
- Reach for omega-3-enriched eggs. Each egg has 0.4 grams of omega-3 fat, 10 times more than a regular egg.

Vitamins and Minerals

When it comes to vitamins and minerals, your diet does influence how much your baby gets. This is especially true for water-soluble nutrients such as the B vitamins and vitamin C. If your diet lacks foods rich in these nutrients, your baby's diet does, too.

During breastfeeding, your requirements for certain vitamins and minerals are increased beyond your pregnancy requirements to meet the demands of milk production.

These notable nutrients include vitamins A, B6, B12, and C, and chromium, selenium, and zinc. Make sure you include good food sources of these nutrients in your daily diet. Your requirement for iron drops considerably when you are breastfeeding. Not until you resume menstruating will your iron needs return to 18 milligrams per day.

The table below shows you how much of each key nutrient you need each day and the best food sources for each. If you compare this with the table for pregnancy in Chapter 7, you'll notice two minerals that you didn't see before—chromium and selenium, minerals that play important roles in lactation.

VITAMIN AND MINERAL RECOMMENDED DIETARY ALLOWANCES (RDAS) DURING BREASTFEEDING

Nutrient	Pregnant	Breastfeeding	Daily Upper Limit[a]	Best Food Sources
Vitamin A	2566 IU	4300 IU	10,000 IU	Butter, cheese, egg yolk, milk
Vitamin B6	1.9 mg	2.0 mg	100 mg	Lean meat, poultry, fish, whole grains, avocado, banana, potato
Vitamin B12	2.6 mcg	2.8 mcg	None established	Meat, poultry, fish, dairy products, eggs, enriched soy or rice beverage
Folate	600 mcg	500 mcg	1000 mcg (1 mg)[b]	Kidney beans, lentils, peanuts, artichoke, asparagus, avocado, spinach
Vitamin C	85 mg	120 mg	2000 mg	Cantaloupe, citrus fruit, kiwifruit, mango, strawberries, broccoli, Brussels sprouts, cauliflower, red pepper, tomato juice
Vitamin D	200 IU	200 IU	2000 IU	Milk, fortified soy and rice beverages, egg yolk, oily fish
Calcium	1000 mg	1000 mg	2500 mg	Cheese, milk, yogurt, calcium-enriched soy milk, calcium-enriched orange juice, tofu, almonds, bok choy, broccoli
Chromium	30 mcg	45 mcg	None established	Fish, poultry breast, oysters, legumes (beans and lentils), brewer's yeast, wheat germ, wheat bran, whole grains, molasses, apples (with skin), green peas, mushrooms, spinach
Iron	27 mg	9 mg	45 mg[c]	Lean beef, baked beans, ready-to-eat breakfast cereals, Cream of Wheat, wheat germ, molasses, dried apricots, raisins, prune juice, spinach

Selenium	60 mcg	70 mcg	400 mcg	Salmon, shrimp, oysters, trout, poultry, wheat bran, whole grains, nuts (especially Brazil nuts), legumes, onion, garlic, mushrooms, Swiss chard, orange juice
Zinc	11 mg	12 mg	40 mg	Lean beef, poultry, pork, seafood, oysters, yogurt, wheat germ, baked beans, chickpeas, pumpkin seeds

a. The upper limit refers to the maximum daily intake of nutrient that is likely to pose no risk of adverse effects. Unless otherwise stated, the upper limit refers to total intake from food, water, and supplements.

b. The upper limit refers to folic acid from supplements and fortified foods.

c. Many prenatal supplements contain 60 milligrams of iron, more than the daily upper limit. For many pregnant women, this amount of iron does not cause stomach upset and is well tolerated. As such, it is safe and appropriate to take 60 milligrams of iron during pregnancy to treat or prevent an iron deficiency.

National Academy of Sciences, Institute of Medicine, Food and Nutrition Board, Committee on Nutritional Status During Pregnancy and Lactation, Subcommittee on Dietary Intake and Nutrient Supplements During Pregnancy, Subcommittee on Nutritional Status and Weight Gain During Pregnancy. *Nutrition during pregnancy.* (Part I—Weight gain. Part II—Nutrient supplements.) Washington, DC: National Academy Press, 1990.

Do You Need a Vitamin Supplement?

Your breastfeeding diet will provide all the nutrients you and your baby need (with the exception of vitamin D, as I discussed earlier in this chapter). However, I do recommend that you take an all-purpose multivitamin and mineral supplement each day to ensure you are getting the nutrients you need, especially folic acid and chromium. Vegetarian women may have difficulty getting vitamins D and B12 and zinc from a diet that contains no animal foods, so a multivitamin is an especially wise idea for these women. When it comes to meeting your calcium needs, you must include three servings of dairy or calcium-enriched soy milk in your daily diet. Multivitamins provide only a small amount of calcium, usually not much more than 100 milligrams.

The good news is that you don't need to take those iron-rich pregnancy vitamins any more. While you're breastfeeding, you need only 9 milligrams of iron each day, an amount that's easily obtained from food. (Vegetarian moms need 16 milligrams of iron.) Ask your pharmacist or health food retailer for advice on choosing a brand.

Fluids

You need to drink 8 to 12 cups (2 to 3 litres) of water each day to stay hydrated. It was once thought that women needed to drink a lot of extra fluid to produce enough breast milk. But the most important factor in determining how much milk you produce is how often you nurse. The more often you breastfeed, the more milk you will have. Now experts believe that you need to drink only to meet your normal fluid requirements and satisfy your thirst (breastfeeding can make you feel thirsty). However, if you exercise, especially in warm or humid weather, you do need to drink more. Drink water while you're breastfeeding if you can, in addition to drinking between feedings.

Caffeine

About 1 percent of the caffeine you consume from coffee, tea, colas, chocolate, and certain medications shows up in your breast milk. Because your baby eliminates caffeine from his body more slowly than you do, the drug stays around longer and has the potential to affect your baby. Caffeine is a stimulant, and for a small baby, a little likely goes a long way. Some mothers have reported that caffeine makes their babies more irritable and restless.

Consuming more than 400 milligrams of caffeine, roughly the amount found in three 8-ounce (250-ml) cups of coffee (or one Starbucks grande-size coffee), might affect your baby. It's best to limit yourself to no more than 300 milligrams of caffeine, or two small cups of coffee, each day. You'll find the caffeine content of common beverages in Chapter 2. If you suspect that caffeine is bothering your baby, eliminate it from your diet for one week to see if it makes a difference. And for each cup of coffee you drink, drink a glass of water to offset the dehydrating effects of caffeine.

Alcohol

You may have heard that drinking a beer helps promote the letdown of milk. But there is not a stitch of scientific evidence to support this notion. Even if beer does increase milk production, research suggests that the presence of alcohol in breast milk can decrease the amount of breast milk an infant drinks by 23 percent.[11]

Once you consume alcohol, it passes into your breast milk at a concentration similar to that found in your bloodstream. Although a nursing infant is exposed to only a fraction of the alcohol a mother drinks, newborns detoxify alcohol much more slowly than adults do. Even a small amount of alcohol, consumed regularly, can affect your baby. Drinking alcohol, even in moderate amounts, can impair a baby's motor development and disrupt his sleep patterns. Drinking large amounts of alcohol can impair the flow of breast milk, as well as the growth and development of your baby.

Occasional drinking while breastfeeding has not been linked with overt harm to infants, but the possibility of adverse effects has not been ruled out either. Until a safe level of alcohol in breast milk is established, it is safest to feed your baby breast milk that does not have any alcohol in it. If you plan to enjoy the occasional drink or two, alter your breast-feeding schedule to allow for the alcohol to be cleared from your bloodstream before you nurse. For each alcoholic drink, wait one hour before feeding your baby. If you drink two drinks, wait two hours. If you're out for an evening that entails a few drinks, make sure you store enough breast milk in advance.

Foods that May Upset Your Baby

Many women can eat anything they like without causing any problems in their infant. But occasionally, a sensitive baby may react to something you've eaten. If your baby is experiencing gas and fussiness, this may be a sign that something in your diet is making its way into your breast milk.

Below is a list of foods that could trigger fussiness. If your baby is fussy 4 to 24 hours after you ate the suspect food, remove it from your diet for at least three days. If this pleases your baby, you've probably found the culprit. Sometimes it's just a matter of eating less of the offending food. Try reintroducing a small amount of the food and monitor your child's behaviour.

- Strongly spiced foods containing chili powder, curry powder, cumin, garlic, onion
- Gas-producing vegetables such as broccoli, Brussels sprouts, cabbage, cauliflower, onion, garlic, peppers, turnip
- Citrus fruits such as grapefruit, lemons, limes, oranges, tangerines
- Chocolate
- Milk, soy, eggs, fish, corn, peanuts, nuts

Prevention of Allergies

If you, the baby's father, or one of your children suffers from allergies, your baby has a higher risk for developing an allergic condition such as eczema, hay fever, asthma, or food allergies. To lessen your child's risk for developing an allergic disorder (atopy), it's wise to eliminate highly allergenic foods from your diet while breastfeeding. A recent analysis of three studies involving 210 allergic mothers found that following an antigen-avoidance diet during breastfeeding protected their children from atopic eczema for the first 12 to 18 months.[12]

Common foods that cause an allergic reaction include cow's milk, egg whites, shellfish, fish, wheat, soybeans, peanuts, and nuts. An allergic reaction can occur when some of the food protein is absorbed from the intestine intact instead of being digested into smaller particles as most proteins are. Once the intact protein is in the bloodstream, your body recognizes it as a foreign invader (an antigen). Your body's immune system then produces antibodies to halt the invasion. As your immune system attempts to fight off the antigen, symptoms appear throughout the body. These symptoms include swelling of the lips, stomach cramps, vomiting, diarrhea, hives, rashes, eczema, and wheezing or breathing problems.

If stray proteins enter your bloodstream, they can make their way into your breast milk. The earlier and more often an infant ingests a protein-rich food, the greater the chance it will become an allergen. That's because a baby's immune system is not functional until six months of age, at which time its digestive system can produce its own immunoglobins to defend against foreign substances. An immature intestinal tract is also more permeable to food allergens, meaning they enter the bloodstream more readily.

In infants, reactions to food most commonly involve the gastrointestinal system and include spitting up, diarrhea (watery loose stools in a greater number and volume than usual), cramping, constipation, gas, and poor weight gain. Skin reactions such as eczema, hives, rash, and itching often occur, too.

If your baby is at greater risk for developing an allergy, you might decide to eliminate potential allergens from your diet while you breastfeed. If you go this route, ensure your nutrient needs are met by including other foods in your diet that provide similar nutrients. The biggest concern is that you meet your daily calcium and vitamin D requirements by using an enriched rice beverage or taking calcium supplements with vitamin D added. I strongly recommend that you consult a registered dietitian to help you map out a healthy meal plan for breastfeeding. To find a dietitian in your area, see the Resources section, page 304.

If there is no history of food allergy in your immediate family, there is no need to avoid allergenic foods while breastfeeding.

Detecting Food Allergies

If you suspect your infant is experiencing an allergic response to a food you are eating, try to determine what that food is. Identifying what food, or foods, your baby is reacting to can be a difficult process, but is definitely worth it. Start by keeping a journal of the foods you eat each day, along with notes about your baby's symptoms. Over time, you may see a connection between certain foods and your baby's behaviour.

If an allergy is present, symptoms generally show up in your baby between 4 and 24 hours after you ate the suspect food. Eliminate the suspect food from your diet for at least seven days and see if symptoms improve. If your baby is allergic, you should notice a distinct improvement within one week. To be certain the food is what's causing your baby's distress, reintroduce it into your diet to see if symptoms return. If your baby reacts again, you've found the culprit. You may then choose to limit your intake of that food or avoid it altogether while breastfeeding.

Herbal Supplements and Herbal Teas

As during your pregnancy, you need to use caution in consuming herbs while breastfeeding. Little research has been conducted about the use of herbs during breastfeeding. We do know that certain herbs may have side effects such as nausea and vomiting, others have drug-like effects, and some can cause reactions in your baby. These herbs are unsafe to use during breastfeeding:

Aloe	Coltsfoot	Fenugreek	Licorice
Buckthorn	Comfrey	Feverfew	Pennyroyal
Burdock	Cornsilk	Ginseng	Sassafras
Cascara	Dong quai	Goldenseal	Senna
Chamomile*	Ephedra	Hawthorn	St. John's wort
Cohosh	Eucalyptus	Horseradish (safe as a food)	Yarrow

*Taken as a tea, chamomile probably poses no danger to your baby.

Major brands of herbal teas, those that contain an herb only for essence, and those that do not contain large amounts of an unusual herb are generally safe to drink when breast-feeding. Brew herbal tea so that it's weak, and don't consume more than 2 cups (500 ml) per day.

Medications

Many over-the-counter and prescription drugs are safe to use during breastfeeding. However, you should avoid radioactive drugs used for certain diagnostic tests, such as thyroid scans, and anti-cancer drugs, such as those used during chemotherapy. If you have cancer, you may need to start treatment as soon as possible, which means you'll have to give up breastfeeding. And, of course, street drugs such as marijuana, ecstasy, cocaine, and heroin should be avoided.

Birth control pills that contain estrogen can decrease your milk production if you start taking them earlier than four months after giving birth. Ask your doctor or pharmacist if the prescription you have is for a pill containing estrogen. However, some women report lower milk production when they start any kind of hormonal birth control. If you find your milk production is reduced, speak to your doctor about another form of birth control.

Always remind your doctor, dentist, and pharmacist that you are breastfeeding. While many medications are considered safe, an alternative drug may be available that has lower risks to your breastfed baby. Using short-acting drugs with minimal side effects right after nursing will reduce your baby's exposure to your medication. When in doubt, consult your doctor first.

12

A Nutrition Plan for Formula-Fed Babies: 4 to 6 Months

With all the promotion of breastfeeding these days, it's hard for moms who go the formula route to find good information, let alone get support. Many women have told me that their decision to use infant formula was agonizing and guilt-ridden. Prenatal educators and hospital nurses made them feel that they were terrible mothers for even considering formula-feeding.

One of my clients, Diana, told me about her experience at prenatal class. She asked, "What if a woman doesn't want to breastfeed?" The instructor, surprised that anyone would ask such a question, asked, "Why would anyone not want to?" Diana replied, already starting to feel guilty, "Let's just say they don't." The reply: "I can't imagine someone not wanting to. . . . It would be almost criminal." Women who had made the decision before delivery not to breastfeed told me they were given little or no instruction in the hospital about choosing the right infant formula.

That many women are made to feel guilty about opting to formula-feed is unfortunate. Many women feel vulnerable after giving birth, especially if it is their first baby. They want to do everything that's best for their newborn. Among all the women I talked with while writing this book, it was evident that it was not a lack of love for their babies that prompted their decisions to feed them formula instead of breast milk.

One of my clients, Lisa, recently had a baby boy. During her pregnancy she was diagnosed with gestational diabetes. Even before she learned she had a problem with her blood sugars, Lisa did everything she could to eat the healthiest diet possible and to exercise. Once she was told she had diabetes, Lisa was more diligent than ever about her diet. She wanted to make sure she protected her unborn baby from any potential problems.

Once her son was born, Lisa started him on infant formula. In Lisa's mind, feeding him formula meant that she could return to her normal self more quickly, and feel less tired and irritable, and much happier. She also wanted her husband to participate in their son's feeding. And she believed that on an emotional level, she would be a better mother if she didn't breastfeed. As her dietitian, I respected her decision.

A small number of women can't breastfeed for medical reasons. Other women stop breastfeeding early because it's too painful, or they return to work—depending on the type of job a woman has and how far from home she works, it may be challenging for her to continue breastfeeding. Some women decide to combine formula-feeding with breastfeeding. How you decide to feed your child is a decision only you can make. It is true that breast milk has plenty of benefits formula can't match. But feeding your baby infant formula does not make you a bad mother—far from it.

Which Formula Is Best for Your Baby?

If you choose to feed your child infant formula, you have many choices. Commercial formulas are continually being developed and reformulated to emulate breast milk in as many ways as possible. Some products are based on cow's milk, soy, or protein hydrosylate. Some are enhanced formulas with added essential fats. And then there's the choice between powdered, concentrated liquid, or ready-to-feed. Here's a closer look at the types of infant formulas available today.

Cow's Milk Protein–Based Formulas

(Mead Johnson's Enfalac with Iron/Regular, Nestlé Good Start, Ross Products' Similac Advance with Iron/Low Iron)
This type of formula is the formula of choice for full-term infants with no family history of food allergy. Cow's milk formulas have been extensively altered so that the proportions of carbohydrate, protein, and fat closely mimic breast milk. This alteration also makes these formulas easier to digest than cow's milk.

Cow's milk formulas contain standard recommended amounts of vitamins and minerals, though not all are high in iron. Some are low iron and contain a similar amount of iron to that found in breast milk; others are iron-fortified. Your baby is born with iron stores that can meet her needs until about 4 to 6 months of age. At this time, she needs to get iron from outside sources, such as an iron-fortified formula and iron-fortified cereal. (You'll learn about introducing solids in Chapter 13.) Although a non-fortified formula can meet your baby's needs until around 4 or 6 months of age, it's easy to forget to then switch to an iron-rich formula. That's why the Canadian Paediatric Society recommends using an iron-fortified formula from birth until your baby is 9 to 12 months old.

Lactose-Free Cow's Milk Protein–Based Formulas

(Mead Johnson's Enfalac LactoFree, Ross Products' Similac Advance LF)
These formulas contain the same ingredients as other cow's milk formulas except that the sugar in them comes from corn syrup solids rather than from lactose. They are useful for babies with lactose intolerance, a condition that occurs when a baby lacks lactase, the enzyme that breaks down the milk sugar lactose. Without lactase, lactose cannot be absorbed into the bloodstream and so remains in the gut. Symptoms include stomach cramps, bloating, watery diarrhea, and excessive gas after drinking more than a small amount of milk. Lactose intolerance in babies is rare; only a small percentage are born with the inability to digest lactose.

Sometimes lactose intolerance can occur in infants as a result of an infection or health condition that damages the intestinal lining (the enzyme lactase is located on the lining of the small intestine). Lactose-free formulas may be useful during a period when babies can't tolerate lactose. Once your baby's intestine heals, you can resume using a regular cow's milk formula.

Specialized Cow's Milk Protein–Based Formulas

(Mead Johnson's Enfamil A+)
Since the late 1980s, the inclusion of special fatty acids, DHA (docosahexaenoic acid) and AA (arachidonic acid), in infant formula has been the subject of much scientific research. Evidence shows that these two fatty acids, which occur naturally in breast milk, have important roles in a baby's brain development, visual acuity, and growth.

When you were pregnant, your baby received DHA and AA directly from you via the placenta. After birth, she continues to receive DHA and AA from human milk if you breast-feed. She will also herself make a small amount of DHA and AA from other fats in breast milk or formula. Once your child begins to eat solid foods, she will get them from fish, eggs, and meats.

For years, scientists thought that infants could metabolize enough DHA and AA from other fats to cover their needs. But now research suggests that this is not the case. Some experts believe that the small amount of DHA and AA produced by an infant is insufficient to meet the high demands of the growing brain and nervous system. Randomized controlled trials have revealed that babies fed a formula supplemented with DHA and AA show better mental development and more mature visual acuity at one year of age compared with infants given formulas lacking these fatty acids.[1] One recent study done at Tayside Institute of Child Health at the University of Dundee in the United Kingdom even found that infants fed a formula supplemented with DHA and AA had lower blood pressure at six years of age compared with those given formula without DHA and AA.[2] With the addition of these fatty acids, such infant formulas offer a composition that's more like breast milk, one which may also support cognitive and visual development.

While not all medical and scientific experts agree that such a formula is necessary, DHA- and AA-enhanced formulas are starting to make their way to stores in Canada. In 2003, Health Canada approved the sale of Mead Johnson's DHA- and AA-supplemented infant formula, Enfamil A+. This is an iron-fortified cow's milk formula with DHA and AA at levels recommended by the World Health Organization. The product is available in powder and concentrated liquid. At the time of writing, no other such products were available. However, Ross Products is apparently adding a DHA- and AA-supplemented formula to its Similac Advance line in early 2004.

Soy Protein–Based Formulas

(Mead Johnson's Enfalac ProSobee, Nestlé Alsoy 1, Ross Products' Isomil)
These formulas include the plant protein soy, modified to make it easier for infants to digest. Soy protein–based formulas also have added vitamins and minerals. These formulas are an alternative for babies who have lactose intolerance, who are vegetarian, or who have galactosemia.

Galactosemia is a rare genetically inherited disorder characterized by the partial or complete lack of an enzyme in the bloodstream that breaks down a sugar called galactose. It's treated by removing all lactose- or galactose-containing foods from the diet. These include breast milk, cow's milk, most legumes, and many other foods. Galactosemia is normally diagnosed through a newborn screening test.

Most babies are put on a soy-based formula because of a perceived or real allergy to cow's milk. This is not recommended, since many babies who are allergic to cow's milk are also allergic to soy protein. It's estimated that up to 40 percent of babies at risk for atopic disease (e.g., someone in the immediate family has an atopic disease) are sensitive to soy protein.[3] If your baby is allergic to cow's milk or is at risk for developing atopy, formulas made from a casein hydrosylate or whey hydrosylate are better tolerated (see below).

Protein Hydrosylate Formulas

(Mead Johnson's Enfalac Nutramigen, Ross Products' Alimentum)
These formulas are intended for babies who cannot tolerate intact cow's milk protein or soy protein. The protein molecules are broken down into very small particles, which make for

easy digestion. Two types of protein hydrosylate formulas are available in Canada. Whey-based hydrosylate formulas are less extensively broken down and are most suitable for babies at risk for atopy. Canadian researchers investigated the link between the type of infant formula and risk of atopic disease in infants with a family history of atopy. Infants were given a formula made from whey hydrosylate, cow's milk, or soy. The researchers also evaluated high-risk infants who were breastfed for at least four months. Upon examining the children five years later, those who received breast milk or the whey hydrosylate formula had the lowest risk of food allergy, eczema, and asthma.[4]

Casein-based hydrosylate formulas are more extensively broken down and are the best choice for infants with a confirmed cow's milk or soy allergy. (Both brands mentioned above are casein hydrosylates.) Despite the fact that babies with food allergies better tolerate these formulas, you still should use them with caution. It is possible that highly allergic babies may react to the broken-down protein.

Follow-up Formulas

(Mead Johnson's Enfalac Next Step, Nestlé Follow-Up, Nestlé Alsoy 2, Ross Products' Similac Advance 2, Ross Products' Isomil 2)

These products are marketed as an alternative in the second six months of life, when babies are starting to eat solid foods but before they are ready to drink cow's milk. The Canadian Paediatric Society recommends that cow's milk not be introduced before 9 to 12 months because it is low in iron, too high in protein and sodium, and hard for your baby to digest. Follow-up formulas available are cow's milk protein–based or soy protein–based. These formulas have more calories, protein, essential fats, calcium, and iron than regular cow's milk– or soy protein–based formulas and may offer growing babies nutritional advantages in their second six months of life.

Preparing Infant Formula

Most formulas come in three varieties: ready-to-use, liquid concentrate, and powder. Aside from cost and convenience, there is no benefit in choosing one over another.

Ready-to-use formulas are the most convenient—all you have to do is open the can and serve. But it is also the most expensive option, and you need shelf space for storing all those cans. As well, once you open a can, you must use its contents within 48 hours. *Liquid concentrate formulas* require that you mix equal parts formula and water. While it's easier to use than powdered formula, it's also more expensive. *Powdered formulas* are the easiest on your budget, but they do take a bit more work to prepare, as you'll need to mix the powder with water. The number of scoops and amount of water per serving will depend on the brand. Powdered formulas last for about one month after the can has been opened. Some parents switch from ready-to-feed to powdered formula after the first few months—there's nothing wrong with this.

It may seem tempting to save money by making homemade formula with canned evaporated milk, but this is not recommended. Evaporated milk, whether it's cow's or goat's milk, is nutritionally incomplete. It is low in essential fatty acids and iron, and the iron is poorly absorbed. There's also the risk that if evaporated milk is not diluted correctly, your baby won't receive appropriate amounts of calories, protein, and carbohydrate.

Whichever type and form of formula you choose, proper preparation is essential to protect the health of your baby. All types of infant formulas have directions for preparing and using the formula—make sure you read this information carefully. Incorrectly mixed formula that's either too diluted or too concentrated can be dangerous for your baby.

Newborn babies have an immature immune system and can't fight off germs as efficiently. The following strategies will help ensure your baby is fed safely:

- Always wash your hands before handling the formula or the utensils you use to prepare it.

- For babies under four months of age, sterilize bottles, nipples, lids, measuring cups, and mixing jugs by placing all equipment in a pot of water. The water should completely cover the equipment. Put the lid on the pot and bring the water to a boil. Boil for five minutes. Let water cool, then remove equipment with sterilized tongs.

- For babies under four months, you must boil the water you use to make the formula, including commercially bottled water. Bring the water (cold filtered tap water or bottled spring water) to a rolling boil for at least two minutes. Boiled water can be stored in a sterilized, tightly sealed container for three days in the refrigerator, or for 24 hours at room temperature. Do not use mineral water or carbonated water to prepare infant formula.

- After opening a can of formula and removing what you will use, promptly close the container and seal it tightly.

- Mix powdered or concentrated liquid formulas with the exact amount of water specified. If using powdered formula, fill the scoop and level off any excess with a spoon. Don't pack the powder in the scoop.

- If you are preparing more than one bottle at a time, put the ones you won't use in the refrigerator as soon as they are prepared. Do not leave prepared formula at room temperature for more than one hour. Unused prepared, refrigerated formula must be used within 24 hours.

- Warm chilled infant formula to room temperature by placing the filled bottle in a pan of hot water and letting it stand for a few minutes. It's not a good idea to warm the baby bottle in a microwave, as the heating is uneven and can cause hot spots. If you can't give up the convenience of a microwave, warm the bottle for only a few seconds on low power. Shake the bottle after warming to evenly distribute the warmed milk. Test the temperature by shaking a few drops on your hand; make sure the formula feels barely warm. Never put a warmed bottle back in the fridge. If your baby doesn't finish the formula, throw out the remainder.

- Never put your baby to bed with a bottle; she may choke on the formula.

How Much Formula Should You Feed Your Baby?

It can be difficult to know how much formula your baby needs. How much formula he needs will depend on his age, weight, and whether he's getting formula only or both breast milk and formula. There are a few general guidelines you can follow, but keep in mind that all babies are different. If you're unsure whether your baby is getting enough to eat, ask your pediatrician for advice.

Baby's Weight

For the first four to six months, when your baby is not eating any solids, the general rule is 2 1/2 ounces (70 ml) of formula per pound (0.5 kilogram) of body weight. So if your baby weighs 9 pounds (4 kilograms), he should drink about 22 1/2 ounces (630 ml) of formula in 24 hours.

Baby's Age

The age of your baby also plays a role in how much formula he needs. When your baby is a newborn, you'll give him a small amount several times per day. As your baby gets older, you'll give him more formula per feeding but fewer feedings will be needed. And as your baby begins to eat more solid foods after six months, he'll need less formula. Here's a guide based on your baby's age.

Age	# Bottles Per Day	Amount in Each Bottle	Total Amount in 24 hours
1–2 weeks	6–10	2–3 oz (60–90 ml)	12–30 oz (340–850 ml)
3–8 weeks	6–8	4–5 oz (110–140 ml)	24–40 oz (680–1140 ml)
2–3 months	5–6	5–7 oz (140–200 ml)	25–40 oz (710–1140 ml)

4–5 months	5–6	5–6 oz (140–170 ml)	25–36 oz (710–1020 ml)
5–7 months	5–6	5–6 oz (140–170 ml)	25–36 oz (710–1020 ml)
7–9 months	4	6–8 oz (170–230 ml)	24–32 oz (680–910 ml)
9–12 months	3–4	6–7 oz (170–200 ml)	21–28 oz (600–800 ml)

Manitoba Health. *Milk … Your Baby's First Food: Infant Formula.* Manitoba, 2001.

Growth spurts will also make your baby hungrier and increase his demand for formula. These typically occur when a baby is two to three weeks, six weeks, and three months. The bottom line: needs and appetites vary from baby to baby. Your own baby's needs will change from day to day and from month to month. It's important to learn his hunger cues (see Chapter 11) and let him be your guide.

Fruit Juices and Other Beverages

A formula-fed baby doesn't need anything but formula for the first four to six months of life. It is not necessary to give your baby fruit juice, vegetable juice, or water. Feeding a baby fruit juice can interfere with his intake of nutrient-rich formula or breast milk. Because fruit juice contains fructose and sorbitol, drinking too much can cause diarrhea, poor weight gain, and failure to thrive.

Giving fruit juice in a bottle is also linked with dental cavities and nursing bottle syndrome. Nursing bottle cavities occur when a baby is allowed to fall asleep with a bottle in his mouth. If the bottle contains a fermentable carbohydrate (like the sugar in soda pop, juice, or milk) and the liquid is allowed to pool around the teeth, the normal bacteria that are present will form acid, eventually leading to tooth decay. Newly erupted baby teeth are not completely hardened and decay more easily. Decay usually starts between the ages of one and four years. The first sign is discolouration of the teeth.

And, of course, soda pops, fruit punches, and sports drinks have a high sugar content and lack important nutrients. Caffeinated drinks, herbal teas, as well as soy and rice beverages, fortified or not, also should never be given to a baby. Because soy and rice beverages do not contain enough protein or calories for infants to grow on, they should not be introduced until after the age of two.

13

⚬⚬⚬

Introducing Your Baby
to Solid Foods: 4 to 12 Months

It's time to bring out the bib and splat mat: introducing your baby to new tastes and textures can be messy. But it's an important part of your child's development—introducing solids stimulates your child to learn how to move things around in her mouth. Every step of the way, you're helping your child develop new motor skills that will allow her to feed herself regular fare.

There is no specific age at which you should introduce solids into your baby's diet. Experts do agree, however, that the transition to solids should not occur before the age of four months. During the first four months, breast milk or formula provide all the calories and nutrients your child needs. Introducing solids too early can increase the risk of infections and allergies since your baby's immune system is still developing. And because solid foods interfere with the absorption of iron in breast milk, introducing solids to a breastfed baby before she is ready can increase the risk of iron deficiency.

It is also important not to introduce solid foods too late—that is, beyond six months. Doing so can result in feeding problems and nutrient deficiencies. Babies may learn to prefer fluids and refuse to progress to foods with different textures.

The time to move on to solids is sometime within the four to six month range. Exactly when depends on your baby's physiological maturation and developmental readiness. All babies develop at different rates. Some are ready for their first spoonful of cereal at four months whereas others are not ready to swallow until the six-month mark. There are a few clues that indicate your baby is ready. Your baby—

• Can sit up alone or with support

• Can hold her head up

• Has doubled her birth weight

• Shows lack of interest in food by keeping her mouth closed and turning her head away

• Makes chewing motions; as she learns to swallow, you may notice less drooling.

• Shows an interest in what you're eating by reaching for food

• Shows an interest in foods by watching the spoon, opening her mouth for the spoon, closing her lips over the spoon, and swallowing

Your Baby's First Foods

4 to 6 Months

The first food to introduce is a *single-grain, iron-fortified cereal*. Because your baby's intestinal tract is still developing and is more susceptible to taking in foreign proteins, it's important to introduce single foods. Offer rice cereal first, then barley or oatmeal. All infant cereals are iron-fortified and play an important role in preventing iron deficiency at a time when your baby's iron stores are running low. Once you know that single grains are tolerated, you can introduce mixed-grain cereals.

Mix the cereal with breast milk or formula. It should be runny. Start with 2 to 3 teaspoons (10 to 15 ml), then progress to 2 to 4 tablespoons (25 to 60 ml) of cereal, twice daily. At first your baby will eat very little cereal. Just be patient and remember he's learning new skills. Use a rubber-tipped spoon to protect your baby's tender mouth (do not feed your baby cereal from a bottle). Continue to feed your infant breast milk or formula on demand.

7 to 9 Months

During these months, your baby's eating and motor skills are progressing. His lips will begin to move while chewing, and he'll begin chewing up and down. He'll play with his spoon and may even help you direct the spoon to his mouth. He will be able to hold his own bottle and will be ready to feed himself foods such as crackers and soft pieces of toast.

Your baby should be eating close to 1/2 cup (125 ml) of iron-fortified cereal each day before moving on to other foods. Continue to feed breast milk or formula on demand.

As your baby's diet expands in these few months, you can expect the number of feedings to decrease slightly. As you gradually add foods to your child's diet, he should be eating 2 to 4 tablespoons (25 to 60 ml) of iron-fortified cereal twice daily. At this point he is ready for cereal that's thick, rather than runny.

Introduce solid foods slowly, one at a time. Add one new food every three to seven days. Introduce single foods first and combination foods last. Not only does this help your little one get used to a new taste and texture, but introducing foods slowly, one at a time, will help you identify any allergic reactions.

After cereal, the next foods to add are *single vegetables and fruit*. Although not proven, it's a good idea to introduce vegetables first so your baby doesn't get stuck on the sweet taste of fruit. If you buy baby food, avoid combination vegetable and meat dinners. Your baby's introduction to meat comes later. Start by offering a few tablespoons of puréed vegetables in the same meal as cereal. Gradually progress to 4 to 6 tablespoons (60 to 90 ml) of soft, mashed vegetables each day (about 2 tablespoons, or 25 ml, at lunch and dinner).

When it comes to fruit, offer puréed cooked fruits or very ripe mashed fruit such as banana. Again, start slowly and progress to 6 to 7 tablespoons (90 to 100 ml) per day (about 2 tablespoons, or 25 ml, at breakfast, lunch, and dinner). By the time your baby reaches 7 to 9 months, you can offer a small amount of fruit juice from a plastic cup. But go easy; offer no more than 4 ounces (125 ml) per day. Unsweetened fruit juice is not necessary, but it can add variety to your baby's diet.

The next food group to introduce is *meats and alternatives,* including puréed meat, poultry, fish, cooked egg yolk, mashed tofu, and well-cooked mashed legumes. If there's a history of any food allergy in your immediate family, hold off on fish and tofu and other soy foods until after your baby is one year old. These protein foods have the potential to cause an allergic reaction. Egg white contains so many different proteins, it should not be given to *any* child until after the age of one, to minimize the chance of an allergic reaction. Work up to 1 to 3 tablespoons (15 to 45 ml) of meats and alternatives per day, offered at one meal, either lunch or dinner.

You can also introduce *dairy products* at this time. Your baby is not ready to drink cow's milk, but he can try yogurt, cottage cheese, or grated hard cheese (try lighter tasting cheeses first such as Monterey Jack, colby, and mozzarella). Yogurt is a great way for your baby to get calcium and the friendly bacteria that keep his intestinal tract healthy. Because your baby's energy needs are high, buy yogurt with 3.25 percent milk fat or higher. Low-fat dairy products should not be introduced until after the age of two. Aim to incorporate 1 to 2 tablespoons (15 to 25 ml) of calcium-rich dairy in your child's daily diet.

Feel free to add other grain products to your child's menu. Dry (unbuttered) toast and unsalted crackers are good items to start off with.

10 to 12 Months

Now your baby is really starting to fine-tune his eating skills. He'll start to make rhythmic biting movements and lick his lips. By this age, your child will be able to hold his bottle well, pick up foods with his fingers or palm, and put foods in his mouth. It's an exciting developmental time in your child's life, but it's also a time that requires careful supervision to ensure he doesn't put an unsafe food in his mouth.

As your baby has become ready to chew, he's ready to move from mashed soft solids to soft, minced, or diced table foods. It's a new world of textures that will help your baby master his eating skills and become interested in more foods. By 10 to 12 months, your child should be eating three meals and two snacks each day. Here's a food guide to help you feel confident you're giving your child enough to eat (these are general guidelines only):

- Breast milk, on demand or about three to four formula feedings in 24 hours
- Iron-fortified cereal at breakfast. For variety introduce other plain cereals, bread, rice, and pasta. About 8 to 10 tablespoons (125 to 150 ml) in total per day.
- Mashed or diced cooked vegetables, about 6 to 10 tablespoons (90 to 150 ml) per day
- Soft fresh fruit that's peeled and seeded, or canned fruit packed in water and diced, about 7 to 10 tablespoons (100 to 150 ml) per day
- Minced or diced cooked meat, fish, chicken, turkey, tofu, beans, or cooked egg yolk, about 3 to 4 tablespoons (45 to 60 ml) per day
- Plain full-fat yogurt, cottage cheese, or other cheese, about 2 to 4 tablespoons (25 to 60 ml) per day.

Introducing Cow's Milk

Provided your baby is eating a variety of different foods, including iron-rich foods such as fortified cereal, meat, fish, legumes, and egg yolk, you can introduce your baby to homogenized (3.25 percent milk fat) cow's milk after 9 months. However, many experts recommend waiting until after the first year of life to minimize the potential for an allergic reaction. If you're breastfeeding, there's no need to add cow's milk now. If you're feeding your baby formula, you might decide you're ready to switch. In this case, feed your child three to four small servings per day.

If you're raising your child to be vegetarian, *do not* substitute a soy or rice beverage for formula. These products do not have enough calories or protein to meet the demands of your growing child. Continue to feed him a soy protein–based formula until the age of two. In the meantime, here are a few creative ways to get him enjoying tofu:

- Offer as a finger food: cut firm tofu into small bite-sized cubes and dust with crushed cheerios, wheat germ, or crushed graham crackers.

- Blend silken or soft tofu with a banana, applesauce, or pears and wheat germ, and spoon-feed.

- Mash firm or soft tofu with cottage cheese to make a sandwich spread, or spoon-feed.

- Blend silken tofu and add soft fruits to create a fruit smoothie.

Preventing Allergies

When it comes to preventing food allergies, eczema, and asthma, there are some foods you might want to hold off introducing until after your child's first birthday, especially if your child was not breastfed. I've already mentioned that you must not offer egg whites until after one year—that's a must-not for every child. Other potentially allergic foods include cow's milk (as mentioned above), nuts and nut butters, soy foods, wheat, corn, fish, seafood, and citrus fruit. If there is an allergy in your baby's immediate family (e.g., you, the baby's father, or a sibling), I recommend that you wait one year before you gradually introduce these foods into your child's diet.

Symptoms of food allergy include stomach pain, diarrhea, vomiting, coughing, wheezing, breathing problems, hives, rash, and eczema. Most allergic reactions to food are relatively mild. But occasionally an allergic reaction can be severe and potentially life-threatening, a condition called anaphylaxis. Anaphylaxis occurs when an offending food causes several parts of the body to experience reactions at the same time—hives, swelling of the throat, and difficulty breathing. If not treated immediately by an injection of adrenalin, this severe form of food allergy can be fatal.

It's rare for a baby to be allergic to more than two or three foods. Most allergies that occur in infants are to milk, eggs, peanuts, nuts, soy, fish, and wheat. If you suspect your baby is reacting to a food, eliminate it from his diet for one to two weeks to see if the symptoms go away. Treatment involves avoiding the food, but keep in mind that many food allergies disappear as your child gets older. For this reason, it's important to rechallenge by offering the offending food at periodic intervals. However, do *not* rechallenge if your child had an anaphylactic reaction to the food. Allergies to peanuts, nuts, wheat, fish, and seafood are the most severe and tend to be lifelong. After your child turns one year old, your doctor can perform a skin-prick test or a blood test known as RAST (radioallergosorbent test) to diagnose a food allergy. If your child is allergic to a number of foods, I recommend that you consult a registered dietitian to help you plan a nutritionally adequate diet.

Laying the Foundation for Healthy Eating Habits

Offer your baby healthy, nutritious snack foods to help set the stage for his future eating habits. Forgo the cookies and junk food. Offer him a small piece of soft fruit or vegetable, a small piece of cheese, well-cooked pasta, unsalted crackers, or a small serving of yogurt instead. There's no need to encourage your child to prefer unhealthy foods.

Don't add sugar or salt to your baby's foods. He doesn't need either. Many commercial single baby foods don't have any salt or sugar added. However, some brands of cereals, dinner combinations, and commercial baby food jars of fruits do, so read labels carefully. And be sure to avoid any commercial baby food that lists hydrogenated vegetable oil on the ingredient list, as this type of oil lacks essential fatty acids.

Making Your Own Baby Food

Every mother wants to feed her baby nothing but the best. With the range of commercial products on the shelves today, including organic offerings, meeting your baby's nutritional needs has never been easier. But many mothers view making homemade baby food as a nutritious and economical option. It also means that your baby can sample a greater variety of foods, including some of those you're enjoying, as long as they're prepared without salt, spices, sugar, or extra fat.

Using standard kitchen equipment, such as mashers, graters, strainers, forks, blenders, and food processors, foods can be prepared in a variety of textures according to your baby's need. Freeze single portions in ice cube trays covered with plastic wrap or in plops on a cookie sheet, then transfer to freezer bags. Label and date each bag.

Here are general guidelines to get you started.

Fruit and vegetables:

- Choose top-quality seasonal produce or unsweetened frozen fruit and unsalted frozen vegetables without added sauces. Do not use canned vegetables; they are laden with sodium.

- When possible, choose organic produce to minimize your infant's exposure to pesticide residues.

- Carefully wash, peel, and remove seeds or pits from produce.

- To preserve vitamins, steam or poach vegetables in a scant amount of water in the microwave or on the stovetop. Mash with a fork, put through a strainer, or purée in a blender or food processor with a small amount of liquid (use the water you cooked with to add back lost vitamins).

- Soft, ripe fruits such as bananas do not need to be cooked.

- To prevent browning of fruit, add a little bit of lemon juice to the purée. The ascorbic acid (vitamin C) aids in the prevention of oxidation reactions that discolour fruit.

Meat, poultry, fish, and alternatives:

- Cook meat, poultry, and fish until well done by baking, poaching, steaming, or boiling in a small amount of water or unsalted vegetable broth. Cook fish until it flakes easily.

- Cook egg yolks until well done.

- Purée in a blender or food processor. Grind the meat first (make sure it's cold) until it's clumpy—no bigger than 1- to 2-inch (2.5- to 5-centimetre) chunks. Then add water, fruit or vegetable water, or natural juices as the liquid.

- When your baby is ready for more texture, mash with a fork or masher rather than puréeing.

Keeping Your Baby's Foods Safe

Babies are less immune to bacteria that enter their digestive tracts than are older children and adults. So it's important to prepare and handle your baby's foods with care to prevent food poisoning. Follow these basic guidelines:

- Wash your hands thoroughly and dry them with a paper towel or clean dishtowel before handling any food.

- If you're making your own baby food, make sure all the equipment you use has been properly cleaned before starting. That includes cutting boards, utensils, and containers to cook, purée, and store the food in.

- Refrigerate or freeze all baby food, whether homemade or store-bought, until you use it. Homemade baby food should be refrigerated or frozen immediately after making it; prepared baby food should not be left to sit at room temperature for longer than one hour.

- Refrigerate homemade foods for only two to three days—no longer.

- Thaw frozen portions of baby food in the fridge or in the microwave at low setting; never thaw at room temperature.

- Use leftover jarred fruits and vegetables within three days. Meats have a shorter shelf life—use the leftovers within two days. If your baby doesn't finish his meal, throw out the leftovers.

- Do not refreeze any baby food that's been thawed.

- When buying commercial baby food, always make sure the safety seal button in the centre of the lid is not broken. The seal should pop up when you open the jar; if it doesn't, throw the food away.

- Never feed your baby food straight from the storage container. Saliva that gets mixed in with the contents can cause the food to spoil quickly. Dish out what you will use, seal the jar, and store the rest in the fridge.

Honey and Eggs: Two Foods to Avoid

Two foods pose a particularly high risk to babies: honey and eggs. Honey may contain *Clostridium botulinum* spores that increase the chance of botulism food poisoning. For this reason, do not give your baby honey, or foods containing honey, until after one year of age.

Eggs are a risk factor for salmonella food poisoning. Sometimes these bacteria can be transferred from infected hens directly into the eggs before the shells are formed. Chances are, you're careful not to eat foods with raw eggs anyway. But your baby must not be fed any raw eggs, or any foods that contain them (no Caesar salad!). Always cook egg yolks before feeding them to your child.

Microwaving Your Baby's Food

Using the microwave is a fast and convenient way to heat your baby's foods. But, a word of warning: because microwave heating is uneven, hot spots can occur in the food, which can then burn your baby's lips and mouth. If you use a microwave, warm food to body temperature by heating for just a few seconds on low power. Stir thoroughly to even out the temperature. Test the temperature of the food on your hand before feeding it to your baby.

Tips for Feeding Success

Introducing your baby to new foods can be challenging at times. Some days your baby won't be in the mood for anything new, her food ending up on the floor. Feeding your baby solids requires patience and perseverance. Here are a few tips that might help her accept a wide variety of foods:

- Offer new foods when your baby is hungry, but not too hungry. Make sure she's seated comfortably in a room free from distractions.

- Initial refusal of new tastes and textures is common. But don't give up. It may take as many as 10 offerings before your baby accepts a new food. Offer the food for three days in a row. If it's still rejected, wait two weeks before trying again. Some parents find their children are more likely to accept a new food if there's only one or two types of food on the plate.

- When offering a new food, start with a small serving size—about 1 to 3 teaspoons (5 to 15 ml) at a time.

- Don't force-feed. If your child is full or not interested, call it a day. Forcing your baby to eat can promote negative feelings about a food and may contribute to overweight.

- Don't bribe or reward your child with food. Use sweets in moderation. Avoid the "no dessert until you clean your plate" mentality. This only suggests to your child that dessert is better than meat and vegetables.

Choking and Gagging

Babies and toddlers can easily choke and gag on foods. While some gagging is normal when new foods are introduced, choking must be prevented. The first step is making sure you supervise your child while she's eating. She should eat sitting upright and not lying down, walking, or running. Eating in the car is off limits too: if your baby chokes while you are driving, it may be difficult to pull over to the side of the road and help her. What's more, she might choke on a food if you have to come to an abrupt stop.

The size, shape, and consistency of the food are the most important factors associated with infant choking. Unsafe foods are those that do not easily dissolve in your child's saliva and can easily block her airways. Foods that are hard, small and round, smooth, or sticky should be avoided. Below is a list of foods your child should not eat until she has enough teeth to chew foods thoroughly.

These foods are considered unsafe to feed to a baby, as they may cause her to choke:

- Apple pieces, raisins, dried cranberries
- Grapes, cherries, berries, unless cut into bite-sized pieces
- Raw carrots, unless grated
- Fish with bones or dry, flaked fish, such as canned tuna
- Hot dogs or veggie dogs, unless diced
- Whole kernels of corn and popcorn
- Nuts and seeds
- Potato chips and pretzels
- Dry flaked cereals (choose O-shaped, low-sugar dry cereal)
- Hard candies

- Marshmallows

- Peanut butter, unless it is spread thinly on a cracker; never serve your baby peanut butter with a spoon

- Snacks using toothpicks or skewers

As you work your way through the feeding stages I've outlined above, your little one will come to enjoy her meals at the table with you. Even if your child eats before you or the rest of the family, include her at the table to stimulate her interest in food. Offer her a piece of cooked vegetable to munch on. By the age of one, your growing child should be eating a wide variety of the foods listed in Canada's Food Guide, in addition to iron-fortified infant cereal and breast milk or formula.

As your child grows and expands her repertoire of tastes in the years to come, continue to offer a steady diet of healthy foods in age-appropriate serving sizes. And most importantly, be a good role model. Make sure your child sees you eating all those healthy foods, too.

14

⚛

Getting Your Figure Back:
Nutrition Strategies
for Weight Loss

Most new moms are anxious to return to their pre-pregnancy weight soon after having their babies. Although the first 20 pounds come off relatively easily, those last 10 or 15 are often stubborn. You need to be patient: you can't expect the weight to come off overnight. After all, it took 9 months to gain those pregnancy pounds. Count on it taking 12 months to return to your pre-pregnancy shape.

For the first six weeks after childbirth, don't even think about cutting back your calories. Having a baby and taking care of a newborn is physically demanding. Let's face it—it's hard work. The first six weeks is your time to regain strength and stamina after the strain of pregnancy and labour. Eating too little can deprive your body of the nutrients and energy it needs to recover. If you had a Caesarean delivery or complications, your recovery may take longer. And the first six weeks is an important time for you and your baby to establish breastfeeding. Whether you breastfeed or formula-feed your newborn, wait at least six weeks after delivery before reducing your calorie intake.

Weight Loss During Breastfeeding

It is possible to lose weight when you're breastfeeding, provided you do so gradually by following a healthy diet and exercising moderately. Most breastfeeding moms lose about 2 pounds (0.9 kilogram) each month, naturally, during the first six months. Some women say they drop twice this each month. However, when the time comes to introduce solid foods into your baby's diet, your milk production slows down. For many women, this means that natural weight loss comes to a halt. This is the time when you might need to downsize your portions and step up activity in order to take off those last few pounds.

Here is a general guide to help you lose weight slowly, without affecting your milk supply or zapping your energy level. (You'll find all the meal plans you need, with corresponding calorie levels, at the end of this chapter.) Since no two women's metabolisms are alike, it may take fine-tuning to get it right.

- For the first six weeks, stick to the 2200-calorie guide I discuss in Chapter 11. This is adequate for most women who were at a healthy weight before pregnancy. If you were underweight prior to pregnancy, or you didn't gain enough during your pregnancy, you may need to eat more calories.

- Stick to this plan for the first four to six months, until you introduce your baby to solid foods. You should be losing 2 to 4 pounds (0.9 to 1.8 kilograms) each month.

- If, after three months, your weight has not changed, follow the 1900-calorie meal plan. And now's the time to add in exercise (more on that later). Don't forget to keep drinking plenty of water to stay hydrated. It is important that you don't eat fewer than 1800 calories each day. Doing so can impair your milk production and drain you of much-needed energy.

- At four to six months, when you introduce your baby to iron-fortified infant cereal, drop your intake to 1900 calories if you have not already done so. Monitor your weight once a week.

- At six to nine months, as your baby's diet expands to include other foods, gradually reduce your calorie intake to 1600. Monitor your weight once a week.

- If you find your weight comes to a standstill, it's time to take a look at your activity level. Are you getting regular, moderate-paced exercise at least four times per week? How quickly are you pushing that stroller? If needed, bump up your exercise level. Monitor your weight for the next four weeks.

- To get those last few pounds off, you may need to follow my 1200 to 1400 calorie plan, especially if you're not physically active.

Advice for Moms Who Aren't Breastfeeding

If you are not breastfeeding, follow these guidelines:

- For the first six weeks, stick to the 2200-calorie plan while you recover and regain your strength.

- After six weeks, reduce your intake to 1600 calories and monitor your weekly weight. Aim to lose 4 to 6 pounds (1.8 to 2.7 kilograms) per month.

- If, after three months, you find that the extra weight isn't coming off, add in moderate exercise four times per week.

- If, after four months, your weight is still stuck, follow the 1200 to 1400 calorie meal plan. And keep exercising.

While you're losing weight, follow the nutrition tips in Chapter 2. Drink plenty of water each day, take a multivitamin and mineral supplement, and make nutritious food choices—you need to restock the nutrient reserves that were used up to support your pregnancy. If you're having difficulty losing your pregnancy weight, consult a registered dietitian, who can customize a healthy weight loss plan for you (see Resources, page 304).

Tips for Successful Weight Loss

There are various reasons why people overeat. Chief among them is an inaccurate perception of what constitutes a one-serving portion.

Size Up Your Portions

Believe it or not, many of us don't know what a serving size is. We've become so used to eating super-sized portions that we've lost touch with what an appropriate serving is. I call this phenomenon portion distortion. American researchers recently studied 16,000 people and the amount of food they consumed at a single serving. Not surprisingly, they found that often the portion an American eats exceeds a Food Guide serving size. French fries are often consumed at almost two and a half servings at a time (10 French fries equals a Food Guide serving of potatoes). By eating a baked potato, most people were eating two or three servings at one sitting. And with pasta, most people were getting about three or four servings on any one eating occasion.[1]

You'll find a range of plans for safe, steady weight loss at the end of this chapter. For each calorie level, I tell you how many servings from each food group you should eat each day, and what constitutes a serving size (also see page 303 for a guide to serving sizes). It is a good idea to measure your foods, at least for the first week. Get to know what 1/2 cup (125 ml) of rice or 1 cup (250 ml) of pasta looks like on your plate. Learn to identify a 3-ounce (90-g) piece of meat. Don't worry; you won't have to measure out portions of foods forever, though it's not a bad idea to refresh your memory every once in a while—portions can easily creep up in size.

A few tricks of the trade will help you practise portion-size self-defence:

- *Buy small packages of food.* Bonus-size boxes of cookies, crackers, pretzels, and potato chips may be a deal at the store, but they encourage overeating. If you resist the more-for-less way of thinking, you'll end up eating less.

- *Serve smaller portions at mealtimes.* If you sit down to a plate overflowing with food, the chances are good that you'll finish it. Most of us have a tendency to clear our plates, a habit rooted in childhood. If you don't serve yourself at dinner, instruct whoever does to put less food on your plate.

- *Use smaller plates.* A few of my clients find this trick really works. Instead of filling a dinner plate with food, they serve less food on a luncheon-sized plate. And guess what? The plate looks full.

- *Plate your snacks.* Never snack out of the bag. When you continually reach your hand into that bag of mini-rice cakes or pretzels, you don't get a sense of how much you're eating, and you end up eating far more than you should. Whether your snack is crackers and low-fat cheese, popcorn, or apples slices, measure out your portion and put it on a plate. And then pay attention to the fact that you're eating.

Get in Touch with Hunger and Satiety

Ideally you should eat when you feel hungry—when your stomach growls, telling you it needs food. Stomach hunger should not be confused with mouth hunger, the desire for food because it will taste good. Eating in response to how good food looks or smells has to do with your appetite, not your hunger.

Some of my clients report never feeling hungry during the day. Yet they eat anyway, either because "it's time to eat" or "the food was there." If you're out of touch with how hunger feels to you, eat according to a schedule for the next two weeks. Eat breakfast, lunch, and dinner at approximately the same time each day. You'll find that you will start to feel hungry before your meals.

Pay attention to your hunger signals and let them dictate how much you eat. When you sit down to a meal, rate your hunger on a scale of 1 to 10—1 being so full you couldn't possibly eat and 10 being ravenously hungry. Halfway through the meal, rate your hunger again. Let your score tell you whether it's time to stop eating.

Learning to stop eating when you feel full can also help you eat less. Feeling full does not mean feeling stuffed. Satiety means that you no longer feel hungry and that, in fact, you feel good. Keep in mind that it doesn't take much to feel satisfied. Sometimes all you need is a small snack to keep hunger at bay.

Recognize What Causes You to Overeat

There are other reasons for eating than just hunger. Some people eat because they feel sad, angry, or bored. Others eat because people around them are eating. And still others reach for the wrong foods simply because those foods are in front of them. It is not within the scope of this chapter to deal with the psychology of eating; however, an important first step is recognizing that these triggers may be part of the reason you are struggling with your weight.

- If negative emotions trigger overeating or binging, I recommend that you seek counselling to help you work through these issues before you embark on a weight loss program.

- If you succumb to unhealthy foods because they surround you, get rid of them. There's a lot to the saying "Out of sight, out of mind." Many of my clients keep a bowl of fresh fruit front and centre at home and at the office.

- If you mindlessly eat because you're not paying attention, take charge. Become aware of the foods you put in your mouth by eating without distractions. Turn off the television or put down the newspaper, and sit down to eat. Watch as the food leaves your plate and makes its way to your mouth. How many times have you eaten while distracted, only to look down at your empty plate, unaware that you had actually finished your meal? Savour each mouthful. You'll feel more satisfied after a meal and won't be inclined to search the cupboards for that elusive something you still crave.

  Recently, a new mom who was having a real battle losing her pregnancy weight came to consult with me. She constantly munched throughout the day, partly because she was bored and partly because food was always within reach. I asked her to keep a notepad on the kitchen counter and record each time she reached for a snack. The first day she kept track, she was shocked to learn that she mindlessly munched 12 times. This awareness was all it took for her to cut out the unnecessary eating. She allowed herself only one planned snack between meals and was able to return to her pre-pregnancy weight.

- If socializing triggers overeating, make a plan. In social settings, people tend to eat more. Eat a snack before you go out so you don't arrived famished. Curb your alcohol intake; alcohol, especially on an empty stomach, can cause food cravings. Plan to sit beside someone you can talk with during the meal. The more talking you do, the less you'll eat. And here's a word of advice—pay attention to the amount of food you eat compared with your male friends. Often I see women who, over time, end up eating the same portion sizes as their male counterparts.

Exercise Advice for New Moms

I hope you were able to put my advice in Chapter 10 on exercising to good use during your pregnancy. If you did exercise your way through pregnancy (at least until your bulging belly got in the way), it will be much easier for you to return to fitness now. But let your body heal first. In the first six weeks after giving birth, take it easy. If you had a Caesarean delivery, you will need to wait until your stitches heal before you do exercise that uses the stomach muscles. At six weeks, it's a good time to discuss with your doctor your plans for getting back to exercise.

There's one exercise that most women can start doing right away, though—the Kegel exercises I mention in Chapter 10. Research has found that working your pelvic floor muscles soon after labour can help reduce the risk of future urinary stress incontinence.[2] Time to start practising! Find your pelvic floor muscles, contract, and hold for up to 10 seconds. Do Kegel exercises several times a day, working up to 25 times daily.

The physical demands of delivery and caring for your new baby may require you to begin exercising at a lower intensity than you were used to nine months ago. And let's not forget the effect of sleep deprivation. You're likely getting less rest each night, so it's only natural that you feel more tired during the day. Even if you're in a hurry to be active again and you feel you're up to it, make sure to take it easy. Start back slowly and gradually increase to a moderate intensity level. If you experience heavy bleeding, pain, or breast infection during or after any exercise, stop and consult your doctor.

Warm-up

Before you jump right into your workout, begin with a 5- to 10-minute warm-up to get your body ready for exercise. Start by walking, cycling, stepping, or swimming at a low intensity. During the last few minutes of your warm-up, gently stretch the leg muscles that you will be working the most during your aerobic workout.

Aerobic Exercise: Four to Seven Days Per Week

The most comfortable aerobic exercise in the early postpartum months is brisk walking. Whether you push your baby in a stroller or carry him in an approved carrier pack, brisk walking gets your heart beating, burns calories, and lets you enjoy the company of other new moms. Activities that require sitting, such as cycling or rowing, are likely to be uncomfortable while the tissues in your pelvic region are healing. Even swimming or water aerobics can cause discomfort. Wait until you are fully recuperated before returning to these activities.

When you start back, exercise three times each week for 15 minutes at a time. Then gradually increase your exercising time to 30 minutes. Once your body feels comfortable exercising, feel free to get back to doing what you were used to. Work up to fives times per week. If your cardio workout of choice is brisk walking, you can do this every day—just make sure you don't feel too tired afterwards. If you do, that means you're overdoing it and need to cut back. To help lose body fat, aim to get moderate aerobic exercise at least four times per week, for 30 to 60 minutes per session.

How hard should you exercise? In Chapter 10, I suggest a few ways to assess your exercise intensity level. You can use the talk test, making sure you can carry on a conversation, although slightly winded, while exercising. Or you can rate your intensity using Borg's rating of perceived exertion (see page 193). Aim for a range of 3 to 5. And, of course, you can always go by your heart rate. To determine your heart rate, follow the instructions in Chapter 10, then use this formula to calculate your target heart rate zone.

Calculate Your Target Heart Rate Zone

You are exercising hard enough if you're working out at between 65 and 90 percent of your maximum heart rate (the maximum number of times your heart can beat in one minute). This is called your target heart rate zone. Beginners should aim to work out at 40 to 50 percent of their maximum heart rate. Here's how to estimate your target heart rate zone:

1. Calculate your estimated maximum heart rate (220 minus your age).

2. Multiply your maximum heart rate by 0.65 for the lower end of your heart rate zone.

3. Multiply your maximum heart rate by 0.90 for the upper end of your heart rate zone.

   For example, here's my target heart rate zone:

1. 220–38 = 182 (my estimated maximum heart rate)

2. 182 × 0.65 = 118

3. 182 × 0.90 = 164

As you can see, my target heart rate zone is 118 to 164 beats per minute. If my heart rate drops below 118, I need to pick up the pace. Conversely, if it exceeds 165, I need to slow down a little. To get a decent workout and help manage my weight, I usually aim for a heart rate of about 140 to 150 beats per minute.

The aerobic portion of your workout must also include a three-minute cool-down to lower your heart rate and get the blood flowing from your working muscles to the rest of your body. To do this, decrease the intensity level or slow the pace of your exercise.

Strength Exercise: Two to Four Days Per Week

Strength training can really get your body back into shape. It helps tone all those muscles that were stretched and pulled during pregnancy and labour. You'll certainly get a good strength workout now that you're carrying a baby around in your arms. (Just wait until your little one gets heavier—I've had plenty of clients show me their impressive biceps!)

Your joints may have seemed loose when you were pregnant; well, they may seem even looser now. That's because hormones associated with breastfeeding can relax your joints. It takes about three months for your joints to return to normal after pregnancy, so it's best to avoid hitting the weight gym until after this time. Doing too much too soon can lead to injury. Start by doing strength exercises at home—exercises that strengthen your chest, shoulders, and back. Make sure your stitches and abdominal wall are healed before you add sit-ups to your routine.

Flexibility Exercises: Four to Seven Days Per Week

Being flexible means that your joints can move fluidly through a range of motion. Gentle reaching, bending, and stretching your muscles keep your joints flexible and your muscles relaxed. The more flexible you are, the less likely it is that you'll get injured during exercise. Stretching also helps reduce muscle soreness after a workout.

Stretch for 5 to 10 minutes each day, holding each stretch for 10 to 30 seconds. Warm up with light activity for 5 minutes before you stretch. This increases your body temperature and range of motion. Or do your stretching after a cardio workout. Stretch slowly and smoothly without bouncing or jerking. Use a gentle continuous movement or stretch-and-hold, whichever is right for the exercise.

There's no need to worry about exercising if breastfeeding. Moderate exercise will not negatively affect your milk flow or the composition of your breast milk. If you work out at higher intensities, the lactic acid your muscles produce during exercise can make its way into your breast milk. This is by no means harmful to your baby, but there's a chance that it might be unpalatable. If you find your baby doesn't feed well after you exercise, try nursing right before your workout. Your breasts will feel better, too. If this isn't possible, postpone feeding until one hour after exercise. You might want to express milk earlier to use after a trip to the gym.

Strategies to Help You Keep the Weight Off

I've helped scores of new moms, breastfeeding or not, return to their pre-pregnancy weight. In most cases it was just a simple matter of paring down portion size, getting back to a regular exercise program, and breaking bad habits (for example, when you're around the house all day, it's easy to mindlessly nibble).

I help my clients lose weight by teaching them what to eat and how to eat—skills we are not taught in school. My philosophy is straightforward: everything you do to lose weight must be everything you do to keep it off. So there is no sense in cutting out your favourite food or exercising fanatically seven days per week: it just won't stick.

Women often ask me what they will do differently once they reach their weight goal. My answer often surprises them: nothing. The only thing (besides pregnancy and breast-feeding) that will dictate how much food healthy people can eat is their level of physical activity and the speed of their metabolism. If a client's exercise increases, I will increase her food plan to help her maintain body weight. If her exercise goes out the window for a period, perhaps because of a busy work schedule or injury, the food plan is revised to decrease food intake. Adjusting one's food intake to match activity level is not automatic for most people. But it's an important skill to learn in order to successfully manage weight over the long term.

But there's more to weight loss success. By studying the habits of successful dieters, researchers have learned key strategies that help keep the weight off. The National Weight Control Registry is a database of more than 2000 people from all over the United States who have successfully maintained a 30-pound (13.5-kilogram) weight loss for at least one year.[3] The average registrant has lost approximately 60 pounds (27 kilograms) and kept it off for about five years. What's more, about half of these people lost weight on their own, without any formal program. What makes these people so successful at weight loss? Here's a look (and while these strategies may not sound sexy, they really do work).

Eat a Low-Fat, High-Carbohydrate Diet

Most people in the registry lost weight and kept it off by following the same eating princi-ples I discuss throughout this book. The average registrant consumes 1400 calories per day, with 24 percent of those calories coming from fat. Successful weight loss maintainers say they don't use fat as a seasoning, avoid frying foods, and substitute low-fat for high-fat foods. Whole grains, legumes, fruit, vegetables, and low-fat dairy products make up the bulk of their diets. But don't forget to monitor your portion sizes of whole grain foods.

Eating larger portions than needed will not help you lose weight—in fact, you'll find it easier to gain!

Keep High-Fat Foods Out of the House

This sounds so simple, yet that's what 85 percent of weight loss registrants say they do to help them stick with their low-fat diet. Almost all say that, to stay on track, they stock their kitchen with plenty of healthy foods, and about one-third say they eat in restaurants less often.

Eat Five Times Per Day

Instead of devouring three big meals, successful dieters eat more often. Spreading out their food keeps their stomach always partly full and prevents overeating at any one time. Plan to eat three meals plus two snacks daily, or divide your calories evenly into five smaller meals eaten every three to four hours.

Don't Deny Yourself

People in the National Weight Control Registry say they don't give up their favourite foods. They continue to enjoy them, but perhaps not as often as they did when they were over-weight. Plan for a treat, be it a decadent dessert or a higher-fat snack food, once per week so you don't feel deprived.

Keep a Food Diary

One-half of the successful weight loss participants say they record their daily food intake and workouts. Doing so provides focus and motivation: you are forced to see, in black and white, the foods you are eating and the foods you are not eating. It will make you think twice about eating that second helping at dinner or that handful of potato chips while watching television.

I encourage you to record your food intake for the next seven days. Each day, take a moment to assess it. What do you notice? No fruit? No vegetables? No breakfast? Too many sweets? Make a plan for change. Each week, set one new goal about changing your diet and write down exactly what you plan to change. Be specific; it's not enough to say that you will eat less fat. How will you do this? By replacing the cream in your coffee with milk, by skipping the butter on your vegetables, or by replacing those afternoon cookies with yogurt and fruit?

Weigh Yourself Often

Almost 80 percent of the registrants weigh themselves on a regular basis, even after six years of maintaining their loss. Monitoring your progress provides motivation and impetus to keep going. It also allows you to nip small weight gains in the bud. Knowing that you've gotten off track and probably put on a few pounds is one thing, but getting on the scale and staring at the result of your indulgences is quite another. You'll be much more likely to do something about it before those 5 pounds turn into 10.

Learn About Nutrition

Seventy-five percent of successful dieters say they buy books and magazines related to nutrition and exercise, and they continue to do so years after they have lost the weight. When you create an environment that fosters healthy eating, you're more likely to stay on track and make these changes permanent.

Get Planned Exercise

I've already discussed the importance of exercise to help you get into shape. Nine out of 10 registrants report getting one hour of scheduled exercise each day. Many participants get their calorie burn from brisk walking—an easy exercise for new moms. Exercise makes you feel good about yourself, making you want to eat healthy. And there's an added bonus: you can enjoy more food if you work out regularly.

Sneak in Activity

Another common denominator among weight loss registrants is that they add little bits of activity to their daily routine. Small changes such as taking the stairs instead of the escalator, parking at the end of the lot, and getting off the bus a few stops early add up.

Expect Failure, but Keep on Trying

People who are successful at losing weight don't expect to be perfect. They consider lapses as momentary setbacks, not the ruin of all their hard work. Whether you have a busy social schedule or you're going on a food-laden vacation, you're bound to put on a few pounds at some point. As I mention above, the key to long-term weight maintenance is all about dealing with small weight gains when they occur. By telling yourself that you're human and it's okay to have slipped a little, you'll be amazed at how easy it is to return to your usual healthy routine.

Weight Loss Plans for the Postpartum Months

Following the guidelines I gave you earlier, choose the meal plan that's right for you. These plans serve as a general guide only. For the first six months after delivery, some women may need more calories. If you were underweight prior to pregnancy, if you had poor weight gain during your pregnancy, or if you are breastfeeding more than one baby, I suggest you consult your dietitian or doctor. Women who are nursing should not eat fewer than 1800 calories per day during the first six months.

2200 CALORIES PER DAY

Breakfast:

Protein servings: 1 (optional)

Starch servings: 2

Fruit servings: 2

Milk servings: 1

Water: 2 cups (500 ml)

Morning Snack:

Fruit servings: 1

Milk servings: 1

Water: 1 to 2 cups (250 to 500 ml)

Lunch:

Protein servings: 3

Starch servings: 2

Vegetable servings: 1 to 2

Fat servings: 2

Water: 2 cups (500 ml)

Afternoon Snack:

Fruit servings: 1

Fat servings: 1

Water: 2 cups (500 ml)

Dinner:

Protein servings: 4

Starch servings: 3

Vegetable servings: 2 to 3

Fat servings: 2

Water: 2 cups (500 ml)

Bedtime Snack:

Grain servings: 1

Milk servings: 1

1900 CALORIES PER DAY

Breakfast:

Protein servings: 1 (optional)

Starch servings: 2

Fruit servings: 1

Milk servings: 1

Water: 2 cups (500 ml)

Morning Snack:

Fruit servings: 1

Milk servings: 1

Water: 1 to 2 cups (250 to 500 ml)

Lunch:

Protein servings: 3

Starch servings: 2

Vegetable servings: 1 to 2

Fat servings: 2

Water: 2 cups (500 ml)

Afternoon Snack:

Fruit servings: 1

Milk servings: 1

Fat servings: 1

Water: 2 cups (500 ml)

Dinner:

Protein servings: 4

Starch servings: 2

Vegetable servings: 2 to 3

Fat servings: 2

Water: 2 cups (500 ml)

1600 CALORIES PER DAY

Breakfast:

Protein servings: 1 (optional)

Starch servings: 1

Fruit servings: 1

Milk servings: 1

Water: 2 cups (500 ml)

Morning Snack:

Fruit servings: 1

OR

Milk servings: 1

Water: 1 to 2 cups (250 to 500 ml)

Lunch:

Protein servings: 3

Starch servings: 2

Vegetable servings: 1 to 2

Fat servings: 2

Water: 2 cups (500 ml)

Afternoon Snack:

Fruit servings: 1

Milk servings: 1

Water: 2 cups (500 ml)

Dinner:

Protein servings: 3

Starch servings: 2

Vegetable servings: 2 to 3

Fat servings: 2

Water: 2 cups (500 ml)

1200 TO 1400 CALORIES PER DAY

Breakfast:

Protein servings: 1 (optional)

Starch servings: 1

Fruit servings: 1

Milk servings: 1

Water: 2 cups (500 ml)

Morning Snack:

Fruit servings: 1

OR

Milk servings: 1

Water: 1 to 2 cups (250 to 500 ml)

Lunch:

Protein servings: 2 or 3

Starch servings: 2

Vegetable servings: 1 to 2

Fat servings: 2

Water: 2 cups (500 ml)

Afternoon Snack:

Fruit servings: 1

AND

Milk servings: 1

Water: 2 cups (500 ml)

Dinner:

Protein servings: 3 to 5

Starch servings: 0 to 2

Vegetable servings: 2 to 3

Fat servings: 1 to 2

Water: 2 cups (500 ml)

Part Four

—⦈⦈⦈—

Leslie's 14-Day
Meal Plan for
a Healthy Pregnancy

Now it's time to put all your newfound nutrition knowledge into action by creating delicious, nutrient-packed meals and snacks. One of the best strategies to help you eat healthy is to cook for yourself, rather than rely on restaurants, take-out places, and processed ready-to-eat meals. Preparing nutritious meals for you and your developing baby is rewarding. Not only will your body feel better for it, your mind will be at ease, too. You'll feel confident knowing that you're nourishing the life inside you with the healthiest of foods. (And, of course, once your baby is born, enjoying these recipes will ensure you're getting the nutrients you need to stay healthy.) You'll see that once you get organized, it's easy to prepare healthy meals.

All the recipes included in the meal plan come from The Test Kitchen at Canadian Living. That means they have been Tested Till Perfect. I had the pleasure of working with Donna Bartolini, a *Canadian Living* magazine contributor, who helped me develop this meal plan, based on my philosophy about healthy eating during pregnancy. The meal plan—

- Follows the principles of a plant-based diet. That means more emphasis is placed on whole grains, vegetables, and beans than on animal foods. You'll find meals based on beans, lentils, and tofu, but you'll also see chicken and meat, just less often.

- Offers fish rich in omega-3 fats two times each week.

- Emphasizes whole-grain choices as often as possible.

- Includes plenty of folate-rich dishes each week. You'll find recipes for lentils and beans, spinach, and other green vegetables.

- Offers recipes that sneak in calcium by using milk, evaporated milk, skim milk powder, and enriched soy milk.

- Offers recipes low in fat (30 percent of calories or less). You needn't avoid those that aren't—it's what you eat over the course of a day that counts, not one single food or meal.

You'll also find plenty of extra recipes that are not part of the 14-Day Meal Plan, to help you eat more vegetables and whole grains, not to mention healthy snacks and desserts. You need more calories when you're pregnant, and this meal plan ensures they're from nutritious treats.

Donna came up with more than 75 dishes that taste great (a top priority), use ingredients that are easy to find, and can be quickly prepared (usually in under 30 minutes). Each recipe includes a nutrient analysis stating the number of calories and grams of protein, fat (including saturated fat), carbohydrate, and fibre per serving. The cholesterol and sodium content is also analyzed. As for key minerals and vitamins, the nutrient analysis details how many milligrams or micrograms of calcium, iron, vitamins A and C, and folate you're getting per serving. You'll see how one serving stacks up in terms of providing the recommended dietary intake for these vitamins and minerals, expressed as "% RDI," so that you can evaluate at a glance the nutrient content of one serving of a recipe. Generally, if one serving provides 15% RDI or higher, it's a good source of that nutrient.

Adjusting the 2200-Calorie Level

The meal plan provides roughly 2200 calories per day from three meals and three snacks. This is an appropriate calorie intake for most women in their second and third trimesters, providing pre-pregnancy weight was maintained on a 1900-calorie diet. You will need to monitor your weight gain to see if you need to eat a little bit more, or less. (See Chapter 7 for tips on adjusting your calorie intake during the first, second, and third trimesters.)

But what about the first trimester, when you really don't need to boost your calorie intake? Women who were underweight prior to pregnancy will do well to follow this plan (again, monitor your rate of weight gain to see if you need to adjust). Other women will likely do well on 1900 calories per day. So all you need to do is reduce the amount of food this plan provides by 300 calories. I suggest you cut out one snack (but do not cut out milk!) and reduce your servings (or portion size) of grain products.

Meal-Plan Strategies

Think of the recipes that follow as your starter kit to eating well throughout your pregnancy. By giving you a two-week plan for breakfast, lunch, and dinner, I've eliminated the first strategy in getting organized: planning your meals. Spending a little bit of time planning your meals in advance makes eating right a breeze. The strategies below will help you put the meal plan into place:

- *Schedule time for grocery shopping once a week.* Read through the recipes and develop your shopping list. If morning sickness is making you feel lousy, send a friend shopping or take advantage of home delivery services.

- *Buy pre-prepped food.* To save time cooking, buy chickpeas, beans, and lentils canned, ready to throw into a recipe. Buy your veggies chopped, ready to throw into salad or steamer basket.

- *Prepare food in advance.* Although each recipe can be easily prepared at mealtime, if you lead a hectic life, like most of us do, consider batch cooking on the weekend and taking advantage of your freezer. Preparing food in advance will be a lifesaver during your busy week. Here are a few time-saving suggestions for using the 14-Day Meal Plan:

- Bake the high-fibre, low-fat quick breads included in Monday breakfasts on Sunday. Freeze what you don't plan to use, to have on hand for another breakfast or a mid-day snack. They make great snacks for kids, too.

- Prepare Monday lunches—20-Minute Chicken Chili and Black Bean Soup—on Sunday. Freeze what you won't eat on Monday in single-serving containers so you'll have a quick meal ready to defrost any day of the week.

- If you work away from the home during the day, make the Lentil Salad with Corn and Red Onion (Week One, Wednesday) and Bulgur Chickpea Tomato Salad (Week One, Thursday) in advance.

- Whenever you have a little extra time, make the delicious Homemade Granola I've planned for Week One, Tuesday. It can be stored in the fridge for up to two weeks. You'll use it again for breakfast the following week in Fruity Yogurt Granola Trifle. You could also bake the Apricot, Oat and Bran Muffins (Week One, Friday) in advance.

- *Have the right tools on hand.* You won't need anything special to cook these healthy recipes. Just some non-stick baking pans (or non-stick cooking spray), pots and pans, a steamer basket, a blender for breakfast smoothies, and standard utensils, including a few sharp knives.

To meet your daily calorie requirements, you'll need to add your own side dishes to many of the meals. But I've made it easy for you by telling you what you need to add. For instance, if I specify a vegetable or grain serving, make your own or try one of the many side dish recipes found on pages 265–274. When soup or salad is on the lunch menu, enjoy a whole-wheat roll, half a pita pocket, or a slice of whole-grain pumpernickel bread. You'll find a guide to serving sizes on page 303.

You don't need to use the meal plan exactly as it's presented. You might not want to adhere to a two-week schedule. Perhaps you'd rather pick and choose recipes to add to your own repertoire of healthy meals. If that's the case, you'll find plenty to choose from. In addition to the 14 breakfasts, lunches, and dinners, I've also provided 39 quick recipes for vegetables, whole grains, snacks, and desserts.

I hope you enjoy all the recipes and make many of them a regular part of your diet. Enjoy.

The 14-Day Meal Plan

WEEK 1

BREAKFAST	LUNCH	DINNER

MONDAY

Two-Grain Cranberry Bread (p. 276)	20-Minute Chicken Chili (p. 290)	Bulgur-Stuffed Red Peppers (p. 266)
Add your own:	*Add your own:*	*Add your own:*
1 milk serving	1 grain serving	Green salad with
1 fruit serving	1 vegetable serving	2 tbsp oil and vinegar dressing*

TUESDAY

Homemade Granola (p. 273)	Salmon Pitas with Celery Heart Salad (p. 264)	Grilled Dijon Herb Pork Chops (p. 292) with Skinny Mashed Potatoes (p. 269)
Add your own:	*Add your own:*	*Add your own:*
1 milk serving	Green salad with 2 tbsp	2 vegetable servings
2 fruit servings	oil and vinegar dressing*	

WEDNESDAY

Fruity Blender Buzz (p. 283)	Lentil Salad with Corn and Red Onion (p. 281)	Spicy Orange Baked Chicken Drumsticks (p. 289) with Roasted Ginger Carrots (p. 268)
Add your own:	*Add your own:*	*Add your own:*
2 grain servings OR	2 grain servings	1 grain serving
Pumpkin, Orange and	1 vegetable serving	1 vegetable serving
Raisin Muffins (p. 300)		

THURSDAY

Hot Almond Honey Multigrain Cereal (p. 273)	Chicken Salad Apple Sandwich (p. 262)	Tofu Vegetable Curry (p. 282)
Add your own:	*Add your own:*	*Add your own:*
1 fruit serving	1 to 2 vegetable servings	1 grain serving
		Green salad with 2 tbsp oil and vinegar dressing*

BREAKFAST	LUNCH	DINNER

FRIDAY

Apricot, Oat and Bran Muffins (p. 275)	Bulgur Chickpea Tomato Salad (p. 280)	Trout Gremolada (p. 287) Grape Tomato Bursts (p. 267) and Grilled Polenta (p. 279)
Add your own:	*Add your own:*	*Add your own:*
1 milk serving	3 protein servings	1 vegetable serving
1 fruit serving	(chicken, tofu, or fish)	

SATURDAY

Whole Wheat Waffles (p. 276) with Chunky Pear Applesauce (p. 298)	Quick Broccoli Soup (p. 261)	Company Sirloin with Grilled Vegetables (p. 291) and Chunky Pear Applesauce (p. 299)
	Add your own:	*Add your own:*
	2 protein servings	1 grain serving
	1 grain serving	2 vegetable servings
	(e.g., 1/2 sandwich)	

SUNDAY

Saucy Tomato Poached Eggs (p. 284)	Bruschetta Steak Sandwich (p. 262)	Chicken with Creamy Pesto Sauce (p. 288)
Add your own:	*Add your own:*	*Add your own:*
1 milk serving	2 vegetable servings	1 grain serving
1 fruit serving		1 vegetable serving

*1 cup (250 ml) raw vegetables and 2 to 4 tablespoons (25 to 50 ml) Herbed White Bean Spread (p. 271), Herbed Yogurt Cheese (p. 299), or Roasted Red Pepper Dip (p. 271) can be substituted for the green salad with oil and vinegar dressing.

WEEK TWO

BREAKFAST	LUNCH	DINNER
MONDAY		
Morning Sunshine Bars (p. 274)	Black Bean Soup (p. 261)	Hoisin Roast Salmon with Orange Spinach Salad (p. 285)
Add your own:	*Add your own:*	*Add your own:*
1 milk serving	2 protein servings	2 grain servings
1 fruit serving	1 grain serving	
	(e.g., 1/2 sandwich)	
TUESDAY		
Tropical Muesli to Go (p. 274)	Salmon Pasta Salad (p. 286)	Vegetarian Tex-Mex Shepherd's Pie (p. 270)
Add your own:		*Add your own:*
1 milk serving		1 vegetable serving
1 fruit serving		
WEDNESDAY		
Fruity Yogurt Granola Trifle (p. 272)	Hummus and Veggie Wrap (p. 263)	Skillet Chicken and Sweet Potatoes (p. 288)
Add your own:	*Add your own:*	*Add your own:*
3/4 cup (175 ml) unsweetened fruit juice	Green salad with 2 tbsp oil and vinegar dressing*	1 vegetable serving
THURSDAY		
Fruity Tofu Smoothie (p. 280)	Smoked Turkey Brown Rice Salad (p. 289)	Sole Pinwheels on Yellow Pepper (p. 286) with Brown Rice with Broccoli (p. 278)
Add your own:		*Add your own:*
2 grain servings		1 vegetable serving

BREAKFAST	LUNCH	DINNER

FRIDAY

Deluxe Porridge (p. 272)	Toaster Oven Salsa Ham Roll-Ups (p. 260)	Mushroom Lentil Patties (p. 281)
Add your own:	*Add your own:*	*Add your own:*
1 milk serving	2 vegetable servings	1 grain serving
2 fruit servings	1 fat serving	2 vegetable servings

SATURDAY

Apple Oatmeal Pancakes (p. 275)	Tofu Burritos (p. 282)	Carrot Steak Stir-Fry on Noodles (p. 291)
Add your own:	*Add your own:*	*Add your own:*
1 milk serving	2 vegetable servings	1 vegetable serving
	1 fat serving	

SUNDAY

Asparagus Frittata (p. 283)	Chicken-Stuffed Focaccia (p. 263)	Rice and Greens with Shrimp (p. 285)
Add your own:	*Add your own:*	*Add your own:*
1 milk serving	1 vegetable serving	1 vegetable serving
1 grain serving		1 fat serving
1 fruit serving		

*1 cup (250 ml) raw vegetables and 2 to 4 tablespoons (25 to 50 ml) Herbed White Bean Spread (p. 271), Herbed Yogurt Cheese (p. 299), or Roasted Red Pepper Dip (p. 271) can be substituted for the green salad with oil and vinegar dressing.

Daily Snack Schedule (Three snacks per day)

Midmorning Snack: 1 fruit and 1 milk serving and 10 unsalted almonds.

Try 1/4 cup (50 ml) Spa Trail Mix (p. 300) with 1 cup (250 ml) of your favourite low-fat yogurt.

Midafternoon Snack:

Option 1: Raw veggies with dip and 1 grain serving.

Try raw veggies with Herbed White Bean Spread (p. 271) with Baked Whole Wheat Pita Chips (p. 271).

Option 2: 2 fruit servings and 1 grain serving.

Try one of the delicious apples from the recipe Granola Baked Apples (p. 294).

Option 3: 2 fruit servings and 1 milk serving.

Try Fruity Blender Buzz (p. 279) or your own homemade smoothie: In the blender, whirl low-fat milk or enriched soy milk, frozen berries, and half a banana. Throw in 1 tablespoon (15 ml) ground flaxseed for an omega-3 boost.

Evening Snack: 1 milk serving and 1 grain serving.

Try:

- 2 Farmland Flax Cookies (p. 298) with 1 cup (250 ml) low-fat milk or calcium-enriched soy milk
- 1 Bodybuilder Cookie (p. 297) with 1 cup (250 ml) low-fat milk or calcium-enriched soy milk
- 2 Apple Crisp Mini-Muffins (p. 297) with 1 cup (250 ml) low-fat milk or calcium-enriched soy milk
- Chocolate Banana Pudding (p. 294)
- Pure and Simple Vanilla Pudding (p. 295)
- Frozen Orange-Vanilla "Cream" (p. 299)

The Recipes

POULTRY

Chicken with Creamy Pesto
    Sauce 288
Skillet Chicken and Sweet
    Potatoes 288
Smoked Turkey Brown Rice
    Salad 289
Spicy Orange Baked Chicken
    Drumsticks 289
20-Minute Chicken Chili 291

MEAT

Carrot Steak Stir-Fry on
    Noodles 291
Company Sirloin with Grilled
    Vegetables 291
Grilled Dijon Herb Pork
    Chops 292

DESSERTS

Rhubarb and Strawberry
    Compote 293
Apricot Compote 293
Chocolate Banana Pudding
    294
Granola Baked Apples 294
Pure and Simple Vanilla
    Pudding 295

Ice and Easy Fruit Sorbets

Simple Syrup 295
Blueberry Frozen Yogurt 295
Canta-Berry Sorbet 296
Lemon Lime Tofu Zinger 296
Peach Sorbet 296
Raspberry Sorbet 296

SNACKS

Apple Crisp Mini-Muffins 297
Bodybuilder Cookies 297
Chunky Pear Applesauce 298
Farmland Flax Cookies 298
Frozen Orange Vanilla
    "Cream" 299
Herbed Yogurt Cheese 299
Pumpkin, Orange and Raisin
    Muffins 300
Spa Trail Mix & Hiker's Happy
    Trail Mix 300–301

SOUPS

Black Bean Soup

Hearty and delicious, this soup looks great, with its spoonful of sour cream swirled into each serving. If you like, purée the soup before adding the coriander; just reserve about 1/4 cup (50 mL) of the whole beans to garnish each bowlful.

1 tbsp	vegetable oil	15 mL
1	onion, chopped	1
3	cloves garlic, minced	3
1	sweet red pepper, chopped	1
1 tsp	ground cumin	5 mL
Pinch	cayenne pepper	Pinch
1	can (19 oz/540 mL) black beans, drained and rinsed	1
2 cups	vegetable or chicken stock	500 mL
2 tbsp	chopped fresh coriander (optional)	25 mL
2 tbsp	lime juice	25 mL
1/4 cup	sour cream	50 mL

In large saucepan, heat oil over medium heat; cook onion, garlic, red pepper, cumin and cayenne, stirring occasionally, for 5 minutes or until onion is softened.

Add black beans and stock; bring to boil. Reduce heat and simmer for 10 minutes. Stir in coriander (if using) and lime juice. Dollop sour cream on each serving.

Makes 4 servings.

Per serving: about 178 cal, 9 g pro, 5 g total fat (1 g sat. fat), 26 g carb, 8 g fibre, 2 mg chol, 687 mg sodium. % RDI: 7% calcium (82 mg), 17% iron (2.4 mg), 12% vit A, 90% vit C (54 mg), 30% folate (65 mcg).

Quick Broccoli Soup

An immersion blender—a long handheld wand with blenderlike blades on the end—is a handy kitchen appliance which allows you to purée soups right in the saucepan. It's even handier later on—for puréeing small amounts of steamed vegetables for your baby.

1 tbsp	butter	15 mL
2	onions, chopped	2
2	potatoes (12 oz/375 g), peeled and coarsely chopped	2
2 cups	vegetable stock	500 mL
1 tsp	each salt and pepper	5 mL
3 cups	frozen broccoli pieces	750 mL
1	can (385 mL) evaporated skim milk	1
2 tbsp	chopped fresh chives or green onions	25 mL

In large saucepan, melt butter over medium heat; cook onions and potatoes, stirring often, until onions are softened, about 10 minutes. Add stock, salt and pepper; bring to boil. Reduce heat to medium; cover and simmer until potatoes are tender, about 15 minutes. Add broccoli pieces; cover and cook for 5 minutes.

In food processor or blender, purée soup until smooth. Return to pan; stir in evaporated milk and heat through. Serve sprinkled with chives.

Makes 4 servings.

Per serving: about 225 cal, 13 g pro, 4 g total fat (2 g sat. fat), 37 g carb, 4 g fibre, 12 mg chol, 1065 mg sodium. % RDI: 34% calcium (374 mg), 10% iron (1.4 mg), 33% vit A, 102% vit C (61 mg), 23% folate (51 mcg).

SANDWICHES AND WRAPS

Bruschetta Steak Sandwich

Enjoy tomatoes for their taste, colour and health bene-fits: they contain a high amount of the carotenoid lycopene, which functions as an antioxidant to help protect against disease.

12 oz	top sirloin grilling steak	375 g
1/2 tsp	salt	2 mL
1/4 tsp	pepper	1 mL
2	plum tomatoes, chopped	2
1/4 cup	chopped fresh parsley	50 mL
1	green onion, chopped	1
1	clove garlic, minced	1
1 tbsp	olive oil	15 mL
2 tsp	wine vinegar	10 mL
1/4 tsp	dried oregano	1 mL
4	kaiser rolls	4
1/2 cup	crumbled feta cheese (optional)	125 mL

Sprinkle steak with half each of the salt and pepper. Place on greased grill over medium-high heat or under broiler; close lid and grill until medium-rare, 4 minutes per side, or until desired doneness. Transfer to board and tent with foil; let stand for 5 minutes. Thinly slice across the grain.

Meanwhile, in bowl, combine tomatoes, parsley, green onion, garlic, oil, vinegar, oregano and remaining salt and pepper. Set aside.

Cut rolls in half horizontally. Place, cut side down, on grill; toast until golden brown, 3 minutes. Sandwich steak, tomato mixture and cheese (if using) in rolls.

Makes 4 servings.

Per serving: about 323 cal, 22 g pro, 10 g total fat (2 g sat. fat), 35 g carb, 4 g fibre, 39 mg chol, 662 mg sodi-um. % RDI: 7% calcium (81 mg), 30% iron (4.2 mg), 4% vit A, 17% vit C (10 mg), 35% folate (76 mcg).

Chicken Salad Apple Sandwich

A chicken sandwich doesn't sound so exciting—until you add a touch of fragrant curry and the sweet crunch of apple to the mix. This chicken salad is also wonder-ful served on a bed of tender baby spinach or spooned into mini-pitas as an hors d'oeuvre.

2	cooked boneless skinless chicken breasts	2
1/3 cup	diced sweet red pepper	75 mL
1/3 cup	diced celery	75 mL
2	green onions, thinly sliced	2
Half	apple	Half
3	multigrain bagels	3
	Leaf lettuce	
Dressing:		
1/3 cup	light sour cream	75 mL
2 tbsp	light mayonnaise	25 mL
1/2 tsp	minced gingerroot	2 mL
1/2 tsp	mild curry paste	2 mL
1/4 tsp	ground cumin	1 mL
1/4 tsp	salt	1 mL
Pinch	pepper	Pinch

In large bowl and using fingers, shred chicken finely to make about 2 cups (500 mL); add red pepper, celery and green onions.

Dressing: In small bowl, stir together sour cream, mayonnaise, ginger, curry paste, cumin, salt and pep-per; add to chicken mixture and stir to combine. (Make-ahead: Cover and refrigerate for up to 24 hours.)

Core apple half; cut into thin slices. Split bagels in half; line bottom halves with lettuce. Spread with chicken salad and top with apple slices.

Makes 3 sandwiches.

Per sandwich: about 422 cal, 31 g pro, 8 g total fat (2 g sat. fat), 60 g carb, 7 g fibre, 83 mg chol, 1062 mg sodi-um. % RDI: 14% calcium (150 mg), 26% iron (3.7 mg), 15% vit A, 62% vit C (37 mg), 10% folate (22 mcg).

Chicken-Stuffed Focaccia

This sandwich is equally good on panini rolls or thick slices of multigrain bread.

1 tbsp	olive oil	15 mL
1	each sweet green and red pepper, thinly sliced	1
1 cup	thinly sliced red onion	250 mL
2	boneless skinless chicken breasts	2
Pinch	each salt and pepper	Pinch
1 loaf	(12 inches/30 cm long) focaccia	1
1 1/3 cups	baby spinach leaves	325 mL
Sauce:		
2 tbsp	low-fat plain yogurt	25 mL
1 tbsp	light mayonnaise	15 mL
1 tbsp	sun-dried tomato pesto	15 mL
Pinch	each salt and pepper	Pinch

In large skillet, heat oil over medium-high heat. Cook green and red peppers and onion for 8 to 10 minutes or until tender. Set aside.

Meanwhile, with knife held horizontally, cut chicken breasts in half; season with salt and pepper. Cook in grill pan or under broiler for 3 to 4 minutes per side or until no longer pink inside.

Sauce: In bowl, whisk together yogurt, mayonnaise, pesto, salt and pepper.

Slice focaccia in half horizontally; cut into quarters. If desired, toast cut sides under broiler. Spread cut side of each bottom piece with sauce. Layer each with one-quarter of the pepper mixture, chicken and spinach.

Makes 4 servings.

Per serving: about 437 cal, 24 g pro, 13 g total fat (2 g sat. fat), 54 g carb, 5 g fibre, 42 mg chol, 747 mg sodium. % RDI: 7% calcium (80 mg), 28% iron (3.9 mg), 26% vit A, 192% vit C (115 mg), 55% folate (120 mcg).

Hummus and Veggie Wrap

Hummus is so easy to make that smart cooks always keep a can or two of chickpeas in the cupboard. Tahini—somewhat less common—can be replaced by peanut butter or sesame oil.

4	large whole wheat tortillas	4
1 cup	shredded romaine lettuce	250 mL
1/2 cup	each chopped tomato, cucumber and green onion	125 mL
Hummus:		
1	can (19 oz/540 mL) chickpeas, drained and rinsed	1
1/4 cup	lemon juice	50 mL
2 tbsp	tahini	25 mL
2 tbsp	chopped parsley	25 mL
2 tbsp	olive oil	25 mL
1	clove garlic, minced	1
1/2 tsp	ground cumin	2 mL
1/4 tsp	each salt and pepper	1 mL

Hummus: In food processor, purée chickpeas. Add lemon juice, tahini, parsley, olive oil, garlic, cumin, salt and pepper; blend, adding a little water to thin, if desired. (Make-ahead: Refrigerate in airtight container for up to 2 days.)

Spread 1/2 cup (125 mL) hummus over each tortilla; sprinkle with lettuce, tomato, cucumber and green onion.

Fold bottom of tortilla up about 1 1/2 inches (4 cm). Roll sides tightly toward centre. Wrap each bundle tightly in plastic wrap.

Makes 4 servings.

Per serving: about 367 cal, 12 g pro, 13 g total fat (2 g sat. fat), 62 g carb, 10 g fibre, 0 mg chol, 708 mg sodium. % RDI: 7% calcium (82 mg), 27% iron (3.8 mg), 7% vit A, 35% vit C (21 mg), 54% folate (119 mcg).

Salmon Pitas with Celery Heart Salad

Grown-ups will love this salmon sandwich flavoured with a vinaigrette. You can mash any soft bones into the salmon for an extra hit of calcium.

2 tbsp	chopped fresh dill	25 mL
2 tbsp	lemon juice	25 mL
1 tbsp	extra-virgin olive oil	15 mL
1/4 tsp	each salt and pepper	1 mL
1	small head celery	1
1/2 cup	thinly sliced radishes	125 mL
1/2 cup	thinly sliced red onion	125 mL
1/4 cup	light sour cream	50 mL
2	cans (each 7 1/2 oz/213 g) salmon, drained	2
4	lettuce leaves	4
4	whole wheat Greek pitas or tortillas	4

In large bowl, whisk 1 tbsp (15 mL) each of the dill and lemon juice, oil and half each of the salt and pepper; set aside.

Remove tough outer stalks from celery to leave 2-inch (5-cm) heart; reserve outer stalks for another use. Trim tops from heart to leave 5-inch (12-cm) long base; reserve tops for another use. Peel outside of celery heart to remove tough strings; trim bottom. Slice celery heart lengthwise into paper-thin slices; cut slices crosswise into thirds. Add to oil mixture along with radishes and onion; toss to coat.

In separate bowl, combine sour cream and remaining dill, lemon juice, salt and pepper. Add salmon, flaking with fork.

Layer lettuce, celery mixture and salmon mixture onto pitas and roll up. (Make-ahead: Wrap in plastic wrap and refrigerate for up to 24 hours.)

Makes 4 servings.

Per serving: about 363 cal, 25.5 g pro, 12 g total fat (3 g sat. fat), 42 g carb, 7.5 g fibre, 27 mg chol, 948 mg sodium. % RDI: 30% calcium (329 mg), 25% iron (3.5 mg), 5% vit A, 28% vit C (17 mg), 48% folate (107 mcg).

Toaster Oven Salsa Ham Roll-Ups

These super easy roll-ups can be made the night before, then wrapped and refrigerated overnight. Choose whole grain tortillas for a fibre boost.

1/2 cup	light cream cheese, softened	125 mL
2	green onions, sliced	2
1/4 tsp	each salt and pepper	1 mL
4	large flour tortillas	4
1/2 cup	salsa	125 mL
12	slices shaved Black Forest ham (6 oz/175 g)	12

In small bowl, combine cheese, onions, salt and pepper; spread evenly over tortillas. Spread with salsa; top each with 3 slices ham and roll up tightly.

Bake on rimmed baking sheet in 400°F (200°C) oven or in toaster oven until ends are golden, 8 to 10 minutes. Cut each diagonally into halves; serve warm.

Makes 4 servings.

Per serving: about 311 cal, 16 g pro, 11 g total fat (4 g sat. fat), 36 g carb, 3 g fibre, 39 mg chol, 1217 mg sodium. % RDI: 7% calcium (79 mg), 19% iron (2.6 mg), 5% vit A, 12% vit C (7 mg), 8% folate (18 mcg).

Tip: For quick hors d'oeuvres when entertaining, thinly slice the roll-ups after heating.

Tip: Choose whole wheat flour tortillas for a fibre boost.

VEGETABLES

A GUIDE TO STEAMING VEGETABLES

This method is most suitable for small quantities of vegetables so that the steam can easily reach each piece and cook evenly. Here's a quick how-to guide.

Method: Prepare vegetables according to directions below. Place vegetables on rack above boiling water. Vegetables should be at least 1 inch (2.5 cm) above surface of water. Cover tightly and steam for time indicated below.

Asparagus
Preparation: Snap off woody stems; peel stems if very thick. Steaming time: 7 minutes.

Beets
Preparation: Remove stems; keep whole and unpeeled until after cooking. Steaming time: 40 minutes.

Bok Choy
Preparation: Trim and chop large head coarsely; for baby bok choy, quarter heads. Steaming time: 5 minutes.

Broccoli
Preparation: Cut into florets; peel and slice stalks. Steaming time: 7 minutes.

Brussels Sprouts
Preparation: Trim off wilted or coarse outer leaves; cut thin end off stem and score shallow X in bottom. Steaming time: 10 minutes.

Carrots/Parsnips
Preparation: Cut into coins, sticks or chunks. Steaming time: 15 minutes.

Cauliflower
Preparation: Cut into florets. Steaming time: 10 minutes.

Corn
Preparation: Husk. Steaming time: 8 to 12 minutes.

Green Beans
Preparation: Cut off stem end. Steaming time: 10 minutes.

Peas
Preparation: Separate pods to shell peas into bowl; for snow peas, pull off vein. Steaming time: 8 minutes.

Potatoes/Sweet Potatoes
Preparation: Peel if directed; cut into similar-size shapes. Steaming time: 30 to 40 minutes for whole new potatoes.

Rutabaga
Preparation: Peel and cube. Steaming time: 15 minutes.

Squash
Preparation: Peel, seed and cut into chunks. Steaming time: 12 minutes.

White Turnips
Preparation: Peel. Steaming time: 15 to 20 minutes.

Basil Roasted Vegetables

Wonderful on the side, Mediterranean-style veggies also make a great stuffing for lunch-box pitas.

2 tbsp	basil pesto	25 mL
1 tbsp	chicken stock or water	15 mL
1	onion, cut in wedges	1
1	large zucchini, cut in 1/4-inch (5-mm) thick diagonal slices	1
1	each sweet red and yellow pepper, thinly sliced	1
1 cup	grape or cherry tomatoes	250 mL
1/2 tsp	salt	2 mL
1/4 tsp	pepper	1 mL

In small bowl, whisk pesto with chicken stock until smooth. In large bowl, toss together onion, zucchini, red and yellow peppers and pesto mixture to coat; spread in 13- x 9-inch (3 L) glass baking dish or greased, rimmed baking sheet.

Roast on top rack of 450°F (230°C) oven for 15 minutes. Stir in tomatoes; roast for 10 minutes or until golden and tender. Sprinkle with salt and pepper.

Makes 4 servings.

Per serving: about 81 cal, 3 g pro, 3 g total fat (1 g sat. fat), 12 g carb, 3 g fibre, 0 mg chol, 382 mg sodium. % RDI: 4% calcium (48 mg), 8% iron (1.1 mg), 26% vit A, 177% vit C (106 mg), 15% folate (32 mcg).

Bulgur-Stuffed Red Peppers

Enjoy this vegetarian main course either hot or at room temperature. Look for firm, unblemished sweet peppers with even bottoms so they'll stay upright during cooking. To serve as a side dish for a family dinner or buffet, halve peppers from top to bottom and serve one half per person.

1/2 cup	bulgur	125 mL
4	sweet red or green peppers	4
4 cups	mushrooms (12 oz/375 g)	1 L
2 tbsp	olive oil	25 mL
1	onion, chopped	1
2	cloves garlic, minced	2
1 tbsp	finely chopped fresh sage (or 1 tsp/5 mL dried, crumbled)	15 mL
3/4 tsp	each salt and pepper	4 mL
1	can (19 oz/540 mL) chickpeas, drained and rinsed	1
1/4 cup	shredded Asiago cheese (optional)	50 mL
1/4 cup	toasted slivered almonds	50 mL
1/4 cup	chopped fresh parsley	50 mL
2 tbsp	lemon juice	25 mL
2	plum tomatoes, seeded and diced	2

In large bowl, pour 1 1/3 cups (325 mL) boiling water over bulgur; cover and let stand for 15 minutes. Drain and press out moisture; return to bowl.

Meanwhile, slice tops off peppers; core and scrape out seeds. Dice tops and set aside.

In food processor or by hand, finely chop mushrooms. In large nonstick skillet, heat half of the oil over medium-high heat; fry diced peppers, mushrooms, onion, garlic, sage and 1/2 tsp (2 mL) each of the salt and pepper until liquid is evaporated, about 10 minutes. Add to bulgur along with chickpeas, cheese (if using), almonds and parsley; toss to combine.

Spoon bulgur mixture into peppers, mounding if necessary. Place peppers, stuffed side up, in 8-inch (2 L) square glass baking dish. Drizzle with lemon juice and remaining oil; top with tomatoes. Sprinkle with remaining salt and pepper.

Cover with foil; bake in 350°F (180°C) oven until peppers are almost tender, about 1 hour. Uncover and bake until tops are crusty, about 30 minutes.

Makes 4 servings.

Per serving: about 360 cal, 12 g pro, 13 g total fat (2 g sat. fat), 54 g carb, 11 g fibre, 0 mg chol, 723 mg sodium. % RDI: 8% calcium (89 mg), 30% iron (4.2 mg), 48% vit A, 353% vit C (212 mg), 52% folate (115 mcg).

5 Ways with Green Beans

Beans need never be boring with this list of quick tosses close at hand.

Toss 1 lb (500 g) green beans, cooked and still hot, with 1 tbsp (15 mL) melted butter or extra-virgin olive oil; pinch each salt and pepper; and one of the following:

- 2 tbsp (25 mL) grated Parmesan or Romano cheese and 1 tbsp (15 mL) chopped fresh basil

- 1/4 cup (50 mL) finely chopped sweet red pepper

- 1 tsp (5 mL) sesame oil and 1 green onion, chopped

- 2 tbsp (25 mL) chopped drained oil-packed sun-dried tomatoes and 2 cloves garlic, minced

- 1/2 tsp (2 mL) caraway seeds, lightly crushed

Makes 4 servings.

Grape Tomato Bursts

Wee oval grape tomatoes are now widely available in produce departments; cherry tomatoes make a good substitute. Either gives superior flavour over full-size tomatoes when the latter are out of season.

In 8-inch (2 L) square glass baking dish, combine 4 cups (1 L) grape tomatoes; 3 cloves garlic, minced; 1 tbsp (15 mL) extra-virgin olive oil; and 1/4 tsp (1 mL) each salt and pepper. Bake in 375°F (190°C) oven until softened but still holding shape, about 8 minutes.

Makes 4 servings.

Per serving: about 57 cal, 1 g pro, 4 g total fat (1 g sat. fat), 6 g carb, 2 g fibre, 0 mg chol, 154 mg sodium. % RDI: 1% calcium (13 mg), 5% iron (0.7 mg), 13% vit A, 30% vit C (918 mg), 4% folate (8 mcg).

Honey Acorn Squash

Try a buckwheat honey or maple syrup for a different flavour. Look for hard-skinned acorn or pepper squash that feel heavy for their size.

Cut 2 acorn squash (2 lb/1 kg total) in half; scrape out seeds. Arrange, cut side down, on rimmed baking sheet. Roast in 375°F (190°C) oven for 30 minutes. Turn cut side up. In each cavity, place 1 tsp (5 mL) each butter and liquid honey; roast until tender and golden, about 15 minutes.

Makes 4 servings.

Per serving: about 125 cal, 1 g pro, 4 g total fat (2 g sat. fat), 24 g carb, 4 g fibre, 10 mg chol, 44 mg sodium. % RDI: 5% calcium (57 mg), 9% iron (1.2 mg), 9% vit A, 23% vit C (14 mg), 11% folate (24 mcg).

Low-Fat Red Pepper Salad Dressing

Puréeing a roasted red pepper gives this salad dressing a supple texture without a lot of oil, and a vibrant, sophisticated flavour. Roast your own or use the jarred variety.

In blender, purée 1 roasted red pepper until smooth. Add 2 tbsp (25 mL) water; 1 tbsp (15 mL) red wine vinegar; 1 tsp (5 mL) Dijon mustard; and 1/4 tsp (1 mL) each salt, pepper and granulated sugar. With motor running, gradually pour in 2 tbsp (25 mL) olive oil.
Makes 1/2 cup (125 mL), enough for 10 cups (2.5 L) of greens.

Per 1 tbsp (15 mL): about 34 cal, 0 g pro, 3 g total fat (trace sat. fat), 1 g carb, 0g fibre, 0 mg chol, 7 mg sodium. % RDI: 0% calcium, 1% iron (0.1 mg), 3% vit A, 27% vit C (16 mg), 0% folate.

Quick Lemony Beets

Usually beets take a long time to cook, but grating them first speeds things up.

1 tbsp	olive oil	15 mL
4	green onions, chopped	4
4	beets (about 1 lb/500 g), peeled and grated	4
2 tbsp	chopped fresh mint or basil	25 mL
1 tbsp	lemon juice	15 mL
1/4 tsp	salt	1 mL
Pinch	pepper	Pinch

In large nonstick skillet, heat oil over medium heat; cook onions for 1 minute. Add beets and 1/2 cup (125 mL) water; cover and cook, stirring occasionally, for about 20 minutes or until beets are tender. Stir in mint, lemon juice, salt and pepper.
Makes 4 servings.

Per serving: about 74 cal, 2 g pro, 4 g total fat (trace sat. fat), 10 g carb, 2 g fibre, 0 mg chol, 214 mg sodium. % RDI: 3% calcium (29 mg), 7% iron (1.6 mg), 2% vit A, 10% vit C (6 mg), 35% folate (77 mcg).

Tip: Grate beets using a food processor or by hand (wear an apron!) using coarse side of box grater.

Roasted Ginger Carrots

Roasting adds depth of flavour and accentuates the natural sweetness of carrots.

2 tbsp	sesame oil	25 mL
1 tsp	grated gingerroot (or 1/2 tsp/2 mL ground ginger)	5 mL
1/4 tsp	each salt and pepper	1 mL
6 cups	thinly sliced carrots	1.5 L
2 tbsp	chopped fresh parsley	25 mL

In large bowl, combine oil, ginger, salt and pepper. Add carrots; toss gently. Transfer to 8-inch (2 L) square glass baking dish. Bake in 425°F (220°C) oven, stirring occasionally, until tender, 20 to 25 minutes. Sprinkle with parsley.
Makes 4 servings.

Per serving: about 137 cal, 2 g pro, 7 g total fat (1 g sat. fat), 18 g carb, 5 g fibre, 0 mg chol, 255 mg sodium. % RDI: 5% calcium (55 mg), 9% iron (1.2 mg), 414% vit A, 10% vit C (6 mg), 12% folate (27 mcg).

Sesame Snow Pea Stir-Fry

A touch of sesame oil adds loads of nutty flavour to sautéed and steamed vegetables alike. Be sure to store it in the refrigerator.
In skillet, heat 1 tsp (5 mL) vegetable oil over medium-high heat. Add 1 lb (500 g) snow peas, trimmed; sauté for 1 minute. Add 1 tsp (5 mL) sesame seeds; 1 tsp (5 mL) water; 1 tsp (5 mL) soy sauce; and 1/2 tsp (2 mL) sesame oil. Cover and steam until snow peas are tender-crisp, about 4 minutes.
Makes 4 servings.

Per serving: about 63 cal, 4 g pro, 2 g total fat (trace sat. fat), 7 g carb, 3 fibre, 0 mg chol, 4 mg sodium. % RDI: 4% calcium (44 mg), 15% iron (2.1 mg), 1% vit A, 82% vit C (49 mg), 14% folate (31 mcg).

Skillet-Steamed Sprouts

Choose tight, bright green brussels sprouts. Smaller sprouts are superior to larger ones, which are older, more strongly flavoured and need the outer leaves trimmed away.

In large skillet, melt 1 tbsp (15 mL) butter over medium heat; cook 1 clove garlic, minced, until fragrant, about 30 seconds.

Add 1 lb (500 g) brussels sprouts, halved; 2 tbsp (25 mL) water; and 1 tbsp (15 mL) soy sauce. Cover and cook, stirring occasionally, until tender-crisp, about 10 minutes.

Makes 4 servings.

Per serving: about 77 cal, 3 g pro, 4 g total fat (2 g sat. fat), 11 g carb, 4 g fibre, 9 mg chol, 314 mg sodium. % RDI: 4% calcium (48 mg), 11% iron (1.6 mg), 12% vit A, 128% vit C (77 mg), 34% folate (75 mcg).

Skinny Mashed Potatoes

Perenially popular mashed potatoes need not be rich with butter or cream to satisfy. Avoid green-tinged potatoes—this indicates the presence of solanine, a naturally occuring toxin produced when potatoes are exposed to light.

2 lb	hot boiled peeled potatoes (4 potatoes)	1 kg
1 cup	buttermilk or low-fat milk	250 mL
4 tsp	butter	20 mL
1/2 tsp	each salt and pepper	2 mL

In saucepan, mash together potatoes, buttermilk, butter, salt and pepper until smooth.

Makes 6 servings.

Per serving: about 139 cal, 4 g pro, 3 g total fat (2 g sat. fat), 25 g carb, 2 g fibre, 9 mg chol, 264 mg sodium. % RDI: 5% calcium (55 mg), 3% iron (0.4 mg), 3% vit A, 25% vit C (15 mg), 6% folate (13 mcg).

Spinach with Almonds

In minutes a mountain of fresh spinach dramatically shrinks into a scrumptious side dish with a delightful nutty taste.

2	bags (each 10 oz/284 g) fresh spinach, trimmed	2
1 tbsp	butter	15 mL
1/4 cup	slivered almonds	50 mL
1	onion, finely chopped	1
2	cloves garlic, minced	2
1/4 tsp	salt	1 mL

Rinse spinach; shake off excess water. In large saucepan with just the water clinging to leaves, cover and cook spinach over medium-high heat, stirring once, for 5 minutes or just until wilted. Transfer to colander; let cool slightly and squeeze out moisture.

In large nonstick skillet, melt butter over medium heat; cook almonds, stirring occasionally, for about 5 minutes or until golden. With slotted spoon, set almonds aside.

Add onion and garlic to pan; cook, stirring occasionally, for about 6 minutes or until softened. Stir in spinach, almonds and salt; cook, stirring, for about 1 minute or until heated through.

Makes 4 servings.

Per serving: about 113 cal, 6 g pro, 7 g total fat (2 g sat. fat), 9 g carb, 4 g fibre, 8 mg chol, 262 mg sodium. % RDI: 18% calcium (198 mg), 34% iron (4.8 mg), 105% vit A, 23% vit C (14 mg), 86% folate (189 mcg).

Vegetarian Tex-Mex Shepherd's Pie

This hearty casserole may take a few steps and ingredients to put together, but its make-ahead one-dish convenience makes it a natural choice when planning a relaxed family supper.

6	Yukon Gold potatoes (2 lb/1 kg)	6
1/4 cup	milk	50 mL
2 tbsp	chopped fresh parsley	25 mL
2 tbsp	butter	25 mL
3/4 tsp	each salt and pepper	4 mL
1 tbsp	vegetable oil	15 mL
2	carrots, diced	2
1	each onion and sweet red pepper, chopped	1
1 tbsp	chili powder	15 mL
1/2 tsp	ground cumin	2 mL
Pinch	cayenne pepper	Pinch
3/4 cup	bulgur	175 mL
2 tbsp	all-purpose flour	25 mL
1 1/2 cups	vegetable stock	375 mL
1	can (19 oz/540 mL) red kidney beans, drained and rinsed	1
1 cup	corn kernels	250 mL

Peel and cut potatoes into 2-inch (5-cm) chunks. In saucepan of boiling water, cover and cook potatoes until tender, about 20 minutes; drain and mash. Blend in milk, parsley, butter and 1/2 tsp (2 mL) each of the salt and pepper.

Meanwhile, in large skillet, heat oil over medium heat; cook carrots, onion, red pepper, chili powder, cumin and cayenne, stirring occasionally, until onion is softened, about 5 minutes.

Add bulgur and flour; cook, stirring, for 1 minute. Gradually stir in stock; cover and cook over low heat until liquid is absorbed, about 10 minutes.

Add kidney beans, corn and remaining salt and pepper. Spread in 8-inch (2 L) square glass baking dish; spread potatoes over top. Broil for 2 minutes or until golden. (Make-ahead: Let cool for 30 minutes; refrigerate until cold. Cover and store up to 24 hours; reheat, covered, in 350°F/180°C oven for 30 minutes or until filling is bubbly.)

Makes 4 to 6 servings.

Per each of 6 servings: about 342 cal, 11 g pro, 8 g total fat (3 g sat. fat), 62 g carb, 11 g fibre, 13 mg chol, 756 mg sodium. % RDI: 6% calcium (69 mg), 20% iron (2.8 mg), 77% vit A, 77% vit C (46 mg), 36% folate (80 mcg).

DIPS

Herbed White Bean Spread

You can make this simple spread at the last minute, or plan ahead to use as the basis of a veggie-filled sandwich.

1	can (19 oz/540 mL) white kidney beans, drained and rinsed	1
1/4 cup	packed fresh parsley	50 mL
2 tbsp	chopped fresh oregano or basil (or 1/2 tsp/2 mL dried)	25 mL
2 tbsp	extra-virgin olive oil	25 mL
2 tbsp	wine vinegar	25 mL
1/4 tsp	each salt and hot pepper sauce	1 mL
1	clove garlic, minced	1

In food processor, whirl together beans, parsley, oregano, oil, vinegar, salt and hot pepper sauce until blended but still chunky. Stir in garlic. (Make-ahead: Refrigerate in airtight container for up to 4 days.)

Makes 2 cups (500 mL).

Per 1 tbsp (15 mL): about 40 cal, 2 g pro, 2 g total fat (trace sat. fat), 5 g carb, 2 g fibre, 0 mg chol, 121 mg sodium. % RDI: 1% calcium (8 mg), 3% iron (0.4 mg), 1% vit A, 3% vit C (2 mg), 6% folate (14 mcg).

Roasted Red Pepper Dip

Serve with crunchy raw vegetables, such as carrots, cucumber, fennel, or spears of lightly steamed asparagus, or with Baked Whole Wheat Pita Chips (recipe, see page 277).

3	sweet red peppers	3
1 tbsp	extra-virgin olive oil	15 mL
1	clove garlic, minced	1
Half	onion, chopped	Half
Pinch	cayenne pepper	Pinch
2 tbsp	fresh bread crumbs	25 mL
1 tbsp	drained capers	15 mL
1/2 tsp	each salt and pepper	2 mL

Place peppers on rimmed baking sheet; roast in 400°F (200°C) oven, turning 4 times, until softened and skins are charred, about 20 minutes. Let cool for 15 minutes; peel, core and seed. (Make-ahead: Refrigerate in airtight container for up to 2 days.)

In small skillet, heat oil over medium heat; cook garlic, onion and cayenne pepper, stirring, until onion is softened, about 2 minutes.

In food processor, purée peppers until smooth. Add onion mixture, bread crumbs, capers, salt and pepper; purée until smooth. (Make-ahead: Refrigerate in airtight container for up to 2 days.)

Makes 1 1/2 cups (375 mL).

Per 2 tbsp (25 mL): about 22 cal, trace pro, 1 g total fat (trace sat. fat), 3 g carb, 1 g fibre, 0 mg chol, 111 mg sodium. % RDI: 0% calcium, 1% iron (0.2 mg), 11% vit A, 82% vit C (49 mg), 3% folate (6 mcg).

GRAIN FOODS

CEREALS

Deluxe Porridge

Here's a hearty, wholesome breakfast cereal with the delicious addition of nuts and raisins.

1 1/2 cups	large-flake rolled oats (not instant)	375 mL
1/3 cup	skim milk powder	75 mL
1/4 cup	packed brown sugar	50 mL
1/4 cup	natural bran	50 mL
1/2 tsp	cinnamon	2 mL
1/4 tsp	each salt and nutmeg	1 mL
2 tbsp	each raisins and chopped pecans	25 mL
2 tbsp	maple syrup	25 mL

In large saucepan, bring 3 1/2 cups (875 mL) water to boil. Using wooden spoon, gradually stir in oats. Reduce heat to medium; cover and simmer for 10 minutes.

Stir in skim milk powder, sugar, bran, cinnamon, salt and nutmeg; cover and cook for about 10 minutes or until porridge is thick enough to mound on spoon.

Spoon into bowls. Top with raisins, pecans and maple syrup.

Makes 6 servings.

Per serving: about 174 cal, 5 g pro, 3 g total fat (trace sat. fat), 34 g carb, 4 g fibre, 1 mg chol, 125 g sodium. % RDI: 7% calcium (78 mg), 11% iron (1.6 mg), 0% vit A, 0% vit C, 4% folate (8 mcg).

Microwave method: In large microwaveable casserole, microwave water at High for 3 minutes. Stir in all ingredients except raisins, pecans and syrup. Microwave, uncovered, at High until thickened, 10 to 12 minutes. Spoon into bowls; add toppings.

OATMEAL TOPPERS

Jazz up your favourite bowl of hot cereal with a tempting topping.

- Dried fruits, such as raisins, cherries, cranberries, chopped apricots, dates or figs
- Fresh or thawed frozen fruits, such as sliced strawberries, raspberries, blueberries, chopped apples or pears (leave the skins on for extra fibre), bananas, sliced plums or peaches
- Chopped toasted nuts or coconut
- Maple or fruit syrup

Fruity Yogurt Granola Trifle

This fun breakfast idea has endless variations. Try cubed cantaloupe, fresh raspberries, pineapple chunks or even your favourite stewed fruit. Of course, you can also use store-bought granola instead of homemade with equally delicious results.

1 cup	low-fat plain or flavoured yogurt	250 mL
1 cup	Homemade Granola (recipe p. 273)	250 mL
3/4 cup	each sliced bananas, kiwifruit and strawberries	75 mL
1 tbsp	liquid honey (optional)	15 mL

Spoon one-third of the yogurt into each of 2 glass dessert dishes. Top with one-third of the fruit, then half of the granola.

Repeat layers, ending with fruit on top. Drizzle with honey, if using.

Makes 2 servings.

Per serving: about 444 cal, 15 g pro, 14 g total fat (2.7 g sat. fat), 66 g carb, 7 g fibre, 7 mg chol, 93 mg sodium. % RDI: 23% calcium (257 mg), 18% iron (2.5 mg), 3% vit A, 70% vit C (42 mg), 34% folate (77 mcg).

Homemade Granola

Granola is almost as easy to make as it is to buy—and you control the ingredients. Customize by adding toasted pecans or almonds, chopped dried papaya or apricots, or flaked coconut with the cranberries.

3 cups	rolled oats	750 mL
2/3 cup	wheat germ	150 mL
1/2 cup	unsalted sunflower seeds	125 mL
1/2 cup	liquid honey	125 mL
1/4 cup	vegetable oil	50 mL
2/3 cup	dried cranberries or raisins	150 mL

In bowl, combine oats, wheat germ and sunflower seeds.

In small saucepan set over medium heat, stir honey with oil just until steaming. Pour over oat mixture, stirring to coat.

Spread mixture on parchment paper–lined baking sheet and bake in 350°F (180°C) oven, stirring frequently, until golden brown, about 15 minutes. Remove from oven; stir in cranberries. Let cool, stirring occasionally to prevent clumping. (Make-ahead: Refrigerate in airtight container for up to 1 month.)

Makes about 4 1/2 cups (1.125 L) or 9 servings.

Per 1/2 cup (125 mL): about 309 cal, 8 g pro, 12 g total fat (1 g sat. fat), 46 g carb, 5 g fibre, 5 mg sodium, % RDI: 2% calcium (21 mg), 15% iron (2.1 mg), 0% vit A, 3% vit C (2 mg), 20% folate (45 mcg).

Hot Almond Honey Multigrain Cereal

Vary the flavour—and boost nutrition—by stirring in a handful of chopped dried fruit, such as dates or figs.

3 cups	low-fat milk	750 mL
1/2 tsp	salt	2 mL
1 cup	multigrain cereal (such as Red River or Sunny Boy)	250 mL
1/2 cup	slivered almonds	125 mL
3 tbsp	liquid honey	50 mL
Pinch	nutmeg or cinnamon	Pinch

In saucepan, bring milk and salt to boil.

Whisk in multigrain cereal, almonds, honey and nutmeg. Reduce heat and simmer, whisking constantly, for 3 to 4 minutes or until desired thickness.

Makes 4 servings.

Per serving: about 349 cal, 14 g pro, 11 g total fat (2 g sat. fat), 53 g carb, 6 g fibre, 8 mg chol, 412 mg sodium. % RDI: 25% calcium (275 mg), 16% iron (2.3 mg), 10% vit A, 3% vit C (2 mg), 12% folate (27 mcg).

Morning Sunshine Bars

Bountifully sized and packed with good things—dates, pecans, bananas and carrots—bars like these can be made on the weekend and frozen, ready for rushed mornings or as a grab-and-go snack.

1 1/2 cups	each all-purpose and whole wheat flours	375 mL
2 tsp	baking powder	10 mL
2 tsp	cinnamon	10 mL
1 tsp	baking soda	5 mL
1/2 tsp	ground ginger	2 mL
1/4 tsp	salt	1 mL
2	eggs	2
1 cup	packed brown sugar	250 mL
1 cup	mashed very ripe bananas (2 large)	250 mL
2/3 cup	plain low-fat yogurt	150 mL
1/3 cup	vegetable oil	75 mL
2 cups	grated carrots (about 4)	500 mL
1 cup	chopped dates or raisins	250 mL
1/2 cup	chopped toasted pecans	125 mL

In large bowl, whisk together all-purpose and whole wheat flours, baking powder, cinnamon, baking soda, ginger and salt.

In separate bowl, whisk together eggs, sugar, bananas, yogurt and oil; pour over dry ingredients. Sprinkle with carrots, dates and pecans; mix just until dry ingredients are moistened.

Spread batter in greased waxed paper–lined 13 x 9-inch (3.5 L) cake pan. Bake in centre of 375°F (190°C) oven for about 30 minutes or until firm to the touch and tester inserted in centre comes out clean. Let cool completely in pan on rack. Cut into bars. (Make-ahead: Store in airtight container for up to 2 days or wrap individually in plastic wrap and freeze in airtight container for up to 2 weeks.)

Makes 16 bars.

Per serving: about 264 cal, 5 g pro, 8 g total fat (1 g sat. fat), 45 g carb, 4 g fibre, 24 mg chol, 171 mg sodium. % RDI: 6% calcium (68 mg), 13% iron (1.8 mg), 32% vit A, 2% vit C (1 mg), 12% folate (27 mcg).

Tropical Muesli to Go

Just measure and mix for an ideal eat-on-the-go breakfast or snack. You can also enjoy it in a bowl with milk or yogurt.

2 cups	cornflakes	500 mL
2 cups	rice crisp or puffed wheat cereal	500 mL
1 1/2 cups	large-flake rolled oats (not instant)	375 mL
1 cup	chopped dried apples or apricots	250 mL
1 cup	banana chips, crushed	250 mL
2/3 cup	raisins	150 mL
1/2 cup	shredded coconut	125 mL
1/2 cup	sliced almonds (optional)	125 mL

In bowl, combine cornflakes, rice crisp cereal, oats, apples, banana chips, raisins, coconut and almonds (if using). (Make-ahead: Store in resealable bag or airtight container for up to 3 weeks.)

Makes 8 cups (2 L).

Per 1 cup (250 mL): about 263 cal, 4 g pro, 7 g total fat (5 g sat. fat), 49 g carb, 5 g fibre, 0 mg chol, 170 mg sodium. % RDI: 2% calcium (20 mg), 23% iron (3.2 mg), 0% vit A, 3% vit C (2 mg), 6% folate (14 mcg).

QUICK BREADS AND PANCAKES

Apple Oatmeal Pancakes

Tender, fluffy pancakes are a snap if you know a few basic rules. Pancake batter should be lumpy; if mixed until smooth, pancakes will be tough. Your skillet should be hot enough that a few drops of cold water bounce vigorously when sprinkled in the pan. Serve with vanilla yogurt and a sprinkle of cinnamon.

3/4 cup	all-purpose flour	175 mL
1/2 cup	whole wheat flour	125 mL
1/3 cup	quick-cooking rolled oats	75 mL
1 tbsp	granulated sugar	15 mL
1 tbsp	baking powder	15 mL
3/4 tsp	cinnamon	4 mL
1/2 tsp	salt	2 mL
1 1/2 cups	low-fat milk	375 mL
1	egg	1
1/4 cup	vegetable oil	50 mL
1 cup	grated peeled apple	250 mL
1/2 cup	raisins	125 mL

In large bowl, whisk together all-purpose and whole wheat flours, oats, sugar, baking powder, cinnamon and salt.

In separate bowl, whisk together milk, egg and oil; add to dry ingredients and mix just until lumpy. Stir in apple and raisins just until incorporated.

Heat nonstick skillet over medium heat. Brush with vegetable oil. Pour in batter by 1/4 cupfuls (50 mL) for each pancake, spreading with spatula if necessary. Cook for 1 1/2 to 2 1/2 minutes or until underside is golden and bubbles break on top. Turn and cook for 1 to 2 minutes or until underside is golden.

Makes 4 servings.

Per serving: about 394 cal, 8 g pro, 16 g total fat (2 g sat. fat), 58 g carb, 5 g fibre, 47 mg chol, 216 mg sodium. % RDI: 10% calcium (115 mg), 21% iron (2.9 mg), 2% vit A, 3% vit C (2 mg), 20% folate (43 mcg).

Apricot, Oat and Bran Muffins

The mild taste of canola oil is ideal for baking. Canola also has the smallest amount of saturated fat of all oils. Whenever vegetable oil is called for, you can use canola.

1/2 cup	natural bran	125 mL
1 1/2 cups	whole wheat flour	375 mL
1 cup	quick-cooking rolled oats (not instant)	250 mL
1/3 cup	wheat germ	75 mL
1 1/2 tsp	baking soda	7 mL
1/2 tsp	salt	2 mL
1 cup	buttermilk	250 mL
3/4 cup	packed brown sugar	175 mL
1/3 cup	vegetable oil	75 mL
1	egg	1
3/4 cup	chopped dried apricots	175 mL

In bowl, mix bran with 1/2 cup (125 mL) boiling water; let cool.

In large bowl, whisk together flour, oats, wheat germ, baking soda and salt. In separate bowl, whisk together buttermilk, sugar, oil and egg; pour over dry ingredients along with bran mixture. Sprinkle with apricots; stir just until combined but still lumpy.

Spoon into greased or paper-lined muffin cups. Bake in centre of 375°F (190°C) oven until tops are firm to the touch, 18 to 20 minutes.

Makes 12 muffins.

Per muffin: about 232 cal, 6 g pro, 8 g total fat (1 g sat. fat), 38 g carb, 5 g fibre, 16 mg chol, 274 mg sodium. % RDI: 5% calcium (53 mg), 15% iron (2.1 mg), 6% vit A, 0% vit C, 8% folate (17 mcg).

Two-Grain Cranberry Bread

You can slice, wrap and freeze individual pieces of this dense loaf for a portable breakfast. Spread it with light cream cheese and add some fresh fruit and a glass of milk for a satisfying breakfast.

1/2 cup	butter, softened	125 mL
2/3 cup	packed brown sugar	150 mL
2	eggs	2
1 cup	rolled oats (not instant)	250 mL
1 cup	all-purpose flour	250 mL
2/3 cup	whole wheat flour	150 mL
1/2 tsp	each baking soda and baking powder	2 mL
1/2 tsp	salt	2 mL
1/4 tsp	ground cloves or cinnamon	1 mL
1 cup	dried cranberries or raisins	250 mL
1/2 cup	chopped pecans, toasted	125 mL
1 1/4 cups	unsweetened applesauce	300 mL

In large bowl, beat butter with sugar until light and fluffy. Beat in eggs, 1 at a time. In separate bowl, whisk together all but 2 tbsp (25 mL) of the rolled oats, the all-purpose and whole wheat flours, baking soda, baking powder, salt and cloves. Add cranberries and pecans. Stir into butter mixture alternately with applesauce, making 3 additions of oat mixture and 2 of applesauce.

Scrape into parchment paper–lined or greased 9- x 5-inch (2 L) loaf pan. Sprinkle with reserved rolled oats. Bake in centre of 350°F (180°C) oven until cake tester inserted in centre comes out clean, about 65 minutes. Let cool in pan on rack for 10 minutes. Turn out onto rack and let cool completely. (Make-ahead: Wrap in plastic wrap and store at room temperature for up to 2 days or overwrap with heavy-duty foil and freeze for up to 1 month.)

Makes 12 slices.

Per slice: about 285 cal, 5 g pro, 13 g total fat (5 g sat. fat), 40 g carb, 3 g fibre, 55 mg chol, 250 mg sodium. % RDI: 3% calcium (34 mg), 11% iron (1.6 mg), 9% vit A, 7% vit C (4 mg), 10% folate (23 mcg).

Whole Wheat Waffles

Serve with: Chunky Pear Applesauce (recipe page 299)

It's easy to feed the whole family nutritiously, even when you're treating them to a special weekend breakfast. Here, whole wheat flour, wheat germ and skim milk powder give fibre and calcium boosts without trading great flavour.

1 1/2 cups	all-purpose flour	375 mL
1/2 cup	whole wheat flour	125 mL
3 tbsp	granulated sugar	50 mL
2 tbsp	each wheat germ and skim milk powder	25 mL
1 tbsp	baking powder	15 mL
1/4 tsp	each salt and ground nutmeg	1 mL
2	eggs	2
2 cups	milk	500 mL
3 tbsp	vegetable oil	50 mL

In bowl, whisk together all-purpose and whole wheat flours, sugar, wheat germ, skim milk powder, baking powder, salt and nutmeg. In separate bowl, whisk together eggs, milk and 2 tbsp (25 mL) of the remaining oil; pour over flour mixture and stir just until combined.

Heat waffle iron; brush lightly with some of the oil. Pour in 1/2 cup (125 mL) batter for each waffle, spreading to edges. Close lid and cook until crisp and golden and steam stops.

Makes 8 waffles, or 4 servings.

Per each of serving (2 waffles = 1 serving): about 471 cal, 15 g pro, 16.5 g total fat (3 g sat. fat), 66 g carb, 5 g fibre, 0 mg chol, 443 mg sodium. % RDI: 26% calcium (287 mg), 24% iron (3.3 mg), 12% vit A, 0% vit C, 35% folate (77 mcg).

Variation: Whole Wheat Pancakes: Heat large nonstick skillet or griddle over medium heat; brush with some of the remaining oil. Using 1/4 cup (50 mL) batter per pancake, pour in batter; cook until bubbles break on top but do not fill in, 2 to 3 minutes. Turn and cook until bottom is golden, about 1 minute. Makes about 18 pancakes.

GRAIN SIDES

Baked Whole Wheat Pita Chips

Here's a lightened-up way to dig into savoury dips and spreads. Let cool; then store in airtight container for up to 1 week.

1 tbsp	vegetable oil	15 mL
2	whole wheat pitas, each split into 2 rounds	2
2 tsp	sesame seeds	10 mL
1/4 tsp	paprika	1 mL

Brush oil on rough sides of each pita round. Combine sesame seeds and paprika; sprinkle over pitas.

Cut each pita into 8 wedges. Place in single layer on baking sheet. Bake in 350°F (180°C) until golden brown and crisp, about 12 minutes.

Makes 4 servings.

Per serving: about 119 cal, 3 g pro, 5 g total fat (trace sat. fat), 17 g carb, 2 g fibre, 0 mg chol, 160 mg sodium. % RDI: 1% calcium (7 mg), 8% iron (1.1 mg), 1% vit A, 0% vit C, 7% folate (16 mcg).

Barley Vegetable Pilaf

Barley is an excellent alternative to rice. It comes with its husk and bran removed, in two forms—pot and pearl—the latter slightly more polished. Use either and enjoy the slightly chewy texture and nutty flavour. If you prefer plain grain side dishes, omit the peas and corn.

1 tbsp	vegetable oil	15 mL
1	small onion, chopped	1
2	cloves garlic, minced	2
2 1/4 cups	chicken stock	550 mL
3/4 cup	pearl barley	175 mL
1/2 cup	each frozen peas and frozen corn	125 mL
1/2 cup	chopped green onions	125 mL
1/4 tsp	each salt and pepper	1 mL

In large saucepan, heat oil over medium heat; cook onion and garlic, stirring often, for 5 minutes or until softened. Stir in stock and barley; bring to boil. Reduce heat to medium; cover and simmer for 30 minutes or until most of the liquid is absorbed. Stir in peas, corn, green onions, salt and pepper; cook for 5 minutes or until barley is tender and liquid is absorbed.

Makes 4 servings.

Per serving: about 226 cal, 7 g pro, 5 g total fat (1 g sat. fat), 40 g carb, 4 g fibre, 0 mg chol, 602 mg sodium. % RDI: 3% calcium (38 mg), 16% iron (2.3 mg), 2% vit A, 8% vit C (5 mg), 19% folate (42 mcg).

Brown Rice with Broccoli

An important consideration when storing whole grains is freshness. If possible, buy grains in amounts you can use within a month. Store in an airtight container in a cool pantry.

2 2/3 cups	water	650 mL
1/4 tsp	salt	1 mL
1 1/3 cups	brown rice	325 mL
3 cups	broccoli florets and chopped peeled broccoli stems	750 mL

In saucepan, bring water and salt to boil; stir in brown rice. Cover and reduce heat to low; simmer for 20 minutes.

Sprinkle broccoli florets and chopped peeled stems over rice; cook, covered, until rice is tender, liquid is absorbed and broccoli is tender-crisp, about 5 minutes. Fluff with fork.

Makes 4 servings.

Per serving: about 246 cal, 7 g pro, 2 g total fat (trace sat. fat), 50 g carb, 5 g fibre, 0 mg chol, 171 mg sodium. % RDI: 5% calcium (51 mg), 10% iron (1.4 mg), 9% vit A, 82% vit C (49 mg), 19% folate (41 mcg).

Couscous with Red Pepper

Couscous, technically a kind of pasta, is a North African staple. Smart cooks keep it on hand to parlay into a quick and simple side dish with maximum versatility. Look for the whole wheat variety for extra fibre.

1 tbsp	olive oil	15 mL
1	small onion, finely chopped	1
Half	sweet red or green pepper, diced	Half
1/4 tsp	dried thyme	1 mL
1/4 tsp	each salt and pepper	1 mL
1 1/2 cups	vegetable stock or water	375 mL
1 cup	couscous	250 mL

In small saucepan, heat oil over medium heat; cook onion, red pepper, thyme, salt and pepper, stirring often for about 5 minutes or until softened.

Add stock; bring to boil. Add couscous; cover and remove from heat. Let stand for 5 minutes. Fluff with fork.

Makes 4 servings.

Per serving: about 221 cal, 6 g pro, 4 g total fat (1 g sat. fat), 39 g carb, 3 g fibre, 0 mg chol, 388 mg sodium. % RDI: 2% calcium (21 mg), 6% iron (0.8 mg), 5% vit A, 482% vit C (25 mg), 13% folate (28 mcg).

Grilled Polenta

Crusty on the outside, soft on the inside, grilled polenta makes a terrific base for a medley of grilled vegetables or for Mediterranean-flavoured grilled or braised meats.

4 cups	water	1 L
1 tsp	salt	5 mL
1 cup	cornmeal	250 mL

In large saucepan, bring water and salt to boil. Whisk in cornmeal in slow steady stream. Reduce heat and simmer, stirring frequently, for 20 to 25 minutes or until polenta mounds on spoon.

Spread in greased 9-inch (2.5 L) square metal cake pan. Refrigerate for 2 hours or until set.

Turn polenta out of pan. Cut into 4 squares; cut each piece diagonally into 2 triangles. Place on greased grill over medium-high heat and cook for 5 minutes per side or until crusty and grill-marked.

Makes 4 servings.

Per serving: about 126 cal, 3 g pro, 1 g total fat (trace sat. fat), 27 g carb, 2 g fibre, 0 mg chol, 581 mg sodium. % RDI: 1% calcium (7 mg), 3% iron (0.4 mg), 1% vit A, 0% vit C, 5% folate (12 mcg).

Tomato Bulgur Pilaf

Cooking bulgur with stock and tomato paste adds flavour without adding fat. This is a great side dish for roast pork, grilled chicken or any vegetarian stew or chili.

In saucepan, heat 1 tbsp (15 mL) extra-virgin olive oil over medium heat. Cook 1 onion, chopped; 3 cloves garlic, minced; and 1/4 tsp (1 mL) each salt and pepper until softened, about 5 minutes.

Add 1 1/2 cups (375 mL) bulgur and 1/4 cup (50 mL) tomato paste; cook for 2 minutes. Stir in 2 cups (500 mL) chicken stock and bring to boil; remove from heat, cover and let stand until tender, about 15 minutes. Stir in 1/3 cup (75 mL) chopped green onions.

Makes 4 servings.

Per serving: about 246 cal, 7 g pro, 2 g total fat (trace sat. fat), 50 g carb, 5 g fibre, 0 mg chol, 171 mg sodium. % RDI: 5% calcium (51 mg), 10% iron (1.4 mg), 9% vit A, 82% vit C (49 mg), 19% folate (41 mcg).

Wheat Berries

Wheat berries are whole wheat kernels with the bran and germ intact. They have the same nutrients as wheat and a wonderful chewy texture. Serve hot or cold, with fresh herbs and enough vinaigrette to moisten. Try them as a substitute for rice or barley in a grain salad.

4 cups	water	1 L
1/2 tsp	salt	2 mL
1 1/2 cups	soft wheat berries	375 mL

In large saucepan, bring water and salt to boil over high heat; add wheat berries. Reduce heat to low; cover and simmer for 45 to 60 minutes or tender but firm.

Makes 6 servings.

Per serving: about 139 cal, 4 g pro, 1 g total fat (trace sat. fat), 31 g carb, 5 g fibre, 0 mg chol, 197 mg sodium. % RDI: 1% calcium (315 mg), 10% iron (1.4 mg), 0% vit A, 0% vit C, 5% folate (12 mcg).

BEANS, LEGUMES AND SOY

Bulgur Chickpea Tomato Salad

This is a terrific weekday lunch—quick to put together in the morning or to make ahead the night before. Bulgur, a staple in Middle Eastern cooking, is made of wheat kernels that have been steamed, dried and crushed. It is usually soaked, not cooked, before eating, making it a thoroughly convenient ingredient.

1 cup	bulgur	250 mL
3	plum tomatoes, chopped	3
3	green onions, chopped	3
1 cup	rinsed drained canned chickpeas (half 19 oz/540 mL can)	250 mL
2/3 cup	finely chopped fresh Italian parsley	150 mL
1/4 cup	shaved Parmesan, Asiago or Romano cheese	50 mL
Dressing:		
3 tbsp	each lemon juice and olive oil	50 mL
3/4 tsp	salt	4 mL
1/4 tsp	pepper	1 mL

In saucepan, bring 1 1/2 cups (375 mL) water to boil; stir in bulgur. Cover and remove from heat; let stand for 20 minutes. Drain in sieve; let stand for 5 minutes.

Dressing: Meanwhile, in bowl, whisk together lemon juice, oil, salt and pepper.

In large bowl, combine bulgur, tomatoes, onions, chickpeas and parsley; drizzle with dressing and toss.

Garnish with Parmesan cheese. (Make-ahead: Cover and refrigerate overnight.)

Makes 6 servings.

Per serving: about 214 cal, 7 g pro, 9 g total fat (2 g sat. fat), 29 g carb, 5 g fibre, 3 mg chol, 471 mg sodium. % RDI: 9% calcium (94 mg), 15% iron (2.1 mg), 7% vit A, 32% vit C (19 mg), 27% folate (59 mcg).

Fruity Tofu Smoothie

Tofu adds protein to this tasty morning drink. Custard-like silken tofu works best.

1 cup	fresh or frozen fruit (such as mixed tropical fruit, peaches or strawberries)	250 mL
1 cup	orange juice	250 mL
1/2 cup	silken or soft tofu	125 mL
1/2 cup	plain low-fat yogurt	125 mL
2 tbsp	lemon juice	25 mL
2 tbsp	liquid honey	25 mL
1	banana	1

In blender, purée together fruit, orange juice, tofu, yogurt, lemon juice, honey and banana until smooth.

Makes 2 servings.

Per serving: about 276 cal, 8 g pro, 3 g total fat (1 g sat. fat), 59 g carb, 4 g fibre, 4 mg chol, 64 mg sodium. % RDI: 13% calcium (147 mg), 7% iron (1 mg), 7% vit A, 103% vit C (62 mg), 35% folate (76 mcg).

Tip: Frozen bananas make smoothies thick and frosty. Wrap peeled ripe bananas tightly in plastic wrap and freeze.

Lentil Salad with Corn and Red Onion

Lentil salads are staples in most Mediterranean countries, though the flavourings and dressings change from nation to nation. In this one, balsamic vinegar and orange rind add depth of flavour; juicy corn and crunchy celery are colourful additions.

1 cup	dried green or brown lentils	250 mL
2 cups	corn kernels	500 mL
1 cup	chopped celery	250 mL
1 cup	chopped fresh Italian parsley	250 mL
1/3 cup	chopped red onion	75 mL
1/4 cup	balsamic vinegar	50 mL
1 tbsp	chopped fresh sage (optional)	15 mL
1 tbsp	extra-virgin olive oil	15 mL
1 tsp	grated orange rind	5 mL
1 tsp	salt	5 mL
1/2 tsp	pepper	2 mL

Sort lentils, discarding any discoloured ones; rinse and drain. In saucepan, cover lentils with water; bring to boil and cook for 25 to 30 minutes or until tender. Drain and let cool. In bowl, combine lentils, corn, celery, parsley, onion, vinegar, sage (if using), oil, orange rind, salt and pepper; toss.

Makes 6 servings.

Per serving: about 197 cal, 11 g pro, 3 g total fat (trace sat. fat), 35 g carb, 6 g fibre, 0 mg chol, 408 mg sodium. % RDI: 4% calcium (44 mg), 29% iron (4.1 mg), 6% vit A, 27% vit C (16 mg), 97% folate (213 mcg).

Mushroom Lentil Patties

A good source of vegetable protein, lentils are low in fat and high in fibre, folate, iron and phosphorus. Serve these patties on whole wheat sesame seed rolls with an array of the usual burger toppings.

3/4 cup	walnuts	175 mL
2 tbsp	vegetable oil	25 mL
4 cups	sliced mushrooms	2 L
1	onion, chopped	1
1	clove garlic, minced	1
1/2 tsp	dried thyme	2 mL
1/4 tsp	each salt and pepper	1 mL
1	can (19 oz/540 mL) lentils, drained and rinsed	1
2 tsp	Worcestershire sauce (optional)	10 mL
1/4 cup	dry bread crumbs	50 mL
1/4 cup	chopped fresh parsley	50 mL

In skillet, toast walnuts until fragrant, about 5 minutes; transfer to food processor. In same skillet, heat 1 tbsp (15 mL) of the oil over medium-high heat; cook mushrooms, onion, garlic, thyme, salt and pepper until liquid is evaporated, about 5 minutes. Add to food processor. Add lentils, and Worcestershire sauce (if using); pulse to combine. Mix in bread crumbs and parsley. Form into eight 1/2-inch (1 cm) thick patties.

In same skillet, heat remaining oil over medium heat; fry patties, in batches, until crusty, about 4 minutes per side.

Makes 4 servings.

Per serving: about 281 cal, 13 g pro, 13 g total fat (1 g sat. fat), 32 g carb, 7 g fibre, 0 mg chol, 473 mg sodium. % RDI: 5% calcium (69 mg), 38% iron (5.3 mg), 2% vit A, 15% vit C (9 mg), 94% folate (207 mcg).

Tofu Burritos

Tofu is a versatile, inexpensive and high-protein ingredient. Because most tofu is coagulated using a calcium compound, the nutritional bonus is that tofu is often rich in calcium. Like chicken, its bland nature means it works well with many different flavourings, like the Tex-Mex seasonings in these burritos.

1	pkg (350 g) extra-firm tofu	1
1 tbsp	vegetable oil	15 mL
1	large onion, chopped	1
1	clove garlic, minced	1
1/2 tsp	each ground cumin and chili powder	2 mL
1/4 tsp	each salt and pepper	1 mL
1	sweet green pepper, chopped	1
1	jalapeño pepper, chopped	1
1 cup	drained chopped canned tomatoes	250 mL
4	large whole wheat flour tortillas	4
3/4 cup	shredded light Cheddar cheese	175 mL

Pat tofu dry; cut into 1/2-inch (1 cm) cubes. Set aside.

In skillet, heat oil over medium heat; cook onion, garlic, cumin, chili powder, salt and pepper, stirring occasionally, until onion is softened, about 3 minutes.

Add tofu cubes, green and jalapeño peppers, and tomatoes; cook until peppers are softened, about 4 minutes.

Spoon about 1 cup (250 mL) of the tofu mixture along centre of each tortilla; sprinkle with one-quarter of the cheese. Fold up bottom edge, then sides; roll up.

Bake on greased rimmed baking sheet in 400°F (200°C) oven until golden and cheese is melted, about 15 minutes. Cut diagonally into halves.

Makes 4 servings.

Per serving: about 334 cal, 22 g pro, 14 g total fat (4 g sat. fat), 43 g carb, 5 g fibre, 13 mg chol, 750 mg sodium. % RDI: 31% calcium (340 mg), 26% iron (3.7 mg), 9% vit A, 62% vit C (37 mg), 50% folate (50 mcg).

Tofu Vegetable Curry

Freshness is essential to tofu. Fresh tofu smells sweet, mild and slightly nutty. Tofu past its prime has a sour odour and should be discarded. Check the best-before date. Serve with a dollop of yogurt.

1	eggplant (about 1 lb/500 g)	1
2	large potatoes (1 lb/500 g)	2
1	pkg (350 g) extra-firm tofu	1
1 tbsp	vegetable oil	15 mL
1	onion, chopped	1
1/2 cup	chopped fresh coriander	125 mL
1 tbsp	mild curry paste	15 mL
1/2 tsp	salt	2 mL
1 cup	vegetable stock	250 mL
1	can (28 oz/796 mL) tomatoes	1
2 cups	small cauliflower florets	500 mL
1 cup	frozen peas	250 mL

Cut eggplant into 1/2-inch (1 cm) cubes. Scrub potatoes; cut into same-size cubes. Set vegetables aside. Pat tofu dry; cut into 3/4-inch (2 cm) cubes. Set aside.

In shallow Dutch oven, heat oil over medium-high heat; cook onion, half of the coriander, the curry paste and salt, stirring occasionally, for 3 minutes. Add eggplant, potatoes and vegetable stock; cook, stirring often, for about 8 minutes or until vegetables are softened.

Add tomatoes; bring to boil, scraping up brown bits from bottom of pan and breaking up tomatoes with back of spoon. Cover and cook, stirring occasionally, for 15 minutes.

Add cauliflower and tofu; cook, covered, for about 7 minutes or until potatoes and cauliflower are tender. Add peas and remaining coriander; cook for 1 minute or until hot.

Makes 4 servings.

Per serving: about 320 cal, 16 g pro, 11 g total fat (1 g sat. fat), 46 g carb, 10 g fibre, 0 mg chol, 794 mg sodium. % RDI: 25% calcium (272 mg), 30% iron (4.2 mg), 16% vit A, 102% vit C (61 mg), 51% folate (113 mcg).

DAIRY AND EGGS

Asparagus Frittata

Asparagus is an excellent source of folate. For this recipe, thick stalks work best; tightly closed tips tinged with purple indicate freshness. You will need about 12 oz (375 g) of asparagus.

1 tbsp	butter	15 mL
2 cups	chopped trimmed asparagus	500 mL
1	sweet red pepper, diced	1
1	clove garlic, minced	1
2 tsp	chopped fresh thyme (or 1 tsp/5 mL dried)	10 mL
1/4 tsp	each salt and pepper	1 mL
8	eggs	8
1/4 cup	milk	50 mL
1/3 cup	crumbled feta cheese	75 mL

In 9- or 10-inch (23- or 25-cm) nonstick ovenproof skillet, melt butter over medium heat; cook asparagus, red pepper, garlic, thyme, salt and pepper, stirring occasionally, until tender-crisp, about 5 minutes.

In bowl, whisk eggs with milk. Stir into asparagus mixture; sprinkle with feta cheese. Cover and cook over medium-low heat until bottom and side are firm but top is still slightly runny, about 7 minutes. Broil until golden and set, about 1 minute.
Makes 4 servings.

Per serving: about 230 cal, 16 g pro, 16 g total fat (7 g sat. fat), 7 g carb, 2 g fibre, 391 mg chol, 425 mg sodium. % RDI: 13% calcium (138 mg), 14% iron (1.9 mg), 35% vit A, 93% vit C (56 mg), 67% folate (148 mcg).

Variation: Broccoli Frittata: Replace asparagus with chopped broccoli florets and peeled stems.

Fruity Blender Buzz

Not always up to eating first thing? Shake things up with a frothy fruit beverage to get your engine running. Instead of berries, you can use sliced peeled pitted peaches or mango.

1 cup	milk or soy beverage	250 mL
2 tbsp	skim milk powder	25 mL
1	ripe banana	1
1 cup	frozen or fresh strawberries, blueberries or raspberries	250 mL

In blender, purée together milk, skim milk powder, banana and berries until smooth. Pour into 2 glasses.
Makes 2 servings.

Per serving: about 155 cal, 6 g pro, 3 g total fat (2 g sat. fat), 28 g carb, 2 g fibre, 10 mg chol, 87 mg sodium. % RDI: 20% calcium (217 mg), 6% iron (0.8 mg), 8% vit A, 62% vit C (37 mg), 14% folate (31 mcg).

Saucy Tomato Poached Eggs

Wake up to a lively breakfast that combines the classic appeal of sunny-side-up eggs with a colourful simmer of tomatoes and zucchini. Serve with whole grain toast and juice.

1 tbsp	olive oil	15 mL
1	onion, chopped	1
1	zucchini, sliced	1
2	cloves garlic, sliced	2
1 tsp	dried Italian seasoning	5 mL
1/4 tsp	each salt and pepper	1 mL
1	can (28 oz/796 mL) tomatoes	1
6	eggs	6

In large skillet, heat oil over medium-high heat; cook onion, zucchini, garlic, Italian seasoning, salt and pepper, stirring often, for 5 minutes or until softened.

Add tomatoes, breaking up with spoon; cook for 20 minutes or until thickened and most of the liquid is evaporated.

Make 6 wells in sauce; gently break egg into each. Cover and cook for 5 minutes or until whites are set, or until desired doneness.

Makes 6 servings.

Per serving: about 135 cal, 8 g pro, 7 g fat (2 g sat. fat), 9 g carb, 2 g fibre, 215 mg chol, 379 mg sodium. % RDI: 7% calcium (71 mg), 13% iron (1.8 mg), 18% vit A, 25% vit C (15 mg), 14% folate (31 mcg).

FISH AND SEAFOOD

Hoisin Roast Salmon with Orange Spinach Salad

When it comes to fish, marinades are for flavour, not tenderness. Marinating fish for more than 45 minutes may allow the acids in vinegar or citrus juice to "cook" the fish, so that when it is heat-cooked, the outside will be dry and woolly.

1	orange	1
1/3 cup	finely chopped green onion	75 mL
1/3 cup	hoisin sauce	75 mL
1/4 cup	rice or cider vinegar	50 mL
4 tsp	soy sauce	20 mL
1/2 tsp	minced gingerroot	2 mL
4	salmon fillets or steaks (1 1/2 lb/750 g total)	4
4 cups	lightly packed fresh spinach	1 L
2 tsp	sesame seeds, toasted	10 mL

Grate rind from orange to make 2 tsp (10 mL); set aside. Cut off ends, remaining rind, pith and outer membrane. Slice orange crosswise and cut slices into quarters; set aside in large bowl.

In dish, whisk together orange rind, onion, hoisin sauce, vinegar, soy sauce and ginger. Remove 2 tbsp (25 mL) and add to orange in bowl.

Add fish to dish, turning to coat. Transfer to foil-lined rimmed baking sheet; pour hoisin mixture over top. Bake in 425°F (220°C) oven until opaque and fish flakes easily when tested, 10 to 15 minutes. Broil for 1 minute or until golden.

Meanwhile, trim spinach; tear into bite-size pieces. Add to orange mixture; toss. Serve with fish. Sprinkle with sesame seeds.

Makes 4 servings.

Per serving: about 275 cal, 23 g pro, 13 g total fat (3 g sat. fat), 18 g carb, 3 g fibre, 56 mg chol, 790 mg sodium. % RDI: 9% calcium (100 mg), 17% iron (2.4 mg), 40% vit A, 65% vit C (39 mg), 73% folate (160 mcg).

Tip: To toast sesame seeds, cook in nonstick skillet over medium heat, shaking pan often, until golden, about 5 minutes.

Rice and Greens with Shrimp

Here's the perfect dish for nights when you want dinner to be a little special but don't have a lot of time.

1 tbsp	extra-virgin olive oil	15 mL
1	onion, chopped	1
4	cloves garlic, minced	4
1/4 tsp	each salt and pepper	1 mL
1 1/3 cups	long grain rice	325 mL
2 2/3 cups	chicken stock	650 mL
1 tsp	grated lemon rind	5 mL
1 lb	large shrimp, peeled and deveined	500 g
3 cups	packed Swiss chard or spinach, coarsely shredded	750 mL
1 tbsp	chopped fresh dill	15 mL
1 tbsp	lemon juice	15 mL
	lemon wedges	

In large saucepan, heat oil over medium heat; cook onion, garlic, salt and pepper, stirring occasionally, until softened, about 5 minutes. Stir in rice. Add stock and lemon rind; bring to boil. Reduce heat, cover and simmer until liquid is almost absorbed, about 15 minutes.

With fork, gently stir shrimp, Swiss chard, dill and lemon juice into rice mixture; cover and cook until shrimp are pink and greens are wilted, about 5 minutes. Serve with lemon wedges.

Makes 4 servings.

Per serving: about 394 cal, 27 g pro, 6 g total fat (1 g sat. fat), 55 g carb, 2 g fibre, 129 mg chol, 821 mg sodium. % RDI: 10% calcium (112 mg), 28% iron (3.9 mg), 37% vit A, 15% vit C (9 mg), 35% folate (77 mcg).

Tip: For more fibre and iron choose brown rice.

Salmon Pasta Salad

Look for whole wheat pastas in your grocery store or at health food stores. Elbow macaroni, farfalle or fusilli would also work well for this salad.

4 cups	small shell pasta	1 L
1 cup	frozen peas	250 mL
1	can (7.5 oz/213 g) sockeye salmon, drained	1
1/2 cup	plain low-fat yogurt	125 mL
1/3 cup	finely diced red onion	75 mL
1/4 cup	light mayonnaise	50 mL
6	radishes, thinly sliced	6
2 tbsp	chopped fresh dill (or 2 tsp/10 mL dried dillweed)	25 mL
1/2 tsp	each salt, pepper and hot pepper sauce	2 mL
12	leaves romaine lettuce	12

In large saucepan of boiling salted water, cook pasta for 7 minutes. Add peas; cook until pasta is tender but firm, about 1 minute. Drain and rinse under cold water; shake out excess water.

Meanwhile, in small bowl, flake salmon with fork, mashing in any bones; remove skin if desired. Set aside.

In large bowl, stir together yogurt, onion, mayonnaise, radishes, dill, salt, pepper and hot pepper sauce.

Tear 4 of the lettuce leaves into bite-size pieces; add to large bowl along with pasta mixture and salmon, and toss to combine. To serve, spoon onto remaining lettuce leaves.

Makes 4 servings.

Per serving: about 484 cal, 24 g pro, 10 g total fat (2 g sat. fat), 74 g carb, 6 g fibre, 26 mg chol, 985 mg sodium. % RDI: 18% calcium (202 mg), 24% iron (3.4 mg), 13% vit A, 25% vit C (15 mg), 87% folate (192 mcg).

Variations: Shrimp Pasta Salad: Replace salmon and peas with cooked salad shrimp and chopped red or yellow pepper.

Crab Pasta Salad: Replace salmon and peas with crabmeat and frozen broccoli florets.

Sole Pinwheels on Yellow Pepper

Serve with: Brown Rice with Broccoli (recipe page 278)

You can use almost any thin fish fillets—red snapper, tilapia or rainbow trout, for instance. For variety, substitute thinly sliced fresh fennel or slices of summer squash for the yellow pepper.

1	sweet yellow pepper	1
1 1/2 cups	cherry tomatoes, halved	375 mL
1	large clove garlic, sliced	2
2 tbsp	extra-virgin olive oil	25 mL
1 tbsp	dried rosemary, crumbled	15 mL
1/2 tsp	each salt and pepper	2 mL
4	sole fillets (1 lb/500 g)	4
2 tbsp	chopped fresh parsley	25 mL
1 tbsp	lemon juice	15 mL

Cut yellow pepper into 1-inch (2.5-cm) strips; place in oval gratin dish. Add tomatoes, garlic, 1 tbsp (15 mL) of the oil, rosemary and 1/4 tsp (1 mL) each of the salt and pepper; toss to coat. Bake in 375°F (190°C) oven until pepper is tender-crisp, about 10 minutes.

Meanwhile, pat sole dry. In small bowl, whisk together remaining oil, salt and pepper, 1 tbsp (15 mL) of the parsley and lemon juice; brush all but 1 tbsp (15 mL) over tops of sole. Starting at 1 short end of each, roll tightly into pinwheel; insert skewer crosswise through sole to hold together. Brush with reserved oil mixture.

Remove dish from oven; place sole on yellow pepper mixture. Bake until fish flakes easily when tested, about 15 minutes. Sprinkle with remaining parsley.

Makes 4 servings.

Per serving: about 186 cal, 22 g pro, 8 g total fat (1 g sat. fat), 5 g carb, 1 g fibre, 54 mg chol, 385 mg sodium. % RDI: 4% calcium (48 mg), 9% iron (1.2 mg), 8% vit A, 90% vit C (54 mg), 10% folate (22 mcg).

Tip: You can use other fresh or thawed frozen thin fish fillets, such as catfish, tilapia, perch or pickerel.

Trout Gremolada

Serve with: Grape Tomato Burst (recipe page 267) and Grilled Polenta (recipe page 279)

Choose two trout fillets that weigh 12 oz to 1 lb (375 to 500 g) each, or four smaller ones. Tilapia or red snapper fillets are other good choices for this recipe.

2 tbsp	finely chopped fresh parsley	25 mL
2 tbsp	grated lemon rind	25 mL
2 tbsp	olive oil	25 mL
1	clove garlic, minced	1
1/4 tsp	each salt and pepper	1 mL
4	rainbow trout fillets, each 6 to 8 oz/175 to 250 g	4

In bowl, combine parsley, lemon rind, oil, garlic, salt and pepper. Pat fillets dry; spread parsley mixture over skinless sides.

Place fillets, skin side down, on greased grill over medium heat; close lid and cook for 8 to 10 minutes or until fish flakes easily when tested with fork.

Makes 4 servings.

Per serving: about 330 cal, 47 g pro, 14 g total fat (2 g sat. fat), 1 g carb, trace fibre, 129 mg chol, 205 mg sodium. % RDI: 15% calcium (161 mg), 32% iron (4.6 mg), 5% vit A, 18% vit C (11 mg), 10% folate (21 mcg).

POULTRY

Chicken with Creamy Pesto Sauce

Standby chicken breasts are elevated to a new level when served with a creamy, elegant sauce. The bonus is that evaporated milk gives rich texture despite its low butterfat content. Try the sauce tossed with linguine and quartered cherry tomatoes.

1 tbsp	vegetable oil	15 mL
4	boneless skinless chicken breasts (1 1/4 lb/625 g total)	4
1	onion, chopped	1
2	cloves garlic, minced	2
3 cups	sliced mushrooms (8 oz/250 g)	750 mL
1 tsp	dried thyme	5 mL
1/2 tsp	salt	2 mL
1/4 tsp	pepper	1 mL
1/2 cup	white wine or chicken stock	125 mL
1 tbsp	all-purpose flour	15 mL
1	can (384 mL) evaporated 2% milk	1
2 tbsp	basil pesto (or 1/3 cup/75 mL chopped fresh basil)	25 mL

In large skillet or shallow Dutch oven, heat oil over medium-high heat; brown chicken, about 10 minutes. Transfer to plate.

Add onion, garlic, mushrooms, thyme, salt and pepper; cook over medium heat until no liquid from mushrooms remains, about 10 minutes.

Add wine to pan; cook, stirring, for 2 minutes. Meanwhile, whisk flour into evaporated milk. Add to pan; cook, stirring, until thickened, about 5 minutes. Stir in pesto.

Return chicken to pan, turning to coat; simmer for 10 minutes or until chicken is no longer pink inside.

Makes 4 servings.

Per serving: about 350 cal, 42 g pro, 11 g total fat (3 g sat. fat), 18 g carb, 1 g fibre, 93 mg chol, 570 mg sodium. % RDI: 31% calcium (339 mg), 19% iron (2.6 mg), 9% vit A, 20% vit C (12 mg), 11% folate (24 mcg).

Skillet Chicken and Sweet Potatoes

Simmering the potatoes right along with the chicken makes for an easy one-pot supper. Sweet potatoes are high in fibre (about 4 g per 1/2-cup/125 mL serving). They are also very high in beta-carotene and are a good source of vitamin C, both of which are antioxidants.

8	bone-in skinless chicken thighs (2 lb/1 kg)	8
1/2 tsp	each salt and pepper	2 mL
2 tsp	canola oil	10 mL
2	onions, sliced	2
2	cloves garlic, minced	2
1/2 tsp	dried thyme	2 mL
1 tbsp	all-purpose flour	15 mL
1 cup	apple cider or juice	250 mL
2	sweet potatoes (about 1 1/2 lb/750 g)	2
1 tbsp	chopped fresh parsley	15 mL

Trim any fat from thighs; sprinkle with salt and pepper. In large skillet, heat oil over medium-high heat; brown thighs. Remove to plate.

Drain any fat from pan. Add onions, garlic and thyme; cook over medium heat, stirring occasionally, until softened, about 5 minutes. Sprinkle with flour; cook, stirring, for 1 minute. Add cider; bring to boil, scraping up any brown bits from bottom of pan. Return chicken, fleshier side down, and any accumulated juices to pan. Reduce heat to medium-low; cover and simmer for 10 minutes.

Meanwhile, peel and cut sweet potatoes into 1-inch (2.5-cm) cubes; add to pan. Turn chicken over; simmer, covered, until juices run clear when chicken is pierced and potatoes are tender, about 30 minutes. Sprinkle with parsley.

Makes 4 servings.

Per serving: about 450 cal, 35 g pro, 11 g total fat (2 g sat. fat), 52 g carb, 5 g fibre, 138 mg chol, 453 mg sodium. % RDI: 6% calcium (70 mg), 24% iron (3.4 mg), 258% vit A, 57% vit C (24 mg), 17% folate (58 mcg).

Smoked Turkey Brown Rice Salad

Like many grain salads, this is a good keeper and will make as popular an appearance at summer barbecues and year-round buffets as it does in take-to-work lunches.

1/4 tsp	salt	1 mL
1 cup	whole grain parboiled brown rice	250 mL
1/4 cup	sesame seeds	50 mL
2 cups	cubed smoked turkey thigh or ham	500 mL
2 cups	bean sprouts	500 mL
1	sweet yellow pepper, diced	1
2	green onions, sliced	2
1/3 cup	raisins (optional)	75 mL
8	leaves Boston lettuce	8
Dressing:		
1/3 cup	orange juice	75 mL
1 tbsp	each soy sauce and sesame oil	15 mL
1 tsp	grated gingerroot	5 mL
1	clove garlic, minced	1
Pinch	each salt and pepper	Pinch

In saucepan, bring 2 cups (500 mL) water and salt to boil; add rice. Cover and reduce heat to medium-low; cook until tender and water is absorbed, about 20 minutes. Remove from heat; let stand for 5 minutes.

Meanwhile, in skillet, toast sesame seeds over low heat until golden; set aside.

Dressing: In large bowl, whisk together orange juice, soy sauce, sesame oil, ginger, garlic, salt and pepper. Add rice, turkey, bean sprouts, yellow pepper, green onions, raisins (if using) and sesame seeds; toss to combine. Serve on lettuce.

Makes 4 servings.

Per serving: about 414 cal, 26 g pro, 15 g total fat (3 g sat. fat), 45 g carb, 4 g fibre, 73 mg chol, 476 mg sodium. % RDI: 7% calcium (77 mg), 28% iron (3.9 mg), 3% vit A, 120% vit C (72 mg), 40% folate (87 mcg).

Spicy Orange Baked Chicken Drumsticks

Serve with: Roasted Ginger Carrots (recipe page 268)

Kids and grown-ups will greet this dinner with equal enthusiasm. The tangy-sweet marinade glazes the chicken, preserving its moisture.

1 tbsp	grated orange rind	15 mL
1/2 cup	orange juice	125 mL
1/3 cup	liquid honey	75 mL
1/2 tsp	hot pepper flakes	2 mL
1/4 tsp	each salt and pepper	1 mL
8	chicken drumsticks (2 lb/1 kg total), skin removed	8

In large bowl, combine orange rind and juice, honey, hot pepper flakes, salt and pepper; add chicken, turning to coat.

Place chicken in single layer in shallow casserole dish; pour marinade over top. Bake in 425°F (220°C) oven, basting twice, until chicken is glossy and golden and juices run clear when chicken is pierced, about 30 minutes.

Makes 4 servings.

Per serving: about 249 cal, 22 g pro, 6 g total fat (2 g sat. fat), 27 g carb, 0 g fibre, 81 mg chol, 228 mg sodium. % RDI: 2% calcium (18 mg), 10% iron (1.4 mg), 3% vit A, 17% vit C (10 mg), 4% folate (8 mcg).

20-Minute Chicken Chili

Here's a quick, warming answer to lunchtime during those chilly months. Double the recipe if you like and serve half for lunch, then freeze the remainder in individual take-along containers for up to 2 weeks. Serve as is or spoon into whole wheat tortillas and sprinkle with cheese to make burritos.

1 lb	boneless skinless chicken breasts	500 g
1 tbsp	vegetable oil	15 mL
1	onion, chopped	1
1	sweet green pepper, chopped	1
1 tbsp	chili powder	15 mL
2 tsp	dried oregano	10 mL
1/2 tsp	salt	2 mL
1/4 tsp	pepper	1 mL
1	can (28 oz/796 mL) diced tomatoes	1
1	can (19 oz/540 mL) black or kidney beans, drained and rinsed	1
1/2 cup	corn kernels	125 mL

Trim any fat from chicken breasts; cut into 1-inch (2.5-cm) cubes. In large heavy saucepan, heat oil over medium-high heat; cook chicken until no longer pink inside, about 5 minutes. Transfer to plate.

Add onion, green pepper, chili powder, oregano, salt and pepper to pan; cook over medium heat, stirring often, until vegetables are softened, about 5 minutes. Add tomatoes and beans; increase heat and boil, stirring often, for 10 minutes. Add corn. Return chicken to pan; heat through.

Makes 4 servings.

Per serving: about 359 cal, 38 g pro, 6 g total fat (1 g sat. fat), 40 g carb, 9 g fibre, 66 mg chol, 929 mg sodium. % RDI: 10% calcium (107 mg), 33% iron (4.6 mg), 21% vit A, 72% vit C (43 mg), 75% folate (165 mcg).

MEAT

Carrot Steak Stir-Fry on Noodles

Orange juice does double duty in this recipe, adding vibrant flavour to the glossy sauce as well as enhancing the body's absorption of iron from the red meat.

3	carrots	3
1	sweet green pepper	1
1 lb	top sirloin grilling steak, thinly sliced	500 g
1/4 tsp	each salt and pepper	1 mL
2 tbsp	vegetable oil	25 mL
1	onion, sliced	1
2	cloves garlic, minced	2
3/4 cup	beef stock	175 mL
1 tsp	grated orange rind	5 mL
1/4 cup	orange juice	50 mL
1 tbsp	cornstarch	15 mL
3/4 tsp	hot pepper sauce	4 mL
1/4 cup	chopped fresh parsley	50 mL
8 oz	linguine	250 g

Thinly slice carrots and green pepper; set aside. Season steak with salt and pepper. In wok or large skillet, heat half of the oil over high heat; stir-fry steak, in batches, until browned but still pink inside, about 2 minutes. Transfer to plate.

Heat remaining oil in wok over medium heat; cook onion and garlic for 2 minutes. Add reserved carrots and green pepper; cook until slightly softened, 4 minutes.

Whisk together beef stock, orange rind and juice, cornstarch and hot pepper sauce; add to wok and bring to boil. Return meat and accumulated juices to wok along with parsley.

Meanwhile, in large pot of boiling salted water, cook linguine for 6 to 8 minutes or until tender but firm; drain and add to wok. Toss to coat well.

Makes 4 servings.

Per serving: about 478 cal, 33 g pro, 12 g total fat (2 g sat. fat), 57 g carb, 5 g fibre, 54 mg chol, 555 mg sodium. % RDI: 6% calcium (69 mg), 34% iron (4.7 mg), 140% vit A, 55% vit C (33 mg), 50% folate (110 mcg).

Company Sirloin with Grilled Vegetables

A large steak is ideal when you're entertaining—it's economical and there's no waste. This one features an Asian blend of chili, garlic and hoisin sauce.

1/3 cup	rice or cider vinegar	75 mL
1/4 cup	hoisin sauce	50 mL
2 tbsp	vegetable oil	25 mL
2	green onions, chopped	2
2	cloves garlic, minced	2
1/2 tsp	Asian chili paste or hot pepper sauce	2 mL
2 lb	sirloin grilling steak (2 inches/5 cm thick)	1 kg
Grilled Vegetables:		
1 tbsp	vegetable oil	15 mL
1 tbsp	sesame oil	15 mL
1 tsp	minced gingerroot	5 mL
1/4 tsp	each salt and pepper	1 mL
5 cups	oyster mushrooms (about 8 oz/250 g)	1.25 L
1	red onion	1
1	bunch asparagus (1 lb/500 g)	1

In shallow glass dish, whisk together vinegar, hoisin sauce, oil, green onions, garlic and chili paste. Add steak, turning to coat. Cover and marinate, turning occasionally, for 4 hours. (Make-ahead: Refrigerate for up to 12 hours.)

Grilled Vegetables: In shallow bowl, whisk together vegetable and sesame oils, ginger, salt and pepper. Lightly brush off any dirt from mushrooms; add mushrooms to bowl. Cut onion into 1/2-inch (1-cm) thick slices; insert toothpick sideways through rings of each slice to hold together. Add to bowl. Snap woody ends off asparagus and discard; add asparagus to bowl. Toss gently to coat. (Make-ahead: Cover and refrigerate for up to 6 hours.)

Reserving half of the marinade, place steak on greased grill over medium-high heat; brush with reserved marinade. Close lid and grill, turning once, until rare, about 20 minutes; medium-rare, about 25 minutes; or to desired doneness. Transfer to cutting board and tent with foil; let stand for 5 minutes. Slice thinly.

Meanwhile, add vegetables to grill; close lid and grill, turning once, until mushrooms and asparagus are lightly browned and tender but firm and onions are tender, 4 to 8 minutes. Remove toothpicks from onions; separate rings. Serve with steak.

Makes 6 servings.

Per serving: about 307 cal, 31 g pro, 14 g total fat (3 g sat. fat), 14 g carb, 3 g fibre, 69 mg chol, 275 mg sodium. % RDI: 4% calcium (47 mg), 29% iron (4.1 mg), 3% vit A, 15% vit C (9 mg), 49% folate (107 mcg).

Grilled Dijon Herb Pork Chops

Serve with: Skinny Mashed Potatoes (recipe page 269)

Either bone-in or boneless chops can be used—the former are less expensive. Be sure to trim away any visible fat before marinating.

1/4 cup	Dijon mustard	50 mL
2 tsp	olive oil	10 mL
2	cloves garlic, minced	2
1/4 tsp	each salt, pepper, and dried thyme	1 mL
1/4 tsp	dried rosemary, crumbled	1 mL
4	pork loin chops, 1/2 to 3/4 inch (1 to 2 cm) thick	4

In shallow glass dish, whisk together mustard, oil, garlic, salt, pepper, thyme, and rosemary. Add chops, turning to coat; let stand for 15 minutes.

Place chops on greased grill or in grill pan over medium-high heat; close lid and cook, turning once, for 8 to 10 minutes or until juices run clear when chops are pierced and just a hint of pink remains inside.

Makes 4 servings.

Per serving: about 216 cal, 30 g pro, 9 g total fat (3 g sat. fat), 1 g carb, 0 g fibre, 80 mg chol, 338 mg sodium. % RDI: 4% calcium (44 mg), 10% iron (1.4 mg), 0% vit A, 2% vit C (1 mg), 2% folate (4 mcg).

DESSERTS

Rhubarb and Strawberry Compote

This springtime compote can be made all year long using frozen rhubarb.

1 cup	granulated sugar	250 mL
1/4 cup	water	50 mL
6 cups	chopped rhubarb (12 large stalks)	1.5 L
1	strip (4 inches/10 cm long) orange rind	1
1 cup	sliced strawberries	250 mL

In top of double boiler over direct heat, bring sugar and water to boil. Place over gently boiling water in bottom of double boiler. Stir in rhubarb and orange rind; cover and cook, without stirring, for 15 to 20 minutes or until tender.

Turn off heat; let cool in pan over hot water. Chill. To serve, remove orange rind; gently stir in strawberries.

Makes 4 servings.

Per serving: about 242 cal, 2 g pro, 1 g total fat (trace sat. fat), 61 g carb, 4 g fibre, 0 mg chol, 9 mg sodium. % RDI: 14% calcium (156 mg), 44% iron (0.5 mg), 2% vit A, 52% vit C (31 mg), 6% folate (13 mcg).

Apricot Compote

This all-season compote can be served at room temperature or warmed on a chilly day. It pairs well with vanilla frozen yogurt or crisp cookies for a special dessert and makes a colourful addition to a brunch buffet.

2 cups	dried apricots (about 11 oz/312 g)	500 mL
1/4 cup	raisins	50 mL
2	sticks cinnamon, broken in half	2
4	strips (6 inches/15 cm long) orange rind	4
1 cup	orange juice	250 mL

In saucepan, combine apricots, raisins, cinnamon sticks, orange rind and juice, and 2 1/2 cups (625 mL) water; bring to boil. Cover, reduce heat and simmer for 20 minutes or until apricots are tender. Discard cinnamon sticks; let cool. Serve at room temperature or chilled. (Make-ahead: Refrigerate in airtight container for up to 2 days.)

Makes 6 servings.

Per serving: about 161 cal, 2 g pro, trace total fat (trace sat. fat), 41 g carb, 5 g fibre, 0 mg chol, 7 mg sodium. % RDI: 3% calcium (29 mg), 19% iron (2.6 mg), 35% vit A, 23% vit C (14 mg), 4% folate (9 mcg).

Chocolate Banana Pudding

A cooked custard pudding, thickened with egg whites and cornstarch, gives the creamy consistency without the rich fat content. For old-fashioned chocolate pudding, omit the banana.

2 1/4 cups	low-fat milk	550 mL
2/3 cup	granulated sugar	150 mL
2	egg whites	2
1/3 cup	unsweetened cocoa powder, sifted	75 mL
3 tbsp	cornstarch	50 mL
2 tsp	vanilla	10 mL
1	banana	1

In medium-size heavy saucepan or double boiler set over medium heat, combine 2 cups (500 mL) of the milk with sugar, stirring often, for about 5 minutes or just until bubbles form around edge of pan.

Meanwhile, in bowl, whisk together remaining milk, egg whites, cocoa powder and cornstarch; gradually whisk into hot milk mixture. Pour into clean saucepan; cook over medium heat, stirring with wooden spoon, for about 10 minutes or until consistency of melted chocolate. Let cool slightly; stir in vanilla.

Place plastic wrap directly on surface of pudding; refrigerate until cold. (Make-ahead: Refrigerate for up to 2 days.) Just before serving, dice banana and stir into pudding.

Makes 4 servings.

Per serving: about 285 cal, 8 g pro, 5 g total fat (3 g sat. fat), 56 g carb, 3 g fibre, 10 mg chol, 152 mg sodium. % RDI: 16% calcium (180 mg), 7% iron (1 mg), 7% vit A, 3% vit C (2 mg), 4% folate (8 mcg).

Granola Baked Apples

Here's a quick dessert that goes with just about anything you have for supper.

4	firm apples (such as Golden Delicious or Northern Spy)	4
1/4 cup	granola or rolled oats	50 mL
1/4 cup	packed brown sugar	50 mL
1/4 cup	dried cranberries	50 mL
1 tsp	lemon rind	5 mL
1/4 tsp	cinnamon	1 mL
2 tbsp	cold butter, cubed	25 mL

Core apples almost to bottom; prick skin all over. Place in pie plate. Combine granola, sugar, cranberries, lemon rind and cinnamon; cut in butter until mixture is crumbly. Stuff into apples. Cover with vented plastic wrap; microwave at High until tender, about 8 minutes. Spoon juices over top.

Makes 4 servings.

Per serving: about 235 cal, 1 g pro, 8 g total fat (4 g sat. fat), 44 g carb, 4 g fibre, 16 mg chol, 67 mg sodium. % RDI: 3% calcium (34 mg), 6% iron (0.8 mg), 6% vit A, 12% vit C (7 mg), 1% folate (3 mcg).

Pure and Simple Vanilla Pudding

Pour warm pudding over raspberries or blueberries in individual dessert bowls for a pretty presentation. Individual servings can also be stored for up to 2 days in the refrigerator for a sweet and creamy calcium boost when you're looking for a snack.

1/2 cup	granulated sugar	125 mL
3 tbsp	cornstarch	50 mL
2 1/4 cups	1% or skim milk	550 mL
2	eggs	2
2 tsp	vanilla	10 mL

In saucepan, whisk sugar with cornstarch; whisk in milk. Stir over medium heat just until steaming.

In bowl, whisk eggs; whisk in half of the hot mixture in slow steady stream. Gradually whisk back into pan; cook over medium-low heat, whisking, for 15 minutes or until thickened. Stir in vanilla.

Transfer to bowl; place plastic wrap directly on surface. Refrigerate for 2 hours or until chilled or for up to 2 days.

Makes 4 servings.

Per serving: about 225 cal, 8 g pro, 5 g total fat (2 g sat. fat), 37 g carb, trace fibre, 103 mg chol, 100 mg sodium. % RDI: 16% calcium (180 mg), 3% iron (0.4 mg), 11% vit A, 2% vit C (1 mg), 8% folate (17 mcg).

Microwave method: In 8-cup (2 L) microwaveable bowl, whisk sugar, cornstarch and milk; microwave at High for 6 minutes or until thickened, stirring every 2 minutes. Microwave at High for 1 minute, stirring twice. Beat eggs; whisk in one-third of the hot mixture. Return to bowl; microwave at High for 1 minute or until bubbly around edge, stirring twice. Stir in vanilla.

ICE AND EASY FRUIT SORBETS

These refreshing fruit ices follow an easy formula based on simple sugar syrup. Choose the flavour that best suits your fancy. Fresh or partially thawed frozen fruits can be used.

Simple Syrup

In saucepan, bring 2/3 cup (150 mL) each granulated sugar and water to boil, stirring, to dissolve sugar. Let cool completely.

Blueberry Frozen Yogurt

3 cups	blueberries	750 mL
1	batch Simple Syrup (recipe above)	1
2/3 cup	plain 2% yogurt	150 mL

In food processor, purée blueberries. Mix in Simple Syrup and yogurt.

Freeze in shallow metal cake pan for about 4 hours or until firm. Break into chunks; purée in food processor. Pack into airtight container and refreeze for 4 hours or until firm or for up to 2 days. (Or freeze in ice-cream machine according to manufacturer's instructions.)

Makes 6 servings.

Per serving: about 135 cal, 1 g pro, trace total fat (trace sat. fat), 33 g carb, 2 g fibre, 1 mg chol, 15 mg sodium. % RDI: 3% calcium (30 mg), 1% iron (0.2 mg), 1% vit A, 17% vit C (10 mg), 3% folate (6 mcg).

Canta-Berry Sorbet

3 cups	cubed cantaloupe, (about 1 small)	750 mL
2 cups	hulled strawberries	500 mL
1	batch Simple Syrup (recipe page 295)	1
2 tbsp	lemon juice	25 mL

In food processor, purée cantaloupe with strawberries. Mix in Simple Syrup and lemon juice.

Freeze in shallow metal cake pan for about 4 hours or until firm. Break into chunks; purée in food processor. Pack into airtight container and refreeze for 4 hours or until firm or for up to 2 days. (Or freeze in ice-cream machine according to manufacturer's instructions.)

Makes 6 servings.

Per serving: about 130 cal, 1 g pro, trace total fat (trace sat. fat), 33 g carb, 2 g fibre, 0 mg chol, 9 mg sodium. % RDI: 2% calcium (17 mg), 3% iron (0.4 mg), 26% vit A, 107% vit C (64 mg), 10% folate (23 mcg).

Lemon Lime Tofu Zinger

1	pkg (12 oz/340 g) soft silken tofu	1
2/3 cup	each lemon and lime juice	150 mL
2	batches Simple Syrup (recipe page 295)	2
1 tbsp	each finely grated lemon and lime rind	15 mL

In food processor, purée tofu and lemon and lime juices. Mix in Simple Syrup and lemon and lime rinds.

Freeze in shallow metal cake pan for about 4 hours or until firm. Break into chunks; purée in food processor. Pack into airtight container and refreeze for 4 hours or until firm or for up to 2 days. (Or freeze in ice-cream machine according to manufacturer's instructions.)

Makes 6 servings.

Per serving: about 221 cal, 3 g pro, 2 g total fat (trace sat. fat), 49 g carb, trace fibre, 0 mg chol, 5 mg sodium. % RDI: 2% calcium (23 mg), 4% iron (0.5 mg), 0% vit A, 23% vit C (14 mg), 2% folate (4 mcg).

Tip: These desserts can be stored in the freezer for 2 days; after that, purée them again in the food processor to enjoy an extra day or two of fresh flavour.

Peach Sorbet

4 cups	peeled sliced peaches (about 6)	1 L
1	batch Simple Syrup (recipe page 295)	1
2 tbsp	lemon juice	25 mL

In food processor, purée peaches. Mix in Simple Syrup and lemon juice.

Freeze in shallow metal cake pan for about 4 hours or until firm. Break into chunks; purée in food processor. Pack into airtight container and refreeze for 4 hours or until firm or for up to 2 days. (Or freeze in ice-cream machine according to manufacturer's instructions.)

Makes 6 servings.

Per serving: about 136 cal, 1 g pro, trace total fat (trace sat. fat), 35 g carb, 2 g fibre, 0 mg chol, 1 mg sodium. % RDI: 1% calcium (7 mg), 1% iron (0.1 mg), 6% vit A, 17% vit C (10 mg), 2% folate (5 mcg).

Raspberry Sorbet

4 cups	raspberries	1 L
1	batch Simple Syrup (recipe page 295)	1
1 tbsp	each corn syrup and lemon juice	15 mL

In food processor or by pressing through sieve with rubber spatula, purée raspberries. Mix in Simple Syrup, corn syrup and lemon juice.

Freeze in shallow metal cake pan for about 4 hours or until firm. Break into chunks; purée in food processor. Pack into airtight container and refreeze for 4 hours or until firm or for up to 2 days. (Or freeze in ice-cream machine according to manufacturer's instructions.)

Makes 6 servings.

Per serving: about 136 cal, 1 g pro, trace total fat (trace sat. fat), 34 g carb, 4 g fibre, 0 mg chol, 5 mg sodium. % RDI: 2% calcium (19 mg), 4% iron (0.5 mg), 1% vit A, 37% vit C (22 mg), 10% folate (22 mcg).

SNACKS

Apple Crisp Mini-Muffins

Lightened up with applesauce instead of more oil, these make healthy snacks for a lunch box—just the right size for small hands. For big kids, make a dozen regular-size muffins and bake for 16 to 20 minutes.

1 1/4 cups	all-purpose flour	300 mL
1 cup	quick-cooking rolled oats	250 mL
1/4 cup	packed brown sugar	50 mL
1 tbsp	baking powder	15 mL
1/2 tsp	each cinnamon and salt	2 mL
1	egg	1
1 cup	grated peeled seeded apple	250 mL
2/3 cup	sweetened applesauce	150 mL
1/3 cup	milk	75 mL
1/4 cup	vegetable oil	50 mL
Topping:		
1/4 cup	each packed brown sugar and quick-cooking rolled oats	50 mL
2 tbsp	butter, melted	25 mL
1/4 tsp	cinnamon	1 mL

Topping: In small bowl, combine sugar, oats, butter and cinnamon; set aside.

In bowl, whisk flour, oats, sugar, baking powder, cinnamon and salt. In separate bowl, whisk together egg, apple, applesauce, milk and oil; pour over dry ingredients and stir just until moistened.

Spoon into greased mini-muffin tins; sprinkle with topping. Bake in centre of 400°F (200°C) oven for 12 to 14 minutes or until tops are firm to the touch. Let cool in pan on rack for 5 minutes. Transfer to rack; let cool completely.

Makes 30 mini-muffins.

Per mini-muffin: about 79 cal, 1 g pro, 3 g total fat (1 g sat. fat), 12 g carb, 9 mg chol, 1 g fibre, 77 mg sodium. % RDI: 2% calcium (22 mg), 4% iron (0.5 mg), 1% vit A, 12% vit C (7 mg), 3% folate (7 mcg).

Bodybuilder Cookies

The surprise ingredient (Cheddar cheese) in these energy-extending morsels may intrigue you, but the delicious taste and crunch will win you over.

3/4 cup	butter or margarine	175 mL
1 cup	packed brown sugar	250 mL
1	egg	1
1 tsp	vanilla	5 mL
1 3/4 cups	all-purpose flour	425 mL
1/2 tsp	each baking powder, baking soda and salt	2 mL
3 cups	flaked bran cereal, slightly crushed	750 mL
1/2 cup	shredded light Cheddar cheese	125 mL
1/2 cup	raisins	125 mL
1/2 cup	chopped toasted pecans or walnuts	125 mL

In large bowl, beat butter with sugar until light and fluffy. Beat in egg and vanilla.

In separate bowl, stir together flour, baking powder, baking soda and salt; stir into butter mixture just until combined. Stir in crushed cereal, Cheddar cheese, raisins and pecans to make slightly crumbly mixture.

Using 1 rounded tablespoonful (15 mL) per cookie, squeeze batter into balls; place about 2 inches (5 cm) apart on ungreased baking sheets. Bake in top and bottom thirds of 350°F (180°C) oven for about 15 minutes or until lightly browned, switching and rotating pans halfway through.

Let cool on pans on racks for 5 minutes. Transfer to racks and let cool completely. (Make-ahead: Store in airtight container at room temperature for up to 1 week or freeze for up to 1 month.)

Makes about 42 cookies.

Per cookie: about 101 cal, 2 g pro, 5 g total fat (2 g sat. fat), 14 g carb, 1 g fibre, 16 mg chol, 122 mg sodium. % RDI: 2% calcium (22 mg), 6% iron (0.9 mg), 3% vit A, 0% vit C, 5% folate (10 mcg).

...r Applesauce

...ce gives applesauce zing, but it
... a more traditional flavour. Use a
...et-tart apple that softens easily, such as Gravenstein
or McIntosh.

2	pears, peeled and cored	2
2	apples, peeled and cored	2
2 tbsp	lemon juice	25 mL
4 tsp	granulated sugar	20 mL
Pinch	salt	Pinch
6	whole cloves	6
2	whole star anise	2
1	stick (about 2 inches/5 cm long) cinnamon	1

Cut pears into bite-size chunks; chop apples. In small
saucepan, combine pears, apples, lemon juice, sugar, salt,
cloves, star anise, cinnamon and 2 tbsp (25 mL) water.
Cover and bring to simmer; cook for 10 minutes.
Uncover; cook until pears are very tender and apples
break down to make thick sauce, 12 to 15 minutes. Let
cool. (Make-ahead: Cover and refrigerate for up to 3 days;
serve at room temperature.)

Makes 2 cups (500 mL).

Per 1/2 cup (125 mL): about 96 cal, 0 g pro, 0 g total
fat (0 g sat. fat), 24 g carb, 4 g fibre, 0 mg chol, 0 mg
sodium. % RDI: 0% calcium, 4% iron (0.4 mg), 0% vit A,
8% vit C (4 mg), 0% folate.

Farmland Flax Cookies

The flaxseed in these wholesome, crunchy cookies is a
source of soluble fibre and alpha-linolenic acid, an
essential fatty acid. Like all nuts and seeds, it should be
stored in the refrigerator.

1/2 cup	butter, softened	125 mL
1/2 cup	packed brown sugar	125 mL
1/3 cup	granulated sugar	75 mL
1	egg	1
1/2 tsp	vanilla	2 mL
1 cup	all-purpose flour	250 mL
3/4 cup	quick-cooking rolled oats	175 mL
2/3 cup	flaxseeds	150 mL
1 tsp	baking soda	5 mL

In bowl, beat together butter and brown and granulated sugars until light; beat in egg and vanilla. In separate
bowl, whisk together flour, oats, flaxseeds and baking
soda; stir into butter mixture until soft dough forms.

Drop by level tablespoonfuls (15 mL), 2 inches (5 cm)
apart, on ungreased rimless baking sheets. Bake in top
and bottom thirds of 350°F (180°C) oven, rotating and
switching pans halfway through, until golden, about
12 minutes. Let cool on pan on rack for 2 minutes.

Transfer cookies to rack; let cool. (Make-ahead: Layer
between waxed paper and freeze in airtight container
for up to 1 month.)

Makes about 40 cookies.

Per cookie: about 69 cal, 1 g pro, 3 g total fat (2 g sat.
fat), 9 g carb, 1 g fibre, 11 mg chol, 57 mg sodium.
% RDI: 1% calcium (12 mg), 4% iron (1.6 mg), 2% vit A,
0% vit C, 5% folate (12 mcg).

Frozen Orange-Vanilla "Cream"

With these frosty treats tucked in your freezer, you can boost your calcium, vitamin C and folate, all while feeling like you're getting away with something.

1 cup	vanilla yogurt	250 mL
1/2 cup	frozen orange juice concentrate, thawed	125 mL
1/3 cup	granulated sugar	75 mL

In bowl, whisk yogurt, orange juice concentrate and sugar until well blended. Divide among 4 empty 6 oz (175 g) yogurt containers or other small freezer-safe containers. Cover with plastic wrap or lids (if available). Freeze for at least 6 hours or until firm. (Make-ahead: Freeze for up to 2 weeks.)

Makes 4 servings.

Per serving: about 185 cal, 4 g pro, 2 g total fat (1 g sat. fat), 39 g carb, trace fibre, 6 mg chol, 39 mg sodium. % RDI: 10% calcium (110 mg), 1% iron (0.2 mg), 2% vit A, 92% vit C (55 mg), 28% folate (62 mcg).

Herbed Yogurt Cheese

Draining the whey from low-fat yogurt gives it a thicker, creamier texture, making it a substitute for higher-fat dairy products. Drained for about 6 hours—or until only half of the volume remains—it has the consistency of sour cream, making it useful in spreads or as a baked potato topping. Yogurt drained for up to 48 hours—until one-third of the volume remains—has the firmer texture of spreadable cream cheese.

3 cups	1% plain yogurt	750 mL
4 tsp	chopped fresh oregano or marjoram	20 mL
1 tbsp	chopped fresh parsley	15 mL
1 tbsp	chopped chives or green onion	15 mL
2 tsp	extra-virgin olive oil	10 mL
1/4 tsp	salt	1 mL

Place yogurt in cheesecloth-lined sieve set over bowl; cover and drain in refrigerator for 48 hours or until reduced to about 1 cup (250 mL).

In bowl, stir together drained yogurt, oregano, parsley, chives, oil and salt. Mound onto plate with spatula or press into serving bowl. (Make-ahead: Cover and refrigerate for up to 2 days.)

Makes 1 cup (250 mL).

Per 1 tbsp (15 mL): about 24 cal, 2 g pro, 1 g total fat (trace sat. fat), 2 g carb, 0 g fibre, 2 mg chol, 52 mg sodium. % RDI: 6% calcium (69 mg), 1% iron (1 mg), 1% vit A, 2% vit C (1 mg), 2% folate (5 mcg).

and Raisin Muffins

re natural flavour partners.

ups	all-purpose flour	500 mL
1 cup	raisins	250 mL
1/3 cup	packed brown sugar	75 mL
1 1/2 tsp	baking powder	7 mL
1 tsp	baking soda	5 mL
1/2 tsp	salt	2 mL
1/2 tsp	cinnamon	2 mL
1/2 tsp	ground ginger	2 mL
1/2 tsp	ground nutmeg	2 mL
1	egg	1
1 3/4 cups	pumpkin purée	425 mL
2 tbsp	coarsely grated orange rind	25 mL
1/2 cup	orange juice	125 mL
1/3 cup	vegetable oil	75 mL

In large bowl, whisk together flour, raisins, sugar, baking powder, baking soda, salt, cinnamon, ginger and nutmeg.

In separate bowl, beat egg; blend in pumpkin purée, orange rind and juice, and oil. Pour over dry ingredients and stir just until moistened.

Spoon into greased or paper-lined muffin cups, filling to top. Bake in centre of 375°F (190°C) oven for about 25 minutes or until tops are firm to the touch. Let cool in pan on rack for 5 minutes; transfer to rack and let cool.

Makes 12 muffins.

Per muffin: about 212 cal, 4 g pro, 7 g total fat (1 g sat. fat), 36 g carb, 4 g fibre, 16 mg chol, 239 mg sodium. % RDI: 4% calcium (43 mg), 14% iron (2 mg), 71% vit A, 10% vit C (6 mg), 11% folate (24 mcg).

Spa Trail Mix

Trail mix is wonderfully easy and portable. Keep a small airtight container at your desk or in your bag for a convenient snack or try sprinkling it over yogurt for a quick breakfast.

4 cups	toasted-oat cereal rounds	1 L
4 cups	waffle-weave wheat cereal squares	1 L
2 cups	multibran cereal flakes	500 mL
1 cup	dried cherries or golden raisins	250 mL
1 cup	whole almonds	250 mL
1 cup	banana chips	250 mL
1 cup	toasted-oat cereal squares	250 mL
1 cup	puffed rice cereal	250 mL
1 cup	dried cantaloupe or pineapple bits	250 mL

In large bowl, gently toss together cereal rounds, wheat cereal squares, multibran flakes, cherries, almonds, banana chips, oat cereal squares, puffed rice and cantaloupe. Store in airtight container at room temperature for up to 1 month.

Makes about 15 cups (3.75 L).

Per 1/2 cup (125 mL): about 259 cal, 6 g pro, 8 g total fat (2 g sat. fat), 45 g carb, 6 g fibre, 0 mg chol, 222 mg sodium. % RDI: 7% calcium (79 mg), 34% iron (4.7 mg), 2% vit A, 0% vit C, 10% folate (23 mcg).

Hiker's Happy Trail Mix

4 cups	toasted-oat cereal rounds	1 L
4 cups	waffle-weave wheat cereal squares	1 L
2 cups	raisins	500 mL
1 1/2 cups	banana chips	375 mL
1 1/2 cups	multibran cereal flakes	375 mL
1 cup	shredded sweetened coconut	250 mL
1 cup	pecan halves	250 mL
1/2 cup	mini chocolate chips	125 mL

In large bowl, gently toss together cereal rounds, wheat cereal squares, raisins, banana chips, multibran flakes, coconut, pecans and chocolate chips. Store in airtight container at room temperature for up to 1 month.

Makes about 15 cups (3.75 L).

Per 1/2 cup (125 mL): about 290 cal, 4 g pro, 11 g total fat (5 g sat. fat), 47 g carb, 6 g fibre, 0 mg chol, 199 mg sodium. % RDI: 3% calcium (33 mg), 31% iron (4.4 mg), 0% vit A, 3% vit C (2 mg), 9% folate (20 mcg).

A Guide to Serving Sizes

Are you wondering what one serving consists of? Here's a selected list to help you determine your food portions. All serving sizes are based on measures *after* cooking.

Protein Foods: 1 serving = 50 to 75 calories

Egg, whole	1
Egg, white	2
Fish, lean meat, poultry, cooked	1 oz (30 g)
Legumes (beans, chickpeas, lentils)	1/3 cup (75 ml)
Soy nuts, roasted	2 tbsp (25 ml)
Tempeh	1/4 cup (50 ml)
Texturized vegetable protein	1/3 cup (75 ml)
Tofu, firm	1/3 cup (75 ml)
Veggie burger	1/2 patty
Veggie dog, small	1

Starchy Foods (choose whole-grain): 1 serving = 85 to 100 calories

Bagel	1/4
Bread, whole-grain	1 slice
Pita pocket	1/2
Roll, large	1/2
Tortilla, 6-inch	1
Cereal, cold flake, or Shreddies	3/4 cup (175 ml)
Cereal, hot	1/2 cup (125 ml)
Cereal, 100% bran	1/2 cup (125 ml)
Crackers, soda	6
Corn	1/2 cup (125 ml)
Corn on the cob	1/2
Grains, cooked	1/2 cup (125 ml)
Pasta, cooked	1/2 cup (125 ml)
Popcorn, plain	3 cups (750 ml)
Potato, white or sweet	1/2 cup (125 ml)
Rice, cooked	1/3 cup (75 ml)

Fruit: 1 serving = 85 to 100 calories

Fruit, medium, whole	1
Fruit, small (plums, apricots)	4
Fruit, sliced or cubed	1 cup (250 ml)
Berries	1 cup (250 ml)
Juice, unsweetened	1/2 to 3/4 cup (125 to 175 ml)

Vegetables: 1 serving = approximately 45 calories

Vegetables, cooked or raw	1/2 cup (125 ml)
Vegetables, leafy green	1 cup (250 ml)

Milk and Alternatives: 1 serving = 90 to 100 calories

Milk, 1% or skim	1 cup (250 ml)
Yogurt, plain, 1% milk fat (MF) or less*	3/4 cup (175 ml)
Cheese, 20% MF or less	1 1/2 oz (45 g)
Rice beverage, calcium-fortified	1 cup (250 ml)
Soy beverage, calcium-fortified	1 cup (250 ml)

*Low-fat fruit-bottom yogurt provides 130 to 150 calories.

Fats and Oils: 1 serving = 45 calories

Avocado	1/8
Butter, margarine, mayonnaise	1 tsp (5 ml)
Nuts and seeds	1 tbsp (15 ml)
Peanut and nut butters	1 1/2 tsp (7 ml)
Salad dressing	2 tsp (10 ml)
Vegetable oil	1 tsp (5 ml)

Breastfeeding

Breastfeeding Referral Service
Toll-free: 1-800-665-4324
National Office
18C Industrial Drive, PO Box 29
Chesterville, Ontario, Canada K0C 1H0
Tel: 613-448-1842
Fax: 613-448-1845

Canadian Lactation Consultant Association
www.clca-accl.ca
Members of this association are affiliated with the International Lactation Consultant Association and the Breastfeeding Committee of Canada. You'll find a list of lactation consultants in Canada on this website.

International Lactation Consultant Association
1500 Sunday Drive, Suite 102
Raleigh, North Carolina, USA 27607
Tel: 919-861-5577
Fax: 919-787-4916
E-mail info@ilca.org
www.ilca.org

La Leche League Canada
Toll-free: 1-800-525-3243
www.lalecheleaguecanada.ca
Founded in 1956, La Leche League's sole purpose is to help breastfeeding mothers. La Leche League groups meet regularly in communities worldwide to share breastfeeding information and mothering experience. Telephone counselling is available, along with access to an extensive library of breastfeeding literature.

Diet and Nutrition

Dietitians of Canada

480 University Avenue, Suite 604
Toronto, Ontario, Canada M5G 1V2
Tel: 416-596-0857
Fax: 416-596-0603
www.dietitians.ca
The Dietitians of Canada is an association of food and nutrition professionals committed to the health and well-being of Canadians. Visit the website to learn about nutrition resources or to find a registered dietitian (RD) in your community.

Canadian Food Information Council

3800 Steeles Avenue West, Suite 301A
Woodbridge, Ontario, Canada L4L 4G9
Tel: 905-265-9124
E-mail: ptanaka@cfic.ca
www.cfic.ca
Launched in 1999, this national, non-profit organization delivers fact-based information on current food, food safety, and nutrition.

The Canadian Partnership for Consumer Food Safety Education

1755 Courtwood Crescent, Suite 500
Ottawa, Ontario, Canada K2C 3J2
www.canfightbac.org
This national association is committed to educating Canadians about the ease and importance of food safety in the home. You'll find plenty of practical information and tips on safe food handling practices in the consumer section of the site.

Health Canada Online

www.hc-sc.gc.ca
Visit Health Canada's main site to find information about nutrition, physical activity, health care, and diseases and conditions. You'll also find the latest headlines and advisories. You can also visit more specific nutrition sites such as www.hc-sc.gc.ca/hppb/nutrition, where you'll find Canada's Food Guide to Healthy Eating and plenty of information on nutrition labelling and healthy weights. For a discussion on the link between folic acid and neural tube defects and useful links to other sources of important information, visit www.hc-sc.gc.ca/english/folicacid.

...formation Council
...enue, NW

...gton, DC, USA 20036
Tel: 202-296-6540
E-mail: foodinfo@ific.org
www.ific.org
The mission of this site is to communicate science-based information on food safety and nutrition. You'll find brochures and fact sheets that discuss pregnancy nutrition, weight management, food additives, infant nutrition, and a lot more. The Q&A centre provides answers to questions about today's food safety issues, from fish and trans fat to pesticides and artificial sweeteners.

National Institute of Nutrition
408 Queen Street, 3rd Floor
Ottawa, Ontario, Canada K1R 5A7
Tel: 613-235-3355
Email: nin@nin.ca
www.nin.ca
This non-profit national organization offers a wealth of nutrition information on topics such as healthy eating, food safety, nutrition labelling, pregnancy, and food allergies. The resource Healthy Bites delivers practical, consumer-friendly facts and tips about healthy eating and active living. These facts sheets separate fact from fiction and provide action-oriented messages to help you adopt healthy lifestyle habits.

Exercise and Fitness

Active Living During Pregnancy: Physical Activity Guidelines for Mother and Baby
This 40-page booklet includes instructions and photos for specific exercises (as well as suggestions for postpartum exercises), and discusses the benefits of exercise during pregnancy, safety considerations, and healthy eating. It's available from:
Canadian Society for Exercise Physiology
185 Somerset Street West, Suite 202
Ottawa, Ontario, Canada K2P 0J2
Tel: 613-234-3755
Toll-free: 1-877-651-3755
Fax: 613-234-3565
www.csep.ca

Canadian Personal Trainers Network
122 D'arcy Street
Toronto, Ontario, Canada M5T 1K3
Tel: 416-979-1654
E-mail: info@cptn.com
www.cptn.com
This network provides referrals for personal trainers who will come to your home.

Health Canada Physical Activity Guide
www.hc-sc.gc.ca/hppb/paguide/index.html
Visit this site to help you make wise choices about physical activity. You'll find a brief guide and an in-depth handbook that list the benefits of physical activity and provide practical suggestions on how to incorporate physical activity into daily routines. Prepared in collaboration with the Canadian Society for Exercise Physiology.

Gestational Diabetes

Canadian Diabetes Association
522 University Avenue, 13th Floor
Toronto, Ontario, Canada M5G 1Y7
Toll-free: 1-800-226-8464
www.diabetes.ca

Midwifery

Canadian Association of Midwives
#207-2051 McCallum Road
Abbotsford, BC, Canada V2S 3N5
Tel: 604-859-0777
Fax: 604-859-0767
E-mail: admin@canadianmidwives.org
www.canadianmidwives.org
The website of this national organization of the midwifery profession is an excellent source of information about midwifery in Canada.

...ada

...asaga Beach, Ontario, Canada L0L 2P0
Tel: 705-429-0901
Toll-free: 1-866-228-8824
Fax: 705-429-9809
E-mail: office@multiplebirthscanada.org
www.multiplebirthscanada.org

Pregnancy & Childbirth

BabyCenter
www.babycenter.com
This U.S.–based resource for new and expecting parents covers everything—nutrition at each stage of pregnancy, pregnancy complications, labour and delivery, breastfeeding, postpartum health, and newborns. The articles are concise and easy to read.

Healthy Beginnings: Your Handbook for Pregnancy and Birth, 2nd edition
This 114-page book offers pregnant women and new mothers a thorough guide to all aspects of pregnancy, from preconception to the first few days at home with the new baby. Advice on exercise and work-related activity is included. It's available for $9.98 from:

Society of Obstetricians and Gynaecologists of Canada
780 Echo Drive
Ottawa, Ontario, Canada K1S 5N8
Tel: 613-730-4192
Toll-free: 1-877-519-7999
Fax: 613-730-4314
www.sogc.org

Mayo Foundation for Medical Education and Research
www.mayoclinic.com
Visit this trusted and reliable source of health information to learn more about pregnancy, breast-feeding, and your baby's health. There's also a great food and nutrition centre that offers tips on healthy eating.

The Society for Obstetricians and Gynaecologists of Canada
780 Echo Drive
Ottawa, Ontario, Canada K1S 5R7
Tel: 613-730-4192 or 1-800-561-2416
www.sogc.org
The public education section of this site offers fact sheets on topics such as HIV testing in pregnancy, managing morning sickness, prenatal testing, and multiple births. You'll also find "Bringing Baby Safely into the World," a brochure that discusses labour and delivery.

Women's Health Matters
www.womenshealthmatters.ca
Developed by women's health experts from Sunnybrook & Women's College Health Sciences Centre and the Centre for Research in Women's Health, this site provides credible and up-to-date information on women's health issues. Visit the virtual Pregnancy Health Centre to learn more about topics ranging from preconception to life with a newborn.

Endnotes

1   Getting Ready for Pregnancy

1. Rogers, I, and the Euro-BLCS Study Group. The influence of birth weight and intrauterine environment on adiposity and fat distribution later in life. *Int J Obes Relat Metab Disord* 2003, 27(7):755–777.

2. Curhan, GC, et al. Birth weight and adult hypertension and obesity in women. *Circulation* 1996, 94(6):1310–1315.

3. Michels, KB, et al. Birthweight as a risk factor for breast cancer. *Lancet* 1996, 348(9041):1542–1546.

2   The "Training" Trimester

1. Hibbeln, JR. Seafood consumption, the DHA content of mothers' milk and prevalence rates of postpartum depression: a cross-national, ecological analysis. *J Affect Disord* 2002, 69(1–3):15–29.

2. Hites, RA et al. Global assessment of organic contaminants in farmed salmon. *Science* 2004, 303:226–229.

3. Decsi T, et al. Inverse association between trans isomeric and long-chain polyunsaturated fatty acids in cord blood lipids of full-term infants. *Am J Clin Nutr,* 2001, 74(3):364–368.

    www.fsai.ie/industry/Dioxins3.htm

4. Jensen, TK, et al. Does moderate alcohol consumption affect fertility? Follow-up study among couples planning for first pregnancy. *BMJ* 1998, 317(7157):505–510.

5. Grodstein, F, et al. Infertility in women and moderate alcohol use. *Am J Public Health* 1994, 84(9):1429–1432.

6. Jensen, TK, et al. Caffeine intake and fecundability: a follow-up study among 430 Danish couples planning their first pregnancy. *Reprod Toxicol* 1998, 12(3):289–295; Grodstein, F, et al. Relation of female infertility to consumption of caffeinated beverages. *Am J Epidemiol* 1993, 137(12):1353–1360; Bolumar, F, et al. Caffeine intake and delayed conception: a European multicenter study on infertility and subfecundity. European Study Group on Infertility Subfecundity. *Am J Epidemiol* 1997, 145(4):324–334.

7. Stanton, CK, and RH Gray. Effects of caffeine consumption on delayed conception. *Am J Epidemiol* 1995, 142(12):1322–1329.

8. Dlugosz, L, et al. Maternal caffeine consumption and spontaneous abortion: a prospective cohort study. *Epidemiology* 1996, 7(3):250–255; Fenster, L, et al. Caffeine consumption during pregnancy and spontaneous abortion. *Epidemiology* 1991, 2(3):168–174.

9. Infante-Rivard, C, et al. Fetal loss associated with caffeine intake before and during pregnancy. *JAMA* 1993, 270(24):2940–2943.

10. Fernandes, O, et al. Moderate to heavy caffeine consumption during pregnancy and relationship to spontaneous abortion and abnormal fetal growth: a meta-analysis. *Reprod Toxicol* 1998, 12(4):435–444.

3   Your Pre-Pregnancy Checklist

1. Romero, BC, et al. Relationship between periodontal disease in pregnant women and the nutritional condition of their newborns. *J Periodontol* 2002, 73(10):1177–1183; Jeffcoat, MK, et al. Periodontal infection and preterm birth: results of a prospective study. *J Am Dent Assoc* 2001, 132(7):875–880.

2. Krejci, CB, and NF Bissada. Women's health issues and their relationship to periodontitis. *J Am Dent Assoc* 2002, 133(3):323–329.

3. Lopez, NJ, et al. Periodontal therapy may reduce the risk of preterm low birth weight in women with periodontal disease: a randomized controlled trial. *J Periodontol* 2002, 73(8):911–924.

4. Freeman, R. Reflections on professional and lay perspectives of the dentist-patient interaction. *Br Dent J* 1999, 186(11):546–550.

5. March of Dimes. Smoking During Pregnancy. February 2003. www.marchofdimes.com professionals/681_1171.asp

6. Association of Ontario Midwives. What is a midwife? 2003. www.aom.on.ca/midwifery/

7. Association of Ontario Midwives. Fact sheets – Overview. 2003. www.aom.on.ca/facts

4   The First Trimester

1. March of Dimes. Miscarriage. 2003. www.marchofdimes.com/pnhec/188_1086.asp.

2. Ibid.

3. Ibid.

4. Ibid.

5   The Second Trimester

1. American Academy of Dermatology. Pregnancy and the skin: medications to avoid, changes to expect. 2000. www.aad.org/PressReleases/pregnancymeds.html

2. Krejci, CB, and NF Bissada. Women's health issues and their relationship to periodontitis. *J Am Dent Assoc* 2002, 133(3):323–329.

3. Society of Obstetricians and Gynaecologists of Canada. Prenatal Diagnosis. 2003. www.sogc. medical.org/pub_ed/prenatalDiagnosis/index_e.shtml

4. Mayo Foundation for Medical Education and Research. Prenatal testing: what's involved and who should consider it. 2002. www.mayoclinic.com/invoke.cfm?objectid=44071E5B -D234-403A-BAD5477EB2F325FE

5. Sunnybrook and Women's College Health Sciences Centre. Women's Health Matters. Screening tests. 2002. www.womenshealthmatters.ca/centres/ pregnancy/pregnancy/screening.html

6   The Third Trimester

1. Mayo Foundation for Medical Education and Research. The third trimester. 2001. www.mayoclinic. com/invoke.cfm?objectid=9C045F97-F0AF-462C- A4714BA8E2C38767

7   Eating Your Way Through Pregnancy

1. Blot, I, et al. Folate and iron deficiencies in mothers and their newborn children. *Blut* 1982,

44(5):297–303; Scholl, T, et al. Anemia versus iron deficiency: increased risk of preterm delivery in a prospective study. *Am J Clin Nutr* 1992, 55(5):985–988; Duthie, SJ, et al. A case controlled study of pregnancy complicated by severe maternal anemia. *Aust N Z J Obstet Gynaecol* 1991, 31(2):125–127.

2. National Academy of Sciences, Institute of Medicine, Food and Nutrition Board, Committee on Nutritional Status During Pregnancy and Lactation, Subcommittee on Dietary Intake and Nutrient Supplements During Pregnancy, Subcommittee on Nutritional Status and Weight Gain During Pregnancy. *Nutrition During.* (Part I—Weight gain. Part II—Nutrient supplements.) Washington, DC: National Academy Press, 1990.

3. Rothman, KJ, et al. Teratogenicity of high vitamin A intake. *N Engl J Med* 1995, 333(21):1369–1373.

4. Klebanoff, MA, et al. Maternal serum paraxanthine, a caffeine metabolite, and the risk of spontaneous abortion. *N Eng J Med* 1999, 341(22):1639–1644.

5. Fernandes, O, et al. Moderate to heavy caffeine consumption during pregnancy and relationship to spontaneous abortion and abnormal fetal growth: a meta-analysis. *Reprod Toxicol* 1998, 12(4):435–444.

6. Fenster, L, et al. Caffeinated beverages, decaffeinated coffee, and spontaneous abortion. *Epidemiology* 1997, 8(5):515–523.

8   Eating Your Way Through a Multiple Pregnancy

1. Multiple Births Canada. General facts and figures. 2002. www.multiplebirthscanada.org/english/facts figures.php.

2. Pederson, AL, et al. Weight gain patterns during twin gestation. *J Am Diet Assoc* 1989, 89(5):642–646.

3. Ho, ML, et al. Changing epidemiology of triplet pregnancy: etiology and outcome over twelve years. *Am J Perinatol* 1996, 13(5):269–275; Crowther, CA, and RA Hamilton. Triplet pregnancy: a 10-year review of 105 cases at Harare Maternity Hospital, Zimbabwe. *Acta Genet Med Gemellol* (Roma) 1989, 38(3–4): 271–278.

4. Luke, B, et al. Maternal nutrition in twin gestations: weight gain, cravings and aversions, and sources of nutrition advice. *Acta Genet Med Gemellol* (Roma) 1997, 46(3):157–166.

5. Dubois, S, et al. Twin pregnancy: the impact of the Higgins Nutrition Intervention Program on maternal and neonatal outcomes. *Am J Clin Nutr* 1991, 53(6):1397–1403.

6. Luke, B, et al. Critical periods of maternal weight gain: effect on twin birth weight. *Am J Obstet Gynecol* 1997, 177(5):1055–1062.

7. Lantz, ME, et al. Maternal weight gain patterns and birth weight outcomes in twin gestation. *Obstet Gynecol* 1996, 87(4):551–556.

8. Luke, B, et al. The association between maternal factors and perinatal outcomes in triplet pregnancies. *Am J Obstet Gynecol* 2002, 187(3):752–757; Luke, B, et al. Prenatal weight gain and the birthweight of triplets. *Acta Genet Med Gemellol* (Roma) 1995, 44(2):93–101.

9. Zeijdner, EE, et al. Essential fatty acid status in plasma phospholipids of mother and neonate after multiple pregnancy. *Prostaglandins Leukot Essent Fatty Acids* 1997, 56(5):395–401; McFadyen, M, et al. Maternal and umbilical cord erythrocyte omega-3 and omega-6 fatty acids and haemorheology in singleton and twin pregnancies. *Arch Dis Child Fetal Neonatal Ed* 2003, 88(2):F134–F138.

10. National Academy of Sciences. *Nutrition during pregnancy.* (Part I—Weight gain. Part II—Nutrient supplements.) Washington, DC: National Academy Press, 1990.

9   Feeling Your Best

1. University of Michigan Health System. Common discomforts of pregnancy. 2003. www.med.umich.edu/1libr/womens/pgprob06.htm

2. Roy-Clavel, E, et al. Induction of intrauterine growth restriction with a low-sodium diet fed to pregnant rats. *Am J Obstet Gynecol* 1999, 180(3 Part 1):608–613.

3. The BabyCenter. Food cravings and what they mean. 2003. www.babycenter.com/refcap/pregnancy/pregnancynutrition/1313971.html

4. Hook, EB. Dietary cravings and aversions during pregnancy. *Am J Clin Nutr* 1978, 31(8):1355–1362.

5. Bayley, TM, et al. Food cravings and aversions during pregnancy: relationships with nausea and vomiting. *Appetite* 2002, 38(1):45–51; Fairburn, CG, et al. Eating habits and eating disorders during pregnancy. *Psychosom Med* 1992, 54(6):665–672.

6. Bowen, DJ. Taste and food preference changes across the course of pregnancy. *Appetite* 1992, 19(3):233–242.

7. Dunbar, P. Gestational diabetes—special delivery. Canadian Diabetes Association. Revised, June 2001. www.diabetes.ca/Section_About/gestational.asp

8. American Diabetes Association. Gestational diabetes. June 2003 (date of access).

www.diabetes.org/main/info/affected/women/gestation_diab.jsp?WTLPromo=SEARCH_diabetes_gestational

9. Berger, H, et al. Screening for gestational diabetes mellitus: SOGC clinical practice guidelines. *JOGC* 2002, 11(121):1–10.

10. Franz, MJ, et al. Effectiveness of medical nutrition therapy provided by dietitians in the management of non-insulin-dependent diabetes mellitus: a randomized, controlled clinical trial. *J Am Diet Assoc* 1995, 95(9):1009–1117.

11. Jenkins, DJ, TM Wolever, and AL Jenkins. Starchy foods and the glycemic index. *Diabetes Care* 1988, 11(2):149–159; Jenkins, DJ, et al. Low-glycemic-index starchy foods in the diabetic diet. *Am J Clin Nutr* 1988, 48(2):248–254; Tsihlias, EB, et al. Comparison of high- and low-glycemic-index breakfast cereals with monounsaturated fat in the long-term dietary management of type 2 diabetes. *Am J Clin Nutr* 2000, 72(2):439–449.

12. University of Michigan Health System. Indigestion or heartburn during pregnancy. 2001. www.med.umich.edu/1libr/womens/pgprob12.htm/

13. MacKay, D. Hemorrhoids and varicose veins: a review of treatment options. *Altern Med Rev* 2001, 6(2):126–140.

14. Lalkin, A, et al. Therapeutic approach to hypertension during pregnancy. Motherisk. 1998. www.motherisk.org/updates/index.php?id=305

15. Helewa, ME, et al. Report of the Canadian Hypertension Society Consensus Conference: 1. Definitions, evaluation and classification of hypertensive disorders in pregnancy. CMJ 1997, 157(6):715–725.

16. Mayo Foundation for Medical Education and Research. Hypertension and pregnancy: careful monitoring is crucial. March 2003. www.mayoclinic.com/invoke.cfm?objectid=473DDAA7-615B-4634-B4FE933382B5401D

17. March of Dimes. Pre-elcampsia (High blood pressure). 2003. www.marchofdimes.com

18. National Heart, Blood and Lung Institute. How common are high blood pressure and pre-eclampsia in pregnancy? 2003. www.nhlbi.nih.gov/hbp/issues/preg/common.htm

19. Helewa, ME, et al. Report of the Canadian Hypertension Society Consensus Conference: 2. Nonpharmacologic management and prevention of hypertensive disorders in pregnancy. *Canadian Medical Association Journal* 1997, 157(7):715–725. http://collection.nlc-bnc.ca/100/201/300/cdn_

medical_association/cmaj/vol-157/issue-7/0907.htm

20. Duley, L. Routine calcium supplementation in pregnancy. Review no. 05938, June 23, 1993. In Enkin, MW, MJNC Keirse, MJ Renfrew, JP Neilson, eds. Cochrane database of systematic reviews. Oxford, UK: Update Software, 1994 (no.1).

21. Bucher, HC, et al. Effect of calcium supplementation and pregnancy-induced hypertension and pre-eclampsia: a meta-analysis of randomized controlled trials. *JAMA* 1996, 275(14):1113–1119.

22. Moutquin, JM, et al. Report of the Canadian Hypertension Society Consensus Conference: 2. Nonpharmacologic management and prevention of hypertensive disorders in pregnancy. *CMAJ* 1997, 157(7):907–919.

23. Zhang, C, et al. Vitamin C and the risk of pre-eclampsia: results from dietary questionnaire and plasma assay. *Epidemiology* 2002, 13(4):409–416.

24. Chappell, LC, et al. Effect of antioxidants on the occurrence of pre-eclampsia in women at increased risk: a randomized trial. *Lancet* 1999, 354(9181):810–816.

25. Makrides, M, et al. Efficacy and a tolerability of low-dose iron supplements during pregnancy: a randomized controlled trial. *Am J Clin Nutr* 2003, 78(1):145–153.

26. Feightner, JW. Routine iron supplementation during pregnancy. Health Canada. Health Care Network. 2003. www.hc-sc.gc.ca/hppb/healthcare/pdf/clinical_preventive/s1c6e.pdf

27. Hammar, M, et al. Calcium treatment of leg cramps in pregnancy: effect on clinical symptoms and total serum and ionized serum calcium concentrations. *Acta obstetricia et gynecologica Scandinavica* 1981, 60(4):345–347.

28. Dahle, LO, et al. The effect of oral magnesium substitution on pregnancy-induced leg cramps. *Am J Obstet Gynecol* 1995, 173(1):175–180.

29. Roffe, C, et al. Randomised, cross-over, placebo controlled trial of magnesium citrate in the treatment of chronic persistent leg cramps. *Med Sci Monit* 2002, 8(5):CR326–CR330.

30. Young, GL, and D Jewell. Interventions for leg cramps in pregnancy. *Cochrane Database Syst Rev* 2002, 1:CD000121.

31. British Columbia Reproductive Mental Health Program. Reproductive mental health: Emotional disorders in pregnancy. 2000. www.bcrmh.com/disorders/pregnancy.htm.

32. British Columbia Reproductive Mental Health Program. Reproductive Mental Health Guideline 3. Identification and assessment of reproductive mental illness during the preconception and perinatal periods. 2003. www.bcrmh.com/docs/Guideline%203%20%20New.Jan.2003.pdf.

33. British Columbia Reproductive Mental Health Program. Reproductive mental health: emotional disorders in pregnancy. 2000. www.bcrmh.com/disorders/pregnancy.htm

34. Society of Obstetricians and Gynaecologists of Canada. Nausea and vomiting during pregnancy. 2003. www.sogc.org/pub_ed/nausea/index_e.shtml

35. Ibid.

36. Ibid.

37. Vutyavanich, T, et al. Pyridoxine for nausea and vomiting of pregnancy: a randomized, double-blind, placebo-controlled trial. *Am J Obstet Gynecol* 1995, 173(3 Part 1):881–884.

38. Sahakian, V, et al. Vitamin B6 is effective therapy for nausea and vomiting of pregnancy: a randomized, double-blind, placebo-controlled study. *Obstet Gynecol* 1991, 78(1):33–36.

39. Fischer-Rasmussen, W, et al. Ginger treatment of hyperemesis gravidarum. *Eur J Obstet Gynecol Reprod Biol* 1991, 38(1):19–24; Vutyavanich, T, et al. Ginger for nausea and vomiting in pregnancy: randomized, double-masked, placebo-controlled trial. *Obstet Gynecol* 2001, 97(4):577–582.

10 Exercising During Pregnancy

1. Kramer, MS. Aerobic exercise for women during pregnancy. *Cochrane Database Syst Rev* 2002, 2:CD000180.

2. Wolfe, LA, et al. Prescription of aerobic exercise during pregnancy. *Sport Med* 1998, 8(5):273–301; Clapp, JF, et al. Exercise in pregnancy. *Med Sci Sport Exerc* 1992, 24(6 Suppl):S294–S300.

3. Marcoux, S, et al. The effect of leisure time physical activity on the risk of pre-eclampsia and gestational hypertension. *J Epidemiol Community Health* 1989, 43(2):147–152.

4. Sorensen, TK, et al. Recreational physical activity during pregnancy and risk of preeclampsia. *Hypertension* 2003, 41(6):1273–1280.

5. Carmichael, SL, et al. Physical activity and risk of neural tube defects. *Matern Child Health J* 2002, 6(3):151–157.

6. Wolfe, LA, and TL Weissgerber. Clinical physiology of exercise in pregnancy: a literature review. *J Obstet Gynaecol Can* 2003, 25(6):473–483.

7. Convertino, VA, et al. American College of Sports Medicine position stand. Exercise and fluid replacement. *Med Sci Sports Exerc* 1996, 28(1):i–vii.

11 Breastfeeding, and a Nutrition Plan for Mom (and Baby, Too)

1. Health Canada. Breastfeeding. Canadian Perinatal Surveillance System. November 1998. www.hc-sc.gc.ca/pphb-dgspsp/rhs-ssg/factshts/brstfed_e.html; McNally, E, et al. A look at breastfeeding trends in Canada (1963–1982). *Can J Public Health* 1985, 76:101–107.

2. Hanson, LA. Breastfeeding provides passive and likely long-lasting active immunity. *Ann Allergy Asthma Immunol* 1998, 81(6):523–533.

3. Schoetazau, A, et al. Effect of exclusive breastfeeding and early solid food avoidance on the incidence of atopic dermatitis in high-risk infants at 1 year of age. *Pediatr Allergy Immunol* 2002, 13(4):234–242; Oddy, WH, et al. Maternal asthma, infant feeding, and the risk of asthma in childhood. *J Allergy Clin Immunol* 2002, 110(1):65–67; Oddy, WH, et al. The effect of respirator infections, atopy, and breastfeeding on childhood asthma. *Eur Respir H* 2002, 19(5):899–905; Oddy, WH, et al. Association between breast feeding and asthma in 6 year old children: findings of a prospective birth cohort study. *BMJ* 1999, 319(7213):815–819.

4. Gdalvevih, M, et al. Breastfeeding and the risk of bronchial asthma in childhood: a systematic review with meta-analysis of prospective studies. *J Pediatr* 2001, 139(2):261–266.

5. McVea, KL, et al. The role of breastfeeding in sudden infant death syndrome. *J Hum Lact* 2000, 16(1):13–20.

6. Wilson, AC, et al. Relation of infant diet to childhood health: seven year follow up of cohort in Dundee infant feeding study. *BMJ* 1998, 316(7124):21–25; Taittonen, L, et al. Prenatal and postnatal factors in predicting later blood pressure among children: cardiovascular risk factors in young Finns. *Pediatr Res* 1996, 40(4):627–632; Bergmann, KE, et al. Early determinants of childhood overweight and adiposity in a birth cohort study: role of breastfeeding. *Int J Obes Relat Metab Disord* 2003, 27(2):162–172; Toschke, AM, et al. Overweight and obesity in 6- to 14-year-old Czech children in 1991: protective effect of breastfeeding. *J Pediatr* 2002, 141(6):764–769;

Armstrong, J, and JJ Reilly. Child Health Information Team. Breastfeeding and lowering the risk of childhood obesity. *Lancet* 2002, 359(9322):2003–2004; Liese, AD, et al. Inverse association of overweight and breast feeding in 9 to 10-year-old children in Germany. *Int J Obes Relat Metab Disord* 2001, 25(11):1644–1650; Gillman, MW, et al. Risk of overweight among adolescents who were breastfd as infants. *JAMA* 2001, 285(19):2461–2467; Bener, A, et al. Longer breastfeeding and protection against childhood leukaemia and lymphomas. *Eur J Cancer* 2001, 37(2):234–238; Infante-Rivard, C, et al. Markers of infections, breastfeeding and childhood acute lymphoblastic leukaemia. *Br J Cancer* 2000, 83(11):1559–1564; Shu, XO, et al. Breastfeeding and risk of childhood acute leukemia. *J Natl Cancer Inst* 1999, 92(20):1765–1772.

7. Oddy, WH, et al. Breast feeding and cognitive development in childhood: a prospective birth cohort study. *Paediatr Perinat Epidemiol* 2003, 17(1):81–90; Mortensen, EL, et al. Breast feeding and intelligence [in Danish]. *Ugeskr Laeger* 2003, 165(13):1361–1366; Gomez-Sanchiz, M, et al. Influence of breastfeeding on mental and psychomotor development. *Clin Pediatr* (Phila) 2003, 42(1):35–42; Horwood, LJ, et al. Breast milk feeding and cognitive ability at 7–8 years. *Arch Dis Child Fetal Neonatal Ed* 2001, 84(1):F23–27; Anderson, JW, et al. Breastfeeding and cognitive development: a meta-analysis. *Am J Clin Nutr* 1999, 70(4):525–535; Jain, A, et al. How good is the evidence linking breastfeeding and intelligence? *Pediatrics* 2002, 109(6):1044–1053. Mortensen, EL, et al. The association between duration of breastfeeding and adult intelligence. *JAMA* 2002, 287(18):2365–2371.

8. Collaborative Group on Hormonal Factors in Breast Cancer. Breast cancer and breastfeeding: collaborative reanalysis of individual data from 47 epidemiological studies in 30 countries, including 50302 women with breast cancer and 96973 women without the disease. *Lancet* 2002, 360(9328):187–195.

9. National Academy of Sciences, Institute of Medicine, Food and Nutrition Board. *Dietary Reference Intakes: Energy, Carbohydrate, Fiber, Fat, Fatty Acids, Cholesterol, Protein, and Amino Acids (Macronutrients).* National Academy Press, Washington, DC, 2002.

10. National Academy of Sciences, Institute of Medicine, Food and Nutrition Board. *Dietary reference intakes for energy: carbohydrate, fiber, fat, fatty acids, cholesterol, protein, and amino acids (macronutrients).* Washington, DC: National Academy Press, 2002.

11. Mennella, JA, and GK Beauchamp. The transfer of alcohol to human milk: effects on flavor and the infant's behavior. *N Engl J Med* 1991, 325(14): 981–985.

12. Kramer, MS, and R Kakuma. Maternal dietary antigen avoidance during pregnancy and/or lactation for preventing or treating atopic disease in the child. Cochrane Methodology Review. In *The Cochrane Library,* no. 4. Chichester, UK: John Wiley and Sons, 2003.

12 A Nutrition Plan for Formula-Fed Babies

1. Birch, EE, et al. A randomized controlled trial of early dietary supply of long-chain polyunsaturated fatty acids and mental development in term infants. *Dev Med Child Neurol* 2000, 42(3):174–181; Hoffman, DR, et al. Visual function in breast-fed term infants weaned to formula with or without long-chain polyunsaturates at 4 to 6 months: a randomized clinical trial. *Pediatr* 2003, 142(6):669–677.

2. Forsyth, JS, et al. Long chain polyunsaturated fatty acid supplementation in infant formula and blood pressure in later childhood: follow up of a randomised controlled trial. *BMJ* 2003, 326(7396):953–957.

3. Chandra, RK, et al. Effect of feeding whey hydrosylate, soy and conventional cow milk formulas on incidence of atopic diseases in high risk infants. *Ann Allergy* 1989, 63(2):102–106; Eastham, EJ, et al. Antigenicity of infant formulas and the induction of systemic immunological tolerance by oral feeding: cow's milk versus soy milk. *J Pediatr Gastroenterol Nutr* 1982, 1(1):23–28.

4. Chandra, RK. Five-year follow-up of high-risk infants with a family history of allergy who were exclusively breast-fed or fed partial whey hydrosylate, soy and conventional cow's milk formulas. *J Pediatr Gastroenterol Nutr* 1997, 24(4):380–388.

14 Getting Your Figure Back

1. Young, LR, and M Nestle. Variation in perceptions of a "medium" food portion: implications for dietary guidance. *J Am Diet Assoc* 1998, 98(4):458–459.

2. Morkved, S, and K Bo. The effect of post-natal exercises to strengthen the pelvic floor muscles. *Acta Obstet Gynecol Scan* 1996, 75(4):382–385; Morkved, S, and K Bo. Effect of postpartum pelvic floor muscle training in prevention and treatment of urinary incontinence: a one-year follow up. *Br J Obstet Gynaecol* 2000, 107(8):1022–1028.

3. Klem, ML, et al. Does weight loss maintenance become easier over time? *Obes Research* 2000, 8(6):438–444; McGuire, MT, et al. Behavioural strategies of individuals who have maintained long-term weight losses. *Obes Research* 1999, 7(4):334–341.

Subject Index

Recipes Index